For EU product safety concerns:
IN TECH d.o.o., Prolaz Marije Krucifikse Kozulić 3, 51000 Rijeka, Croatia,
info@intechopen.com or visit our website at intechopen.com.

Meet the editor

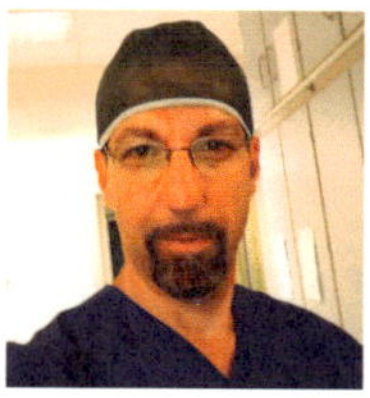

Giuseppe Lo Giudice obtained an MD from the University of Messina, Italy. He completed his ophthalmological residency at the Department of Ophthalmology, University of Padua, Italy, after residency training. He was a fellow in the Ophthalmology Department of the Gironcoli Ophthalmic Center, Italy from 2002 to 2004. He was an assistant in ophthalmology at Conegliano Hospital Conegliano, Italy from 2004 to 2007. Since 2007, Dr. Lo Giudice has been a surgeon and vice director at San Antonio Hospital, University of Padua. His major fields of interest are treatments for retinal diseases (proliferative retinopathies, age-related macular degeneration, and diabetic retinopathy) and vitreoretinal surgery. He has more than 25 years of experience in clinical research as well as in clinical trials and laboratory research. He performed more than 9000 anterior segment surgeries (cataract surgery, glaucoma surgery, corneal transplantation) in the last 5 years and more than 3000 vitreoretinal surgeries for several vitreoretinal diseases (ocular trauma, complicated cataract surgery, retinal pucker, retinal detachment, and vitreoretinal proliferative disease) in the last 3 years.

Contents

Preface

Research has yielded major discoveries about the etiology, pathophysiology, and treatment of several ocular diseases over the last decade. Basic science and translational research in every field of ophthalmology and for retinal disease have accelerated. The resultant novel discoveries have improved and will continue to improve the daily lives of our patients, also giving us the opportunity to better understand what we must know and what we need to do. Novel therapies offer not only sight-saving, less destructive forms of treatment for several retinal diseases but also treatments that can improve visual acuity in many cases. In addition, preventive treatments are being developed. This book presents the latest information on the pathophysiology, diagnosis, management, and surgical treatment of several retinal diseases.

The first section focuses on vitreous and macular diseases. Chapters in this section discuss the clinical findings seen in the vitreoretinal interface, macular hole pathogenesis, and treatment. Each chapter in this section includes color pictures, tables, and figures. The chapters also examine surgical approaches to the treatment of medical retinal diseases by exploring the latest advances in ophthalmologic surgical treatment. While traditional medical therapies such as intravitreal injections have been effective in treating these conditions, the development of new surgical interventions offers the potential for longer-lasting solutions.

The next sections present in-depth information on current and experimental forms of treatment for vitreous retinal disease, glaucoma, ocular tumors, and inflammation. Chapters discuss mechanisms of action, clinical treatment techniques, target patient population, expected outcomes, and both the positive and negative aspects of each treatment. One chapter is dedicated to the progress in optogenetic retinal prostheses. Optogenetics has emerged as a revolutionary technology that enables circuit-specific restoration of neuronal function with millisecond temporal resolution. Restoring vision is one of its most promising applications. These areas of research may one day lead to future treatments that help to overcome visual loss and damage. Progress in these areas renews our hope for future generations afflicted with some retinal diseases. As in the case of the first edition, this volume does not compile and analyze all the existing knowledge of retinal disease.

I hope that the information presented herein continues to incite inquiry and ignite research that may unearth those enigmatic answers to questions about the etiology of and cure for some very complicated diseases.

Giuseppe Lo Giudice
San Paolo Ophthalmic Center,
San Antonio Hospital,
University of Padua,
Padova, Italy

Section 1

Vitreous and Macular Disease

Chapter 1

Introductory Chapter: Treatment of Medical Retinal Diseases by Surgical Approaches – Mini-Review of the Latest Advances in the Field of Ophthalmology

Giuseppe Lo Giudice, Alessandro Galan and Irene Gattazzo

1. Introduction

Medical retinal disease, such as diabetic retinopathy (DR) and age-related macular degeneration (AMD), are leading causes of vision loss worldwide. While traditional medical therapies such as intravitreal injections have been effective in treating these conditions, the development of new surgical intervention offers the potential for longer-lasting solutions.

With this mini-review, we will explore the latest advances in the field of ophthalmology for the surgical treatment of the main retinal diseases.

2. Neovascular age-related macular degeneration

Since 1985, the therapy for neovascular AMD has rapidly evolved. Initially, it was primarily parasurgical utilizing argon laser treatment and photodynamic therapy, as well as surgical with subretinal choroidal neovascular membrane removal, macular translocation, and surgical transplantation of the retinal pigment epithelium (RPE).

Macular translocation surgery, which was first proposed by Lindsey in 1983, aims to relocate the fovea from a severely diseased subretinal bed to a new location with healthier subretinal tissues to preserve and improve functional central vision [1]. The original technique involved a pars plana vitrectomy (PPV) under general anesthesia and the induction of a retinal detachment through transscleral injection of subretinal fluid. Subsequently, a 360° retinectomy was performed and the subretinal blood and choroidal neovascularization (CNV) were removed. After a partial filling with silicone oil, retinal translocation was performed and the silicone oil filling was completed. Finally, laser retinopexy was performed [1].

With the approval of Pegabtanib as first anti-angiogenic therapeutic for ocular neovascularization in 2004, the role of the macular surgery decreased, and medical approaches became predominant [2]. However, recent developments in the field of surgical strategy are bearing fruit. The food and drug administration (FDA) authorized the port delivery system (PDS) for ranibizumab in October 2021 (Susvimo, Genentech/

Roche), expanding our arsenal of clinical tools for wet AMD. Additionally, new treatments, such as gene therapy, are revolutionizing the treatment of retinal diseases [3].

One such example is RGX-314 (REGENXBIO Inc.), which uses adeno-associated virus serotype 8 vector to deliver a gene encoding an anti-VEGF antigen-binding fragment similar to ranibizumab. It is intended to produce ongoing anti-VEGF therapy through subretinal and suprachoroidal delivery for the treatment of DR and wet AMD, resulting in a stable antibody production and a reduced number of required injections [4–6]. This technique involved the formation of a subretinal bleb with a 41-gauge needle after a PPV, which is necessary for subretinal administration.

Data from a two-year Phase I/IIa trial of RGX-314 are now available. The trial has enrolled 42 patients with wet AMD in five cohorts, receiving increasing doses of the subretinal delivery system, to investigate its safety and efficacy. The six patients in cohort 3, who received a dose of 6×10^{10} GC/eye, showed an improvement of best-corrected visual acuity (BVCA) of + 14 letters from baseline. Furthermore, when compared to the 12 months before receiving RGX-314 therapy, Cohort 3 exhibited a 66.7% lower rate of yearly anti-VEGF injections. Similarly, Cohort 4 and Cohort 5 patients presented a 58.3% and 81.2% reduction, respectively, at 1.5 years. Both cohorts showed stable vision and decreased central macular thickness. No abnormal immune response, drug-related ocular inflammation, or postsurgical inflammation have been reported, highlighting a profile of safety and good tolerability [7]. However, 20 serious adverse events have been reported in 13 patients, predominantly mild postoperative side effects such as conjunctival hemorrhages (67%), inflammation (36%), visual acuity reduction (17%), irritation, and pain. Only one patient in the high-dose Cohort 5 presented a significant decrease in vision possibly drug-related [8]. Furthermore, retinal pigmentary changes have been found at the site of the subretinal bleb in 67% of the patients. Therefore, modifications to the surgical approach should be considered to prevent macular abnormalities.

The study has been extended to a five-year follow-up and other studies are derived from this. While subretinal injections of RGX-314 for nAMD patients are being clinically evaluated in the pivotal ATMOSPHERE trial, the suprachoroidal route is being evaluated in the Phase 2 Trials AAVIATE and ALTITUDE for neovascular AMD and diabetic retinopathy, respectively.

3. Geographic atrophy (GA)

Dry AMD accounts for almost 85–90% of all AMD cases and is characterized by irreversible RPE cell degenerations, loss of retinal photoreceptors, and GA formation, leading to permanent vision loss. The development of the disease is thought to be linked to an abnormality in the complement system [9].

To address this issue, GT005 (Gyroscope Therapeutics) uses an adeno-associated virus to deliver a plasmid that encodes for Complement Factor I (CFI), a natural inhibitor of the complement system [10].

GT-005 is currently being evaluated for safety and efficacy in multiple Phase 1 (FOCUS) and Phase 2 (HORIZON and EXPLORE) clinical trials, using either a transvitreal approach or a suprachoroidal cannulation through the Orbit Subretinal Delivery Device System (Gyroscope Therapeutics) [11]. Preliminary results have demonstrated both efficiency, with an increase in vitreous CFI levels, and safety of GT005, as no significant ocular inflammatory events have been reported [12]. Twelve patients presented mild postsurgical adverse effects, and only two patients had an increase in intraocular pressure, one of which has self-resolved [13]. As the follow-up is still going on, trials will provide long-term data.

Another possible surgical option is represented by the transplantation of induced pluripotent stem cell-derived RPE [14]. These cells are derived from the somatic cells of patients with GA, which differentiate into RPE cells and grow on a monolayer of biodegradable polylactic-co-glycolic acid scaffold. Their subretinal transplantation would avoid further degradation of the overlying neurosensory retina [14–16]. The surgical technique consists of performing a PPV, creating a planned retinotomy to place the pluripotent stem cells, and tamponading with gas [14]. The feasibility and safety are being evaluated in phase 1/2a clinical trial at the National Eye Institute.

Similarly, a different trial called OpRegen is evaluating the subretinal transplantation of human embryonic stem cell-derived RPE cells in patients with GA. To date, phase 1/2a trial shows the safety of the treatment, with no unexpected adverse events reported, nor inflammatory events. The efficiency data look promising, with a statistically significant improvement in BCVA compared with the fellow eyes and a resolution of outer retinal atrophy at optical coherence tomography (OCT) scans [17].

4. Routes of delivery

With the development of anti-VEGF and intraocular steroids, intravitreal injection has become the most common option for intraocular delivery due to their ability to enter the vitreous cavity using a needle in an outpatient clinical setting. However, this delivery route is not free from complications such as endophthalmitis, retinal detachment, hemorrhages, and cataract and ocular hypertension in the case of intravitreal steroids. There is also a risk of triggering host immune responses if the injected substance exits into the systemic circulation, as in the case with certain AAV subtypes [18]. Furthermore AAV subtypes are blocked from the internal limiting membrane (ILM); thus, they do not penetrate into the neurosensory retina [12].

4.1 Subretinal injections

To overcome the ILM barrier and deliver therapeutic agents directly to photoreceptors and RPE cell in focal regions of the retina, subretinal injections have been developed. This route of delivery is less immunogenic than intravitreal injections due to the presence of the outer blood-retina barrier [19]. There are two routes for subretinal injections: transscleral and transvitreal. The transscleral route uses a microneedle through the choroid, and the transvitreal route is performed with a PPV. The latter is more common in humans, but it is not free form complications, such as hemorrhage, cataract, endophthalmitis, and retinal detachment [20].

4.2 Suprachoroidal injections

The suprachoroidal route is a new method for delivering drugs to the posterior retina while minimizing exposure of anterior structures [21, 22]. Microneedles have been developed to access this space, which is located between the scleral wall and choroidal vasculature and to advance into the suprachoroidal space [23], avoiding the need of invasive vitreoretinal surgery [20]. However, larger particles such as steroids, viral particles, or nanoparticles should avoid rapid egress from the high blood flow suprachoroidal space [24]. Moreover, as the suprachoroidal space is outside the outer blood-retina-barrier, there is a potential risk for host immune responses to the viral particle or transgene [25].

5. Diabetic retinopathy

DR represents one of the leading causes of blindness among industrial countries with a worldwide prevalence of 34.6% (93 million people), becoming a relevant socioeconomic problem [26]. Therefore, research in this field is focused on both improving existing treatments and investigating new delivery systems. Several approaches to anti-VEGF therapy are currently being investigated, including sustained delivery, high-dose therapeutics, and a novel antibody biopolymer conjugate platform, in addition to exploring new treatments beyond anti-VEGF agents [27].

In the PANORAMA clinical trial, monthly injections of aflibercept (Eylea, Regeneron) were found to significantly reduce the occurrence of vision-threatening complication in both moderate severe and severe non-proliferative DR without center-involving diabetic macular edema (DME). The consequences related to proliferative DR, including vitreous hemorrhage and tractional retinal detachments, usually require surgical intervention [28].

Aflibercept is also being investigated in high-dose (8 mg) in PHOTON trial, which has demonstrated that, administered at intervals of 12 or 16 weeks, it provides non-inferior BCVA compared to standard 2 mg aflibercept dosed every 8 weeks [29].

Moreover, a novel anti-VEGF, tarcocimab, is being investigated in phase 3 GLEAM and GLIMMER trial to evaluate the efficacy and safety of the intravitreal administration of 5 mg in the treatment of naïve DME in comparison with aflibercept [30, 31]. This new drug is a bioconjugate of a recombinant, full-length humanized anti-VEGF monoclonal antibody and a phosphorylcholine biopolymer.

Other potential intravitreal anti-VEGF therapies are currently in phase 2 and 3 trials including faricimab (Genentech/Roche), RC28-E (RemeGen), conbercept (Chengdu Kanghong Biotech), OPT-302 (Opthea), KSI-301 (Kodiak), and GB-102 (Graybug Vision). Furthermore, there are several novel targets in phase 2 trials: UBX1325, a senolytic Bcl-xL inhibitor, THR-149 (Oxurion), a bicyclic peptide that selectively inhibits human plasma kallikrein, and D-4517.2 (Ashvattha Therapeutics), a tyrosine kinase inhibitor. Many of these seem to offer increased durability or sustained release for the treatment of both DR and neovascular AMD [27].

On the other hand, the surgical treatment of DME has gained significant attention with the approval of the PDS with ranibizumab (Susvimo 100 mg/mL, Genentech/Roche) in October 2021 [31]. The PDS is a permanent, refillable intraocular implant that is placed in the supero-temporal quadrant of the eye. The surgical technique consists of a 6 × 6 mm conjunctival peritomy and dissection, followed by scleral hemostasis, which allows for a full-thickness scleral incision of 3.5 mm in length, of 4 mm from the limbus. Laser is applied to the pars plana, which is then opened to release the SUVISMO implant. This PDS continuously releases ranibizumab over time and can be refilled in the office [32].

Two phase 3 randomized trials, PAGODA and PAVILION, evaluate the PDS with ranibizumab in the treatment of diabetic retinopathy in patients respectively with and without center-involving DME, respectively. Refill-exchange procedures occur every 24 and 36 weeks, respectively [33–35].

6. Conclusions

As new therapeutic approaches emerge, the treatment of retinal diseases will inevitably continue to shift between medical and surgical interventions. The initiation of various trials facilitates the advancement of retina and enhances patient care. These trials provide opportunities for collaboration among researchers, clinicians, and industry partners, which could lead to the development of more effective treatments and therapies. With the introduction of novel treatments, including several surgical options, there is hope for longer-lasting and even permanent solutions to these challenging conditions.

Author details

Giuseppe Lo Giudice[1*], Alessandro Galan[1] and Irene Gattazzo[2]

1 San Paolo Ophthalmic Center, San Antonio Hospital—University Hospital, Padova, Italy

2 NESMOS Department, Ophthalmology Unit, St. Andrea Hospital, University of Rome "La Sapienza", Rome, Italy

*Address all correspondence to: giuseppe.logiudice@aopd.veneto.it

References

[1] Vander JF. Macular translocation. Current Opinion in Ophthalmology. 2000;**11**(3):159-165. DOI: 10.1097/00055735-200006000-00001

[2] Gragoudas ES, Adamis AP, Cunningham ET Jr, Feinsod M, Guyer DR. VEGF inhibition study in ocular neovascularization clinical trial group Pegaptanib for neovascular age-related macular degeneration. The New England Journal of Medicine. 2004;**351**:2805-2816

[3] Deaner J, Vajzovic L. Surgical Innovations to Treat Medical Retinal Disesases. Retina Today; 2021. pp. 34-36. Available from: https://retinatoday.com/articles/2021-nov-dec/surgical-innovations-to-treat-medical-retinal-diseases

[4] Avery RL. Two-year results from the subretinal RGX-314 gene therapy phase 1/2a study for the treatment of nAMD, and an update on suprachoroidal trials. [Paper presentation]. In: Retina subspecialty day, American Academy of Ophthalmology, 125 th Annual Meeting, New Orleans, LA, United States; 12 November 2021

[5] RGX-314 Gene Therapy Administered in the Suprachoroidal Space for Participants with Neovascular Age-Related Macular Degeneration (nAMD) (AAVIATE). Available from: http://www.clinicaltrials.gov/ct2/show/NCT04514653 [Accessed: October 29, 2021]

[6] RGX-314 Gene Therapy Administered in the Suprachoroidal Space for Participants with Diabetic Retinopathy (DR) without Center Involved-Diabetic Macular Edema (CI-DME) (ALTITUDE). Available from: http://www.clinicaltrials.gov/ct2/show/NCT04567550 [Accessed: October 29, 2021]

[7] REGENXBIO Announces Additional Positive Interim Phase I/IIa and Long-Term Follow-up Data of RGX-314 for the Treatment of Wet AMD. Available from: http://www.prnewswire.com/news-releases/regenxbioannounces-additional-positive-interim-phase-iiia-and-long-term-follow-up-dataof-rgx-314-for-the-treatment-of-wet-amd-301228344.html [Accessed: April 1, 2021]

[8] Siddiqui FA, Aziz AA, Khanani AM. Gene therapy for neovascular AMD an update on ongoing clinical trials. Retinal Physician. 2020;**17**:36-39. Available from: https://www.retinalphysician.com/issues/2020/special-edition-2020/gene-therapy-for-neovascular-amd

[9] Bahadorani S, Singer M. Recent advances in the management and understanding of macular degeneration. F1000Research. 2017;**6**:519

[10] Dreismann AK, McClements ME, Barnard AR, Orhan E, Hughes JP, Lachmann PJ, et al. Functional expression of complement factor I following AAV-mediated gene delivery in the retina of mice and human cells. Gene Therapy. 2021;**28**:265-276

[11] Grishanin R, Vuillemenot B, Sharma P, Keravala A, Greengard J, Gelfman C, et al. Preclinical evaluation of ADVM-022, a novel gene therapy approach to treating wet age-related macular degeneration. Molecular Therapy. 2019;**27**:118-129

[12] Kiss S, Oresic Bender K, Grishanin RN, Hanna KM, Nieves JD, Sharma P, et al. Longterm safety evaluation of continuous

intraocular delivery of aflibercept by the intravitreal gene therapy candidate ADVM-022 in nonhuman primates. Translational Vision Science & Technology. 2021;**10**:34

[13] Waheed NK. FOCUS interim results: GT005 gene therapy phase I/II study for the treatment of geographic atrophy. [PowerPoint slides] Virtual presentation at Angiogenesis, Exudation, and Degeneration. 12 February 2021. Available from: chrome-extension://efaidnbmnnnibpcajpcglclefindmkaj/https://www.gyroscopetx.com/wp-content/uploads/2021/02/Waheed-Focus_FINAL.pdf

[14] A Phase I/IIa Trial for Autologous Transplantation of Induced Pluripotent Stem Cell-Derived Retinal Pigment Epithelium for Geographic Atrophy Associated with Age-Related Macular Degeneration. Available from: http://www.clinicaltrials.gov/ct2/show/NCT04339764 [Accessed: July 15, 2021]

[15] Ohmine S, Dietz AB, Deeds MC, et al. Induced pluripotent stem cells from GMP-grade hematopoietic progenitor cells and mononuclear myeloid cells. Stem Cell Research & Therapy. 2011;**2**(6):46

[16] Buchholz DE, Hikita ST, Rowland TJ, et al. Derivation of functional retinal pigmented epithelium from induced pluripotent stem cells. Stem Cells. 2009;**27**(10):2427-2434

[17] Ip M. OpRegen trial: Phase I/IIa dose escalation study of human embryonic stem cell-derived retinal pigment epithelium cells transplanted subretinally in patients with advanced AMD. [Paper presentation]. In: Retina subspecialty day, American Academy of Ophthalmology, 125 th Annual Meeting, New Orleans, LA, United States. 12 November 2021

[18] Peng Y, Tang L, Zhou Y. Subretinal injection: A review on the novel route of therapeutic delivery for vitreoretinal diseases. Ophthalmic Research. 2017;**58**:217-26.2442

[19] Khanani AM, Thomas MJ, Aziz AA, Weng CY, Danzig CJ, Yiu G, et al. Review of gene therapies for age-related macular degeneration. Eye (London, England). 2022;**36**(2):303-311. DOI: 10.1038/s41433-021-01842-1

[20] Yiu G, Chung SH, Mollhoff IN, Nguyen UT, Thomasy SM, Yoo J, et al. Suprachoroidal and subretinal injections of AAV using transscleral microneedles for retinal gene delivery in nonhuman primates. Molecular Therapy-Methods & Clinical Development. 2020;**16**:179-191

[21] Moisseiev E, Loewenstein A, Yiu G. The suprachoroidal space: From potential space to a space with potential. Clinical Ophthalmology. 2016;**10**:173-178

[22] Emami-Naeini P, Yiu G. Medical and surgical applications for the suprachoroidal space. International Ophthalmology Clinics. 2019;**59**:195-207

[23] Yiu G, Pecen P, Sarin N, Chiu SJ, Farsiu S, Mruthyunjaya P, et al. Characterization of the choroid-scleral junction and suprachoroidal layer in healthy individuals on enhanced-depth imaging optical coherence tomography. JAMA Ophthalmology. 2014;**132**:174-181

[24] Shen J, Kim J, Tzeng SY, Ding K, Hafiz Z, Long D, et al. Suprachoroidal gene transfer with nonviral nanoparticles. Science Advances. 2020;**6**(27). DOI: 10.1126/ sciadv.aba1606

[25] Chung SH, Mollhoff IN, Mishra A, Sin T-N, Ngo T, Ciulla T, et al. Host immune responses after suprachoroidal delivery of AAV8 in nonhuman

primate eyes. Human Gene Therapy. 2021;**32**:682-693

[26] Flaxel CJ, Adelman RA, Bailey ST, Fawzi A, Lim JI, Vemulakonda GA. Ying G-s, diabetic retinopathy preferred practice pattern®. Ophthalmology. 2019. DOI: 10.1016/j.ophtha.2019.09.025

[27] Kiryakoza L, Sridhar J. DR Rearch Roundup: Phase 2 and 3. Retina Today; November/December, 2022. pp. 42-44. Available from: https://retinatoday.com/articles/2022-nov-dec/dr-research-roundup-phase-2-and-3

[28] National Center for Chronic Disease Prevention and Health Promotion. Diabetic Retinopathy. Available from: http://www.preventblindness.org/wp-content/uploads/2017/10/factsheet.pdf [Accessed: September 8, 2022]

[29] Boyer DS. Treatment of moderately severe to severe nonproliferative diabetic retinopathy with intravitreal aflibercept injection: 52-week results from the phase 3 PANORAMA study. Investigative Ophthalmology & Visual Science. 2019;**60**(9):1731-1731

[30] Aflibercept 8 mg Meets Primary Endpoints in Two Global Pivotal Trials for DME and wAMD, with a Vast Majority of Patients Maintained on 12 and 16-Week Dosing Intervals [Press Release]. Regeneron. Available from: http://www.investor.regeneron.com/newsreleases/news-release-details/aflibercept-8-mg-meets-primary-endpoints-two-global-pivotal; [Accessed: September 8, 2022]

[31] A Trial to Evaluate the Efficacy, Durability, and Safety of KSI-301 Compared to Aflibercept in Participants with Diabetic Macular Edema (DME) (GLEAM). [Updated: June 6, 2022]. Available from: http://www.clinicaltrials.gov/ct2/show/NCT04611152 [Accessed: October 12, 2022]

[32] A Study to Evaluate the Efficacy, Durability, and Safety of KSI-301 Compared to Aflibercept in Participants with Diabetic Macular Edema (DME) (GLIMMER). [Updated: June 6, 2022]. Available from: http://www.clinicaltrials.gov/ct2/show/NCT04603937 [Accessed: July 28, 2022]

[33] Ranade SV, Wieland MR, Tam T, et al. The port delivery system with ranibizumab: A new paradigm for long-acting retinal drug delivery. Drug Delivery; 2022;**29**(1):1326-1334

[34] This Study Will Evaluate the Efficacy, Safety, and Pharmacokinetics of the Port Delivery System with Ranibizumab in Participants with Diabetic Macular Edema Compared with Intravitreal Ranibizumab (Pagoda). Available from: http://www.clinicaltrials.gov/ct2/show/NCT04108156.4

[35] A Multicenter, Randomized Study in Participants with Diabetic Retinopathy without Center-Involved Diabetic Macular Edema to Evaluate the Efficacy, Safety, and Pharmacokinetics of Ranibizumab Delivered Via the Port Delivery System Relative to the Comparator Arm (PAVILION). Available from: http://www.clinicaltrials.gov/ct2/show/NCT04503551

Chapter 2

Perspective Chapter: The Vitreous Body Visualization Technique in Diagnosis and the Classification of Idiopathic Macular Holes

Natalia Kislitsyna and Sergei Novikov

Abstract

Application of the developed technology of vitreous body visualization in patients with macular holes (MH) of different sizes provides a principally new approach to clinical and diagnostic examination based on the development (depending on the stage of the pathological process) of basic classification anatomical and morphological signs (elongation of the vitreous cisterns in anteroposterior direction, violation of the integrity of the vitreous cistern wall and probability of staining composition exit beyond stained cavities, the degree of adhesion of the vitreous body on the internal limiting surface, etc). and characterized by advantages over traditional MH classifications, which in general (based on the outlined recommendations) makes it possible to significantly increase the clinical effectiveness of vitreoretinal surgical intervention in comparison with traditional classifications.

Keywords: vitreocontrast, macular holes, vitreous anatomy, macular surgery, body visualization technique

1. Introduction

Currently, researchers show big interest to the study of vitreoretinal interface, its components, adhesion mechanisms, processes leading to their disorder, and subsequent anatomic functional changes. Up till now, the role of cortical vitreous and retinal vitreous layers interrelation in the aspect of pathogenesis and full classification of idiopathic macular holes has been insufficiently disclosed [1–7]. The development of the new ways of intravital imaging of the structural components of the vitreous body and vitreoretinal interface is an important tool to improve clinicians' knowledge of the pathogenesis of various vitreoretinal diseases in order to improve the methods and quality of treatment [7–9]. New staining solutions provide an opportunity to study anatomic topographic changes in the structures of the vitreous body (VB) and vitreoretinal interface (VRI) during surgical intervention with possible subsequent histological and ultrastructural studies [1, 10]. All this contributes to the development of innovative methods and modernization of existing approaches for the treatment of diseases of the posterior segment of the eyeball [4–6, 11–15].

The aim of this work was to study the anatomical and topographic specifics of changes in the vitreous body and vitreoretinal interface at different stages of idiopathic macular holes (MH). We followed up 143 patients (143 eyes), 105 females, 38 males, aged 51–78 years (mean age 64.8 ± 5.3 years). Inclusion criteria for patients were the presence of MH, transparent optical medium, the absence of diabetes mellitus, and other systemic diseases and ophthalmic surgical procedures in the medical history. The study exclusion criteria for patients were high myopia and traumatic MH. All the patients were divided into the following three groups according to the traditional classification of the International Vitreomacular Traction Study Group (2013) [13]:

- patients with small (≤ 250 μm) diameter MH (40 patients, 40 eyes);
- patients with MH of medium (>250—≤400 μm) diameter (58 patients, 58 eyes);
- patients with large (>400 μm) diameter MH (45 patients, 45 eyes).

At the same time (according to the classification), in all the cases this was a primary MH without vitreomacular traction .

Vitreoretinal intervention was performed using vitreocontrastography technique, a distinctive feature of which was the use of Vitreocontrast suspension to highlight VB and VRI structures in order to study their topographic anatomy [1, 2].

The VRI topographic anatomy was assessed and intraoperatively video recorded.

When cortical layer remnants were visualized on the retinal ILM surface, their topography, area, and configuration were assessed followed by photo and video recording of changes in VRI anatomy and determination of the borders of abnormal posterior vitreous detachment (PVD).

Application of the developed technology of vitreous body visualization in patients with macular holes (MH) of different sizes provides a principally new approach to clinical and diagnostic examination based on the development (depending on the stage of the pathological process) of basic classification anatomical and morphological signs (elongation of the vitreous cisterns in anteroposterior direction, violation of the integrity of the vitreous cistern wall and probability of staining composition exit beyond stained cavities, the degree of adhesion of the vitreous body on the internal limiting surface, etc.) and characterized by advantages over traditional MH classifications, which in general (based on the outlined recommendations) makes it possible to significantly increase the clinical effectiveness of vitreoretinal surgical intervention in comparison with traditional classifications.

2. Experimental study 1

Currently, glucocorticosteriod (GC) (triamcinalone acetonide (TA), Kenalog-40) suspensions are widely used as contrast staining agents for the structures of the vitreous body [8, 12, 16, 17]. In ophthalmology, these substances have been used since 1950s to suppress intraocular pressure and the proliferation of fibroblasts. In 1974, R. O. Graham described their intravitreal use for the treatment of experimentally induced endophthalmitis [18]. In 1988, Machemer R. confirmed the effectiveness of the intravitreal introduction of GC crystal forms for the local suppression of intraocular inflammatory and proliferative processes [16, 17]. Currently, GC is used to inhibit inflammatory processes in diabetic macular edema and cystic macular edema caused by the central retinal vein occlusion, subretinal neovascularization, and other vitreoretinal diseases. However, these medicine remedies may have such side effects as lens opacification, elevated intraocular pressure, and endophthalmitis [19].

In 2000, Peyman G. for the first time described TA as a vital dye for chromo-vitrectomy. During the study, it was found that the particles of the vital dye penetrate between the vitreous cortex fibers staining them, thus enabling their better visualization and facilitating the removal of these tissues [12]. Besides, not being a true dye but a suspension it settles on the VB in the form of precipitates, thus making it possible to easily distinguish VB from surrounding intraocular structures [20]. The staining agent precipitates on the surface of epiretinal membranes (ERMs) facilitating their subsequent removal [12, 21]. Clinical studies confirmed TA efficacy as a staining contrast agent for intraocular structures. Matsumoto H. et al proved that the removal of vitreous posterior cortical layers during vitrectomy is safer with the use of TA than without the use of the vital dye [22]. Enaida H. et al studied 177 eyes of 158 patients who had chromo-vitrectomy for rematogeneous retinal detachment, macular hole, proliferative diabetic retinopathy with TA and without it. The authors did not find any difference in the visual acuity in both groups. However, the number of retinal detachment recurrences that required repeated surgery was lower in the group where vitrectomy was performed with the use of TA [23]. The authors did not find any statistically significant difference in the occurrence of complications after the surgical intervention with the use of TA and without it [17]. Horio N., Furino et al. used TA to facilitate the removal of ILM and epiretinal membranes during vitrectomy. In all the cases, there was visual acuity improvement and no complications in the postoperative period [20, 21]. Nevertheless, some authors mention difficulties in ILM removal when TA is used as a staining agent. Due to the size of its particles, the dye spreads over the retinal surface making the macular tissue invisible, the manipulation is poorly controlled, and the risk of iatrogenic retinal damage increases [4]. The TA injectable form present at the domestic pharmacological market is Kenalog-40 suspension (Bristol-Myers Squibb., Italy). A dose of the drug for intravitreal injection contains 4 mg of TA active substance in 0.1 ml of solution. The suspension contains 40 mg of TA and 9.9 mg of benzyl alcohol in isotonic sodium chloride solution.

According to a number of authors, it is the benzyl alcohol contained in Kenalog-40 suspension that can have a toxic effect on the retina. The preservative contained in the suspension can cause necrosis of retinal pigment epithelial cells (PECs) and have a damaging effect on glial cells as opposed to TA in physiological solution. The toxic effect depends on the dose and exposure time of the solution. The TA crystals themselves have no cytotoxic effect on PEC cells. Nevertheless, Narayanan R. et al. refuted the data that the preservative contained in the suspension Kenalog-40 (Bristol Meyers Squibb., USA) has a toxic effect on retinal cells [24]. The TA and benzyl alcohol toxic effect on the structures of the posterior segment of the eye has been studied in the experiment on animals. The results of these studies are also contradictory. A number of researchers did not reveal the damaging effect of TA on the retina of rabbits [5, 25], while others demonstrated the toxic effect of the main substance and the preservative [24, 26]. Therefore, in order to avoid morphofunctional changes in the posterior segment structures during vitreoretinal intervention, it is recommended to use TA solution without a preservative, and the exposure time of the solution should not exceed 5 min. Thus, the use of TA facilitates the removal of VB and VRI structures during chromo-vitrectomy. However, this suspension has a number of side effects and can have a toxic effect on the structures of the posterior segment of the eye. The undeniable advantages and effectiveness of chromo-vitrectomy technology make scientists continue their research in this area.

At the S. Fedorov Eye Microsurgery Complex of the Russian Ministry of Health, Vitreocontrast suspension has been used for the intraoperative visualization of the vitreous body structures and the VRI since 2009. This staining agent (TU No. 9398-017-29039336-2009) is an ultradisperse suspension based on barium sulfate, insoluble in water and physiological liquids, a neutral nontoxic inorganic salt in an isotonic solution with osmolarity of 300–350 mOsm. Barium sulfate is a white crystalline substance with a molecular weight of 233.43 g/mol, particle size in Vitreocontrast suspension less than 5 μm, and density of 4.4 g/cm^3 [27–30].

Each 1.0 ml of sterile solution contains 140 mg of dry substance (barium sulfate) [6, 13, 15]. Various experimental studies have confirmed the safety of intraocular administration of the suspension [6, 13, 15]. Vitreocontrast is currently used to stain VB and VRI for retinal detachments, proliferative diabetic retinopathy, macular holes, and idiopathic epiretinal membranes.

Thus, both vital dyes have similar physical and chemical characteristics. They are biologically inert substances used to stain intraocular structures in different vitreoretinal pathologies. In order to choose the optimum vital dye, we carried out experimental staining of VRI by suspensions «Kenalog-40» and «Vitreocontrast», which made it possible to assess their main characteristics and to choose intraoperative staining of the eye posterior segment, to evaluate the results of the comparative staining by suspensions Kenalog-40 and Vitreocontrast in the PVD induction during the experimental study [27, 31–33].

The study was performed on 20 cadaveric human eyes. Kenalog-40 glucocorticoid suspension and Vitreocontrast suspension were chosen as VB staining agents. The staining ability of the proposed compositions was assessed on the VB macro preparation. A set of microsurgical ophthalmological instruments including: scissors, needle-holders, eye microsurgical forceps, ophthalmosurgical knives, insulin syringes, 27 G, 30 G needles, 25 G ports (Alcon, USA), and 25 G endovitreal forceps (Alcon, USA) were used to prepare eyeball and VB. In all the groups, non-fixed eyeballs were dissected in several stages according to the suggested original technology. Initially, the sclera was incised with scissors 4 mm from the limbus in a circle, leaving the anterior segment of the eye intact (cornea, iris, and lens). Then the sclera was cut between the rectus muscles not reaching the projection of the yellow spot and the place of optic disc exit forming scleral petals (**Figure 1a** and **b**).

The scleral petals were cut off leaving a part of sclera with a dimeter from 10 to 11 mm in the posterior pole of the eye, which included the projection zone of the macula and the optic nerve. Then, with the help of the razor and the anatomical forceps, choroid petals were formed and also cut off (**Figure 2a–c**)

The next step was to form retinal petals with the help of anatomical forceps, separate them from the VB surface leaving them fixed to the anterior segment and the posterior pole of the eyeball. Then the retina was separated from the VB surface, thus modeling the PVD. The VB and retina were examined to detect concomitant pathology.

Using a 25 G cannula and a 2.0 ml disposable syringe, 1.0 ml of Kenalog-40 suspension was applied on the vitreous surface and separated retina, then the surface was washed with saline to remove excess dye. The surface of VB and separated retina was photographed immediately after staining after 3, 5, 15, and 30 minutes. The staining intensity of the vitreoretinal interface structures was assessed visually. Then

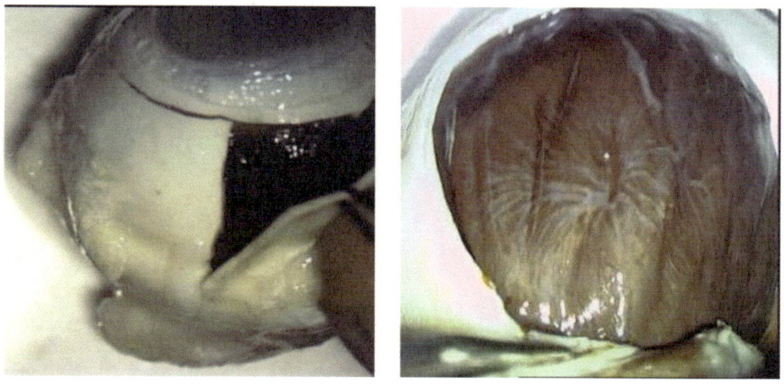

(a) (b)

Figure 1.
(a, b) Stages of preparation of eyeballs. a. Formation of scleral petals. b. Exposure of the choroid.

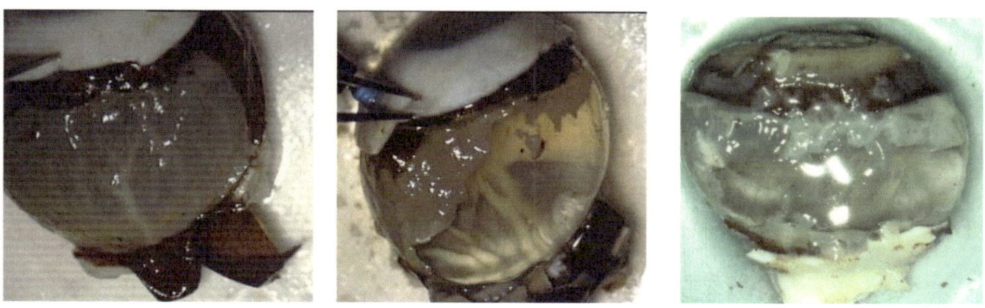

(a) (b) (c)

Figure 2.
The eyeball during the stages of preparation. a. Forming and cutting off scleral petals. b. Forming and cutting off choroid petals. c. Induction of posterior vitreous detachment by forming retinal petals and separating them from the vitreous.

Vitreocontrast suspension was applied on the same area of the VB surface and separated retina, the surface was also washed, photographed, and the staining intensity was assessed visually. Next, the stained retinal sections and VB cortical layers were cut using Vanasse scissors, separated using scissors and anatomical forceps, and sent for histological examination. Morphological examination of stained VRI structures—retina and vitreous cortex—was done. For this purpose, the material was fixed in 10% neutral formalin solution, washed with running water, dehydrated in ascending alcohols, and embedded in paraffin. Then we made a series of histological sections using hematoxylin-eosin and Van Gieson staining and alcian blue staining. The preparations were studied under a Leica DMLB2 microscope at ×50, ×100, ×200, and ×400 magnification followed by photographing. Photographic registration was performed using a DFC-320 digital color camera included in the kit. After the instillation of glucocorticoid suspension Kenalog-40 on the retinal surface, not having sufficient degree of adhesion, the particles freely rolled off the surface of the retina and VB. In all the cases, the retinal surface remained visually unchanged, the vitreous surface was shiny smooth and completely transparent (**Figure 3a–c**). Repeated application of Kenalog-40 suspension on the surface of VB and retina did not change the results obtained earlier.

The application of Vitreocontrast suspension on the vitreous surface and corresponding separated retinal lobes made it possible to visualize the sites of split cortical layers after experimental PVD induction. At these sites, a thin vitreous

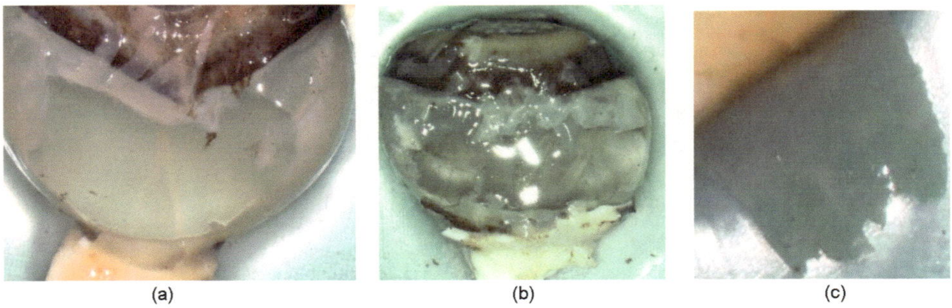

Figure 3.
The eyeball after instillation of Kenalog-40 suspension. a, b. The surface of the vitreous. c. The surface of separated retinal fragment.

layer was detected on the retinal surface, and the vitreous surface corresponding to the retina was covered with a layer of Vitreocontrast suspension particles. At other sites, the vitreous surface remained smooth, shiny, and transparent, and the corresponding retinal sites also remained visually unchanged. The degree of suspension adhesion did not change over time, and vitreous fibers were clearly visualized on the retinal surface.

Thus, in case of true PVD and complete separation of VB from the retinal ILM, VB remained smooth, transparent, and shiny, Vitreocontrast particles did not adhere to its surface. In case of the tight adhesion of VB cortical layers to the retinal ILM during PVD induction, they split (vitreoschisis). In this case, the VB layer was visualized on the ILM surface (**Figure 4a–d**).

The areas of the retina stained by Vitreocontrast suspension were excised and histologically examined to identify the stained layer.

On the histological preparation, cortical VB layers stained by Vitreocontrast suspension were visualized on the retinal surface of the donor eyeball. The retinal structure was unchanged. No visible artifactual damage was detected. There were signs of autolytic processes: moderate edema and loss of some nuclear layers, destruction of photoreceptor layer with elements of pigment granules (remnants of pigment epithelium), and fragmentary ILM detachment that were not aggravated by dispersed particles in the vitreal cavity (**Figure 5a** and **b**)

The experimental study confirmed the possibility of vitreous cortical layers splitting in induced PVD. It should be noted that it was impossible to assess this condition when using Kenalog-40 suspension as a contrast staining agent. Not having sufficient degree of adhesion glucocorticoid suspension particles did not allow for the visualization of vitreous layer or the remnants of vitreous fibers on the retina. Thus, it was impossible to determine the areas of true PVD and the areas of vitreous stripping. On the contrary, the use of Vitreocontrast suspension as a contrast staining agent made it possible to visualize the areas of laminated vitreous cortex during PVD induction. The sites of the retina, on the surface of which the VB layer was stained, were sent for histological examination that confirmed the presence of the VB layer on the retinal tissue specimen after PVD induction.

The study revealed that during PVD, some cortical layers may completely detach from the retinal surface, while others, having a higher degree of fixation to the retinal surface, may split, thus forming an abnormal PVD. Today, Vitreocontrast suspension has a sufficient degree of adhesion and allows visualization of this condition—areas of true and abnormal PVD. Vitreocontrast has a number of advantageous properties.

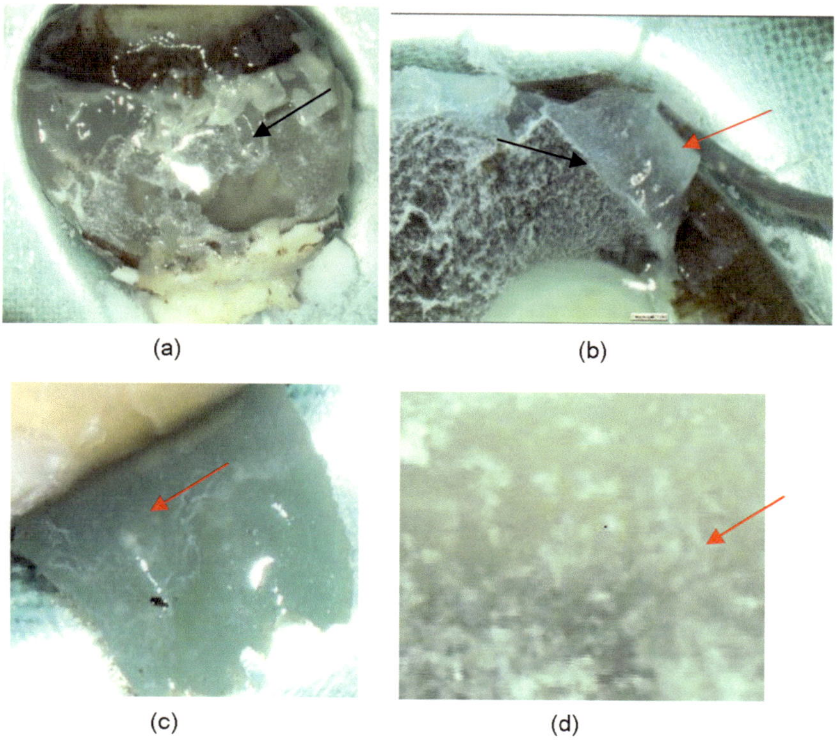

Figure 4.
The eyeball after the instillation of the Vitreocontrast suspension. Splitting of the cortical layers of the vitreous body during the induction of PVD. a and b. The surface of the vitreous body (black arrows). b and c. The retinal surface (red arrows).
The arrows indicate the vitreous fibers that were not contrasted during the instillation of Kenalog-40 suspension and which were contrasted after the instillation of the Vitreocontrast suspension.

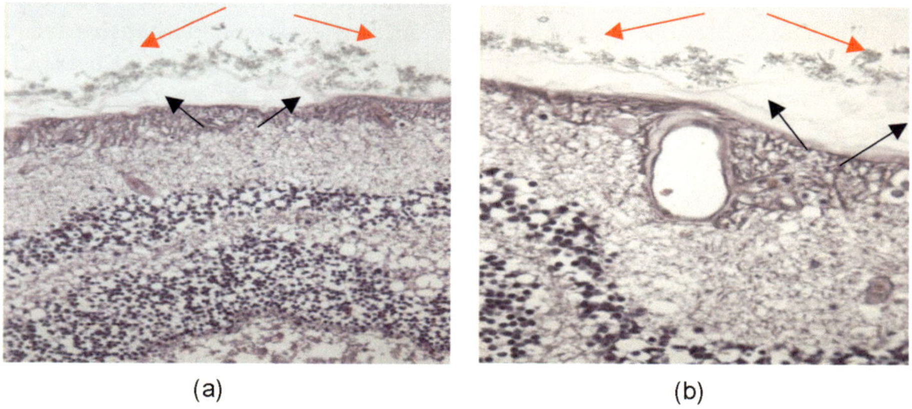

Figure 5.
Micro photography. Fragments of the vitreo-retinal interface, split cortical layers of the VB (black arowws) with adhered particles of Vitreocontrast suspension (red arrows), the structure of the retina is unchanged.

It stains VB structures in isolation, has high adhesion, due to which the intensity of staining of intravitreal structures does not change over time. Besides, it is a biologically inert substance. These characteristics indicate the feasibility of its introduction into ophthalmological practice in order to use it as a staining agent for VB structures and vitreoretinal interface during vitrectomy.

Comparative staining by Vitreocontrast and Kenalog-40 suspensions revealed that Vitreocontrast, due to its properties, determined by its physical and chemical characteristics did not stain only all intravitreal structures but also revealed the areas of cortical layer splitting in PVD. And the staining intensity of studied VB structures did not change with time.

The experimental study confirmed the possibility of splitting of cortical layers during PVD with the development of abnormal PVD. Under cortical layer splitting, a thin vitreous layer was visualized on the retinal surface, and the adhered particles of Vitreocontrast suspension remained on the corresponding laminated section of the vitreous.

3. Experimental study 2

The study was carried out on 40 cadaveric human eyes. In 14 cases, the vitreous body was stained by specialized contrast staining agent Vitreocontrast. The control group included the 14 eyes where Kenalog-40 suspension was instilled.

Simultaneous (comparative) contrast staining by Kenalog-40 + Vitreocontrast was performed in 12 cases.

Antegrade and retrograde dye injections were used.

In the control group, it was revealed that Kenalog-40 stains vitreous fibers but has a low-grade adhesion to the structural elements of the vitreous body. When Kenalog-40 was injected into the vitreous canals, it did not stay in their cavities. Vitreocontrast showed well-expressed adhesion to the VB structural elements (canals, cisterns, and their anastomoses), the degree of adhesion did not change with time. When injected in the projection area of VB canals, the dye settled on the walls of cisterns.

For the first time, a specialized contrast staining agent Vitreocontrast was developed, which due to its high mechanical adhesion, particle size, and intensive dye accumulation on VB structures made it possible to visualize not only VB fibers but also intravitreal channels, cisterns, and their relations.

One of the urgent issues of modern vitreoretinal surgery is intraoperative visualization of the vitreous body (VB), staining of its native structures and pathologically changed areas. The quality of the removal of transparent VB structures and the atraumatism of the intervention determine the anatomical and functional prognosis of the procedure. In this respect, the issue of VB structure undoubtedly remains important.

In 1973, J.Worst and Makhacheva Z.A. anatomical carried out functional studies of VB with the use of vital dyes that gave new understanding of its structure. Three rows of cisterns (the circle of equatorial, retrociliary and petaliform cisterns): canals (lentico-macular, optico-ciliary canal) and other VB structural elements were discovered and described [7]

Selection of perfect contrast staining agent still remains a topical problem due to the specific requirements (high dispersity, easy instillation and elimination, possibility of elimination via natural outflow ways, lack of side effects, etc.) imposed by surgeons.

Today, various vital dyes are used to identify the transparent structures of the posterior segment of the eye. These are triamcinolone acteonid (TA), trypan blue,

[34–36] membrane blue (0.15%), fluorescein, and indocyanine green [15, 21, 23, 37]. At the same time, none of the vital dyes allows for the antemortem identification of intravitreal structures described in the works by J. Worst [7].

A number of researchers showed that modern vital dyes due to their nonselective diffusion stained not only VB but the surrounding intraocular structures too, which impaired the identification of VB. Besides, the abovementioned agents have a number of side effects (cytotoxic, phototoxic, cataractgenic action, elevated intraocular pressure, and pharmacological activity) [6, 11, 15, 16].

Staining by TA is more effective because being not a true vital dye but a suspension it settles on VB as precipitates and VB can be easily distinguished from surrounding intraocular structures [22, 23, 38, 39]. That is why we chose this agent to stain VB in the control group.

The purpose of this study is to develop a specialized contrast staining agent for the intraoperative vitreous body structures visualization.

The study was carried out on 20 cadaveric human eyes. Researchers used specialized agent Vitreocontrast and triamcinolone acteonid or kenalog-40 to stain vitreous structures.

Preliminarily, VB was completely dissected from the overlying membranes (conjunctiva, sclera, choroid, and retina) (**Figures 6** and 7).

In 14 cases, staining was performed by Vitreocontrast intravitreal injection.

The control group consisted of 14 eyes, in which kenalog-40 suspension was injected. Simultaneous (comparative) staining by Kenalog-40 + Vitreocontrast was performed in 12 cases.

Antegrade and retrograde methods of contrast staining agent injection were used.

We managed to stain the structures described in the works by J.Worst and Z.A. Makhacheva [7] staining VB structures with Vitreocontrast suspension retrograde injection. These were the circle of equatorial, petaliform and retrociliary cisterns, optociliary and lentico-macular canals, and premacular bursa (**Figure 8a–c**). Vitreocontrast showed pronounced adhesion to VB structural elements that did not change over time.

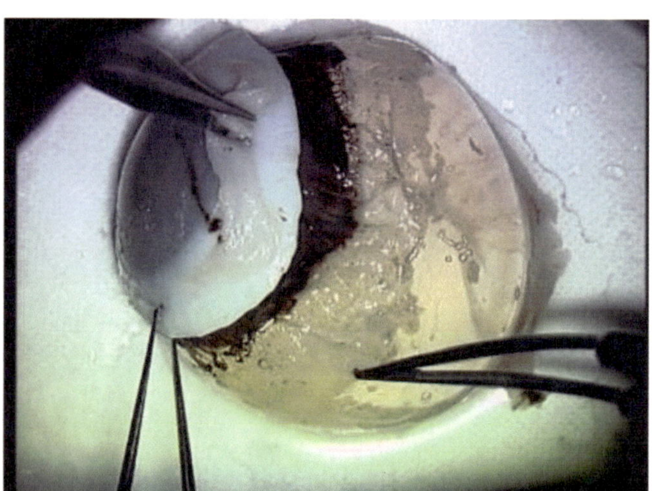

Figure 6.
The eyeball dissection. Sclera, choroid, and retina sequential removing.

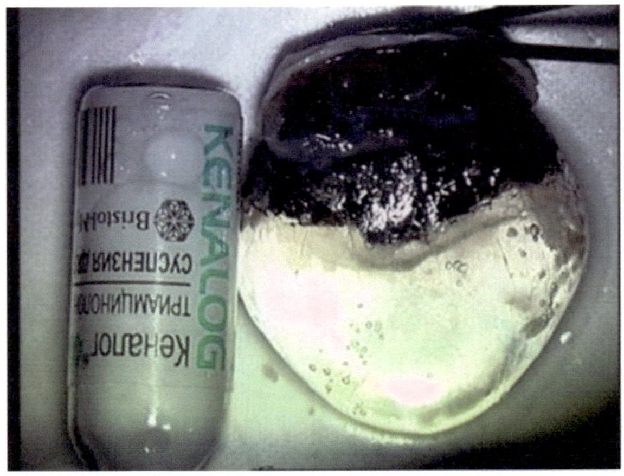

Figure 7.
The eyeball after dissection.

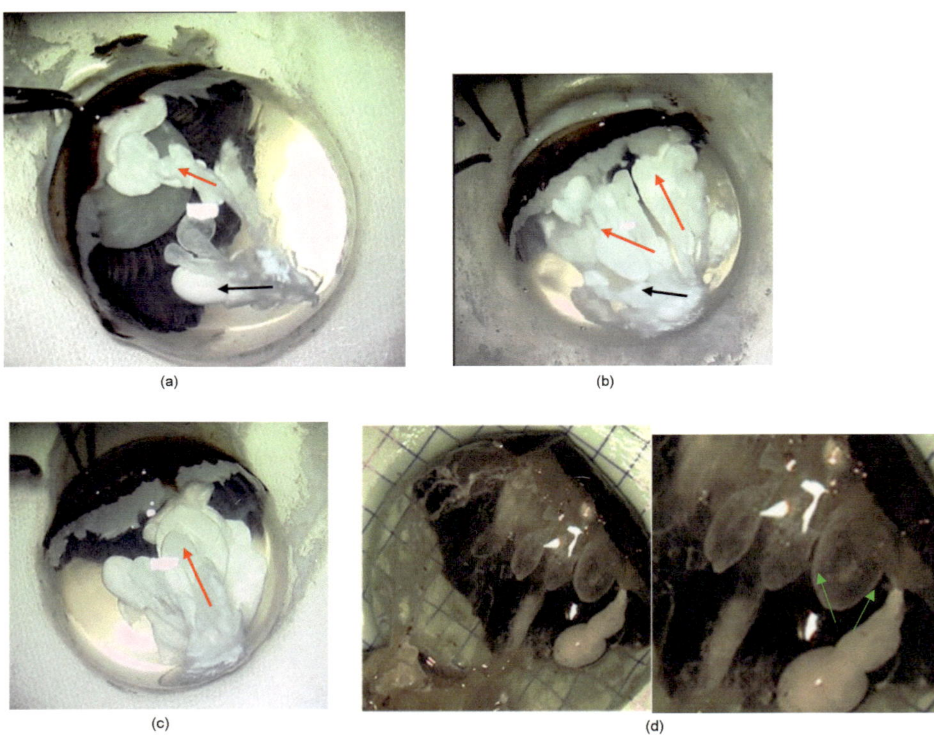

Figure 8.
(a-d) Vitreal body structures contrasting by the Vitreocontrast suspension (retrograde injection). Equatorial cysterns (red arrows) and lenticular cysterns (black arrows), retrociliary cisterns (green arrows) earlier J. Worst described.

The size of intravitreal structures was determined during the study (average size of retrociliary cisterns was 10–12 mm, equatorial cisterns were 15–17 mm, petal-like cisterns were 8–10 mm)

When staining with Kenalog-40 antegrade injection in the projection of lentico-macular canal was used the walls of the canal were not clearly visualized, the vital dye did not stay in the canal cavity gradually settling into the posterior hyaloid (**Figure 9a–c**).

Under the comparative contrast staining of VB structures, Vitreocontrast was injected in the lentico-macular canal in the macular projection after the administration of kenalog-40 suspension. Vitreocontrast stained this canal, anastomoses with the cisterns surrounding it, and the premacular bursa (**Figure 9a–c**).

For the first time, a specialized contrast staining agent Vitreocontrast was developed, which due to its high mechanical adhesion, particle size, and intensive dye accumulation on more loose structures made it possible to visualize not only VB fibers but also intravitreal canals, cisterns, and their relations (**Figures 10–13**).

The new contrast staining agent is not toxic that allows us to recommend it for the further use in diagnosis and treatment of vitreoretinal diseases after its clinical approbation.

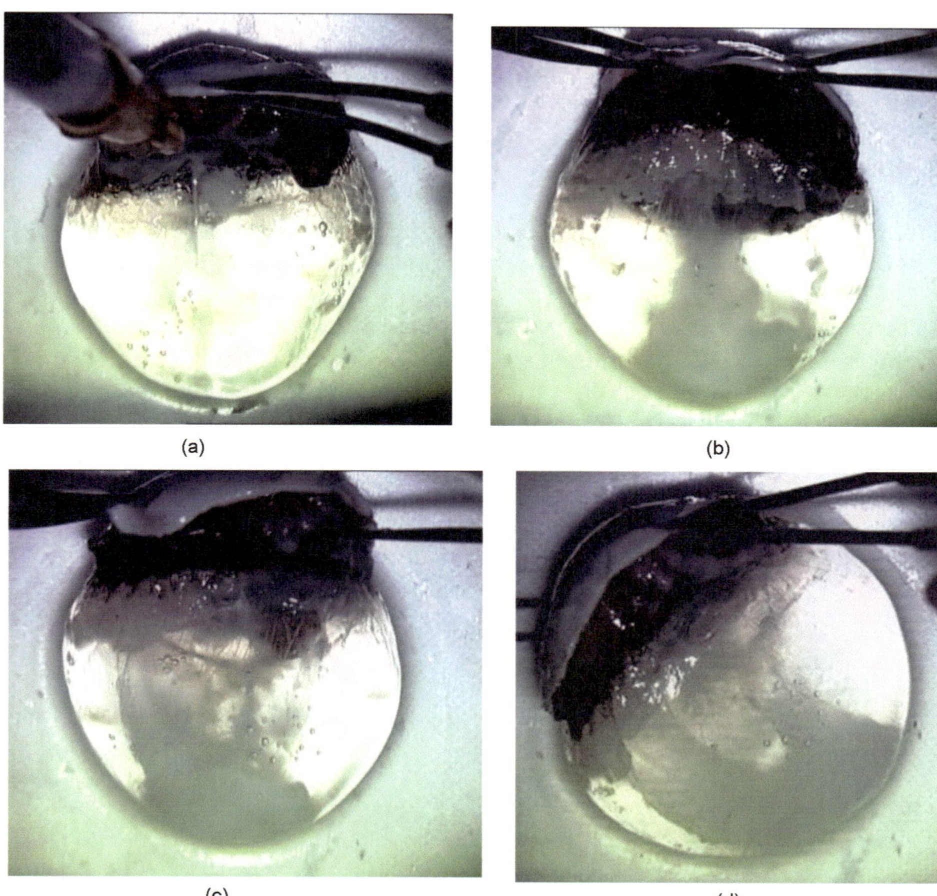

Figure 9.
a. Kenalog-40 injection (anthegrade injection). b in the projection zone of lentico-macular the walls of the canal are not clearly visualized, the suspension settles in the VB hyaloid layers. c and d. Kenalog-40 particles settled on the vitreous cortical layers. The channels and ci sterns (their walls) not visualized. Retrograde administration of Kenalog-40 in the projection zone of lentico-macular canal, the walls of the canal are not clearly visualized, the suspension settles in the VB hyaloid layers.

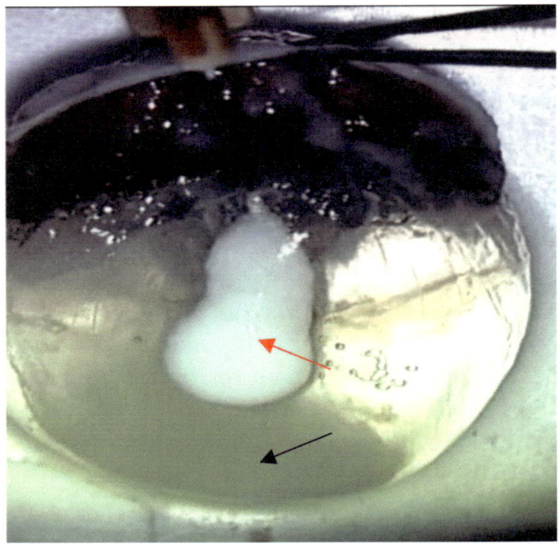

Figure 10.
Vitreocontast suspension injection (red arrow) and Kenalog-40 injection (black arrow) in comparative vitreous structures contrasting.

4. Clinical study

4.1 Methods and results of the application of the developed technique of vitreous body visualization in the diagnosis of idiopathic macular holes

This aim of this work was to study the anatomical and topographic specifics of changes in VB and VRI at different stages of idiopathic macular holes (MH).

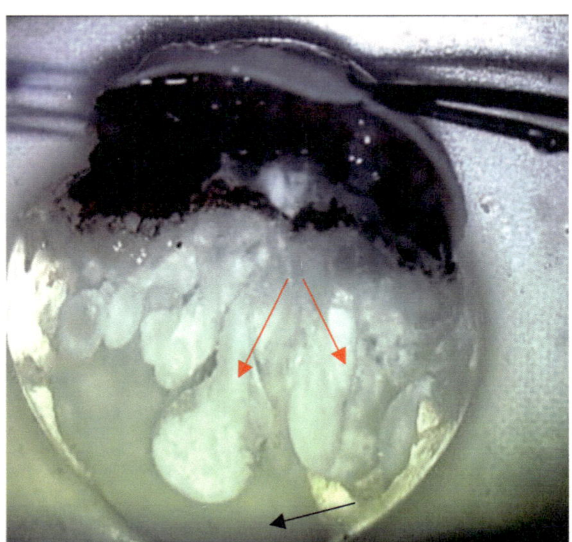

Figure 11.
Vitreocontrast injection (red arrow) and Kenalog-40 (black arrow) in the comparative vitreous structures contrasting. The Vitreocontrast suspension provides retrociliar (red arrow) and equatorial cisterns (red arrow) contrasting.

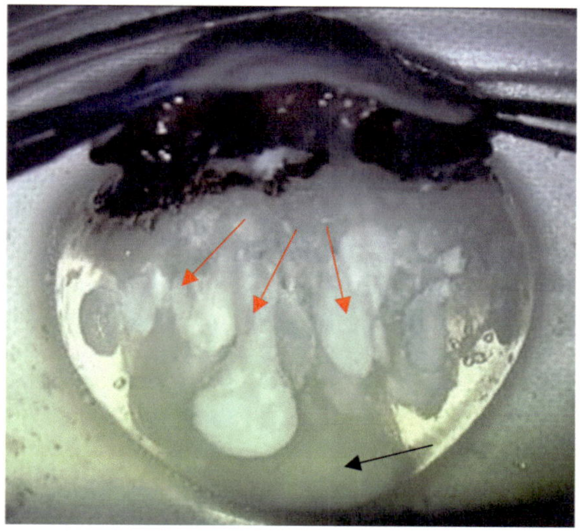

Figure 12.
Vitreocontrast injection (red arrow) and Kenalog-40 (black arrow) in the comparative vitreous structures contrasting. The Vitreocontrast suspension provides retrociliar (red arrow) and equatorial cisterns (red arrow) contrasting.

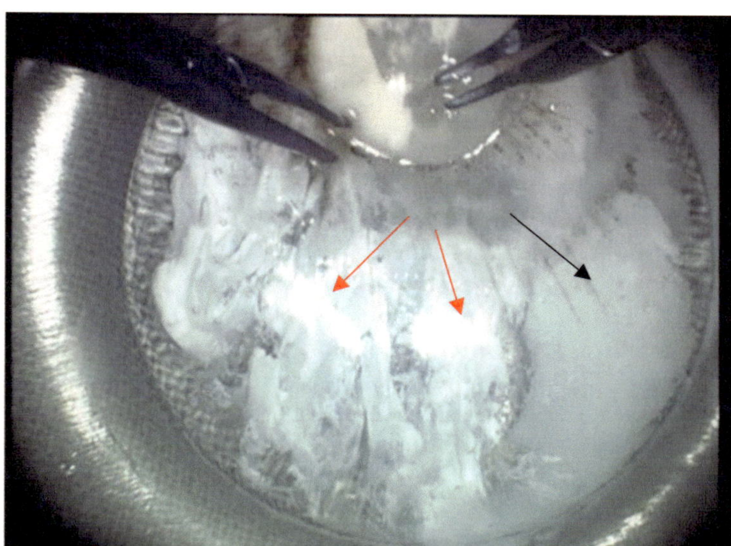

Figure 13.
Vitreocontrast suspension injection (red arrows) and Kenalog-40 (black arrow) suspension in comparative vitreous structures contrasting.

We followed up 143 patients (143 eyes), 105 females, 38 males, aged 51–78 years (mean age 64.8 ± 5.3 years). Inclusion criteria for patients were the presence of MH, transparent optical medium, the absence of diabetes mellitus and other systemic diseases and ophthalmic surgical procedures in the medical history. The study exclusion criteria for patients were high myopia and traumatic MH. All patients were divided into the following three groups according to the traditional classification of the International Vitreomacular Traction Study Group (2013) [1]:

- patients with small (≤250 μm) diameter MH (40 patients, 40 eyes);
- patients with MH of medium (>250–≤400 μm) diameter (58 patients, 58 eyes);
- patients with large (>400 μm) diameter MH (45 patients, 45 eyes).

At the same time (according to the classification), in all the cases this was a primary MH without vitreomacular traction [33, 40].

The preoperative examination of patients was performed using traditional methods (visometry, tonometry; biomicroscopy of anterior segment, vitreous body and ocular fundus; B-scan, electroretinography and spectral optical coherence tomography (OCT). All the patients had a penetrating retinal defect in the macular area and increased (due to edema) retinal thickness along the MH edge. Besides, ocular fundus photography was made by MAIA fundus microperimeter (CenterVue, Italy) combining a black and white fundus camera with an image angle of 45° in addition to the perimeter. All the stages of the surgery including IIM peeling were recorded using a digital video camera Panasonic LQ-MD800E (Panasonic Corporation, Osaka, Japan) connected to operating microscope OMS-800 OFFISS (Topcon, Japan). Before each imaging session, routine exposure adjustment and calibration were performed by adjusting the white balance of the recording system to a standardized sample (Xpo-Balance, Lastolight Ltd., Coalville, Leicestershire, United Kingdom).

The intraoperative Vitreocontrastography was performed using regional infiltrational block anesthesia with central potentiation. Three-port vitrectomy was performed using 25 Short Totalplus Vitrectomy Pak under operating microscope Topcon OFFISS OMS 800 (Japan) on surgical machine Constellation (Alcon, USA). The ports were placed 4 mm from the limbus. BSS irrigation solution (Alcon Laboratories Inc., USA) was used to maintain the vitreous cavity volume during the procedure. Sterile air was used for postoperative tamponade of the vitreous cavity. All the patients underwent standard three-port 25G closed vitrectomy, a distinctive feature of which was the use of Vitreocontrast suspension for highlighting of VB and VRI structures in order to study their topographic anatomy. At the first stage, 3 25G ports were set at a distance of 4 mm from the limbus in the planar ciliary body projection at 2.30, 4.00, and 9.30 o'clock. Staining of the vitreous structures was performed sequentially through each port in order to visualize their preservation, size, topographic anatomy of intravitreal structures, and the degree of its destruction. In order to do this, we injected 0.1 ml in all the accessible quadrants using a 30G needle and stained the VB structures with Vitreocontrast suspension. After highlighting of intravitreal structures in all the segments and the video registration of anatomical topography of the VB condition, a three-port 25 G vitrectomy was performed using standard technique. The next stage was highlighting of the vitreous cortical layers. Then intraoperative induction of PVD and the removal of vitreous cortical layers with a vitreotome needle were performed in an aspiration mode. Then Vitreocontrast suspension was reapplied on the retinal surface, its excesses were removed by passive aspiration. The VRI topographic anatomy was assessed and video-recorded. If there were the remnants of cortical layers or vitreous fibers on the retinal ILM surface, their topography, area, and configuration were assessed. There were photo recording and video recording of changes in ILM topographic anatomy—abnormal PVD. In order to assess the degree of the adhesion of cortical layers to the retinal ILM surface, attempts to remove them by 25G endovitreal forceps were made. We also assessed the possibility of the cortical layer removal separately from the ILM, the degree of the adhesion, and the link of cortical layers to the MH edges. After the maximum possible removal of the vitreous cortical layers from the retinal surface, Vitreocontrast suspension was reapplied and the VRI topography was evaluated. After the mechanical removal of all the possible vitreous fibers, the retinal ILM was stained using 25G end-gripping Constellation Grieshaber forceps and the ILM around the MH was peeled. The proposed suspension made it possible to visualize the residual fibers on the ILM surface and to remove the ILM only within this area. As soon as the suspension settled on the ILM surface, the excess agent was immediately removed by passive aspiration. After the visual inspection of the macular area, we proceeded to the formation of ILM fragments using 25G end-gripping forceps. The formation of an ILM flap was started at 2.0–2.5 mm to the superior temporal arcade from the hole edge. Using micro forceps, an ILM section was separated from the retina by a pinch at the indicated point; then, gripping the ILM tip by forceps the membrane was cut off along 2–3 hourly meridians in a motion directed along the arc of an imaginary circle with MH in the center while making sure that there was no separation of the ILM from the hole edge. Then we intercepted the ILM separated along the arc at the end point and continued cutting off the ILM. By successive intercepting of the separated ILM section edges by forceps, we performed a circular separation of the ILM around the MH without the complete detachment of the fragment. Then we used a vitreotome in a "shave" mode to trim the edges of the dissected circular fragment of the ILM that were facing the vitreous cavity. After that, the ILM flap was placed in an inverted manner without mechanical impact on the foveola area.

The results of the study indicated that in the first group of patients in 64% of the cases the vitreous cisterns were elongated in the anteroposterior direction extending toward the posterior pole. The size of the cisterns was 6.5 mm in length; 8 mm in width; in 45% of cases there was disruption of the cistern wall integrity and the exit of the contrast composition outside the stained cavities that was determined from the viewpoint of VB destruction in general (64% of cases) (**Figure 14**).

After staining of cortical layers, intraoperative PVD induction with the presence of a Weiss ring was performed. At the current stage of research, this is a confirmation of the complete separation of cortical layers from retinal ILM. However, after the application of contrast suspension on retinal ILM in all the cases, a vitreous layer was highlighted on the retinal surface in the macular area that proved to the abnormal PVD and vitreoschisis (**Figure 15**).

Topographically, this vitreous layer is located in the center of the retina (macular area) and is of medium size, with 95% of cases characterized by a low degree of adhesion to the underlying tissues, friability and possibility of mechanical separation (**Figure 16**).

Upon the repeated Vitreocontrast suspension application, the retinal ILM was visualized, but in 45% of the cases, no formed vitreous cortical layer was visualized on its surface. However, the ILM itself was visualized as a result of the adhesion of particles but as a thin "dusting" since the surface is rough. In 35% of the cases, residual vitreous fibers were visualized as separate areas, half of which could be difficult to remove mechanically.

In 45% of the cases, VB was visualized on the ILM surface in the central zone, but the layer was ultrathin. In cases when residual vitreous fibers or layers were present, we performed classical circular ILM peeling with obligatory capturing of pathologically changed ILM zones characterized by the presence of ILM areas with the tight adhesion of vitreous residues, which is a risk factor for ERM formation and proliferation.

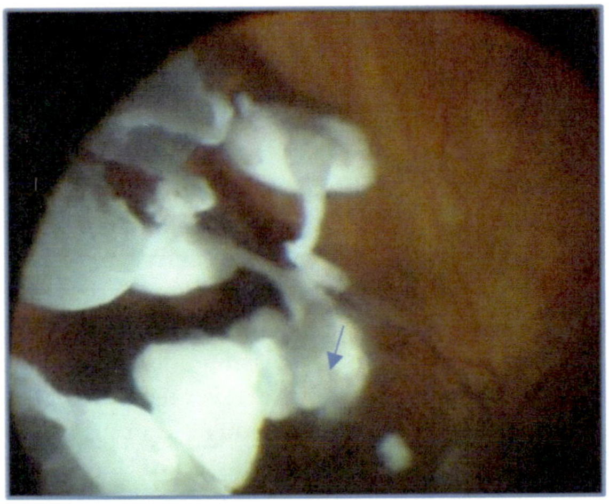

Figure 14.
Visualization of intravitreal structures. The cisterns are elongated up to 10–12 mm, the contrast suspension out of the cavity can be seen (marked with an arrow), small MH, Group 1 patients.

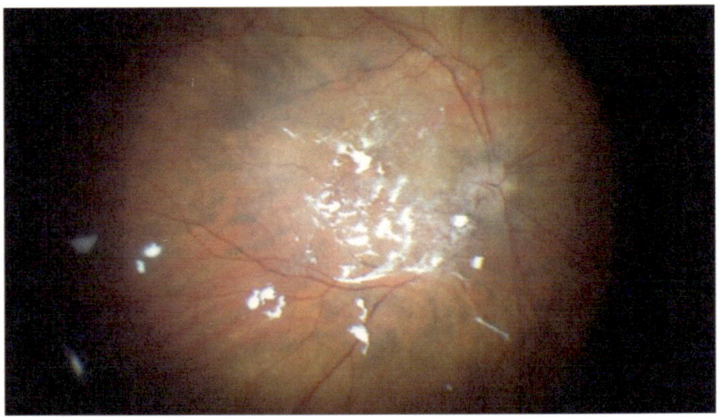

Figure 15.
A vitreous layer on the retina after the PVD induction. On the retinal surface in the macular area, one can see a vitreous layer (vitreoschisis) with clear borders (small MH, I group patients).

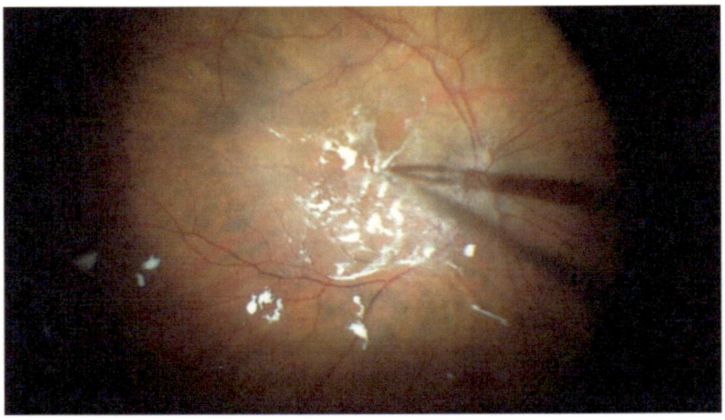

Figure 16.
Mechanical removal of the stained vitreous layer (small MH, I group patients).

The results of the study in the second group of patients evidenced that the destruction of the VB (changes in its shape, size, and integrity) was observed in 78% of the cases and was expressed in the elongation (up to 10 mm) of equatorial and retrociliary cisterns, which in 68% of cases was accompanied by the exit of the contrast agent from the cistern cavity and its settling in the macular projection zone. After staining of cortical layers and the intraoperative PVD induction, a suspension was applied on the retinal surface, and in 100% of cases, the vitreous layer was visualized on the ILM surface only in the macular area. No adhesion of the contrast suspension particles was observed throughout the rest of the retinal surface that indicated to the abnormal PVD with a vitreoschisis zone in the macular area. The vitreous layer visualized in the central zone of the retina (macular area) was of medium size. In 60% of the cases, it was characterized by a low degree of adhesion to the underlying tissues, friability and the possibility of mechanical separation (**Figures 17–19**).

In the third group of patients, the VB destruction (changes in shape, size, and integrity) was observed in all the cases and was expressed in the elongation (up to 12 mm) of equatorial and retrociliary cisterns; in 95% of cases, it was accompanied by the exit of the contrast agent from cistern cavity and its settling in the macular projection zone (**Figure 20**).

The vitreous layer visualized in the center of the retina (macular area) is medium sized. In 15% of the cases, it was characterized by the low degree of adhesion to the underlying tissues, friability and the possibility of mechanical separation (**Figure 21a** and **b** and **22a** and **b**).

Discussing the results presented, the following four main points should be mentioned. The first one is related to the choice of the basic classification of MH. In this regard, it should be noted that the concept, according to which the leading role in IMH pathogenesis is attributed to tangential vitreomacular traction (VMT), is currently generally accepted. The essence of the concept is that the radial vitreous fibers left on the perimacular surface after PVD are reduced, which gradually leads to a round-shaped retinal tear in the macular area. This theory was proposed by J. Gass [3]. And

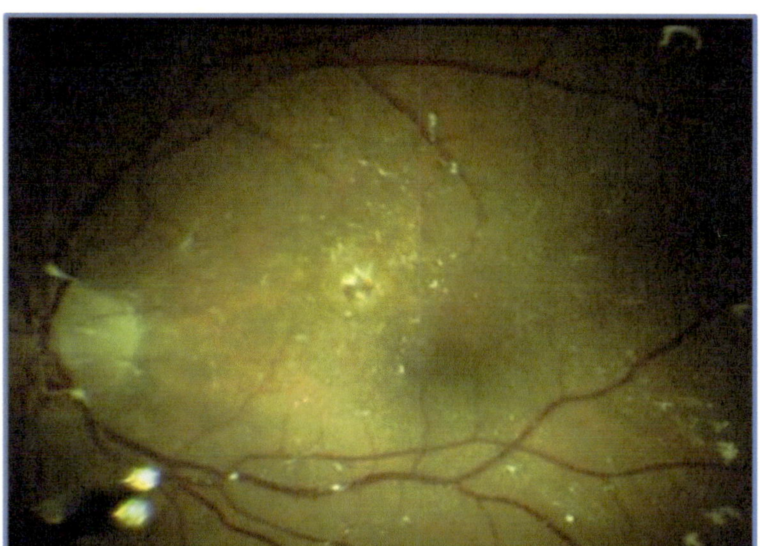

Figure 17.
Macular hole contrasted.

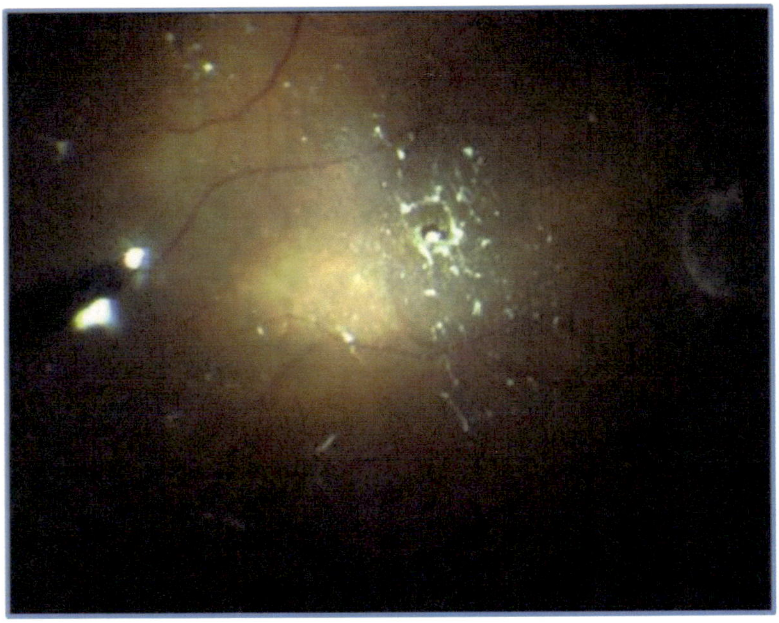

Figure 18.
Contrasted macular hole area.

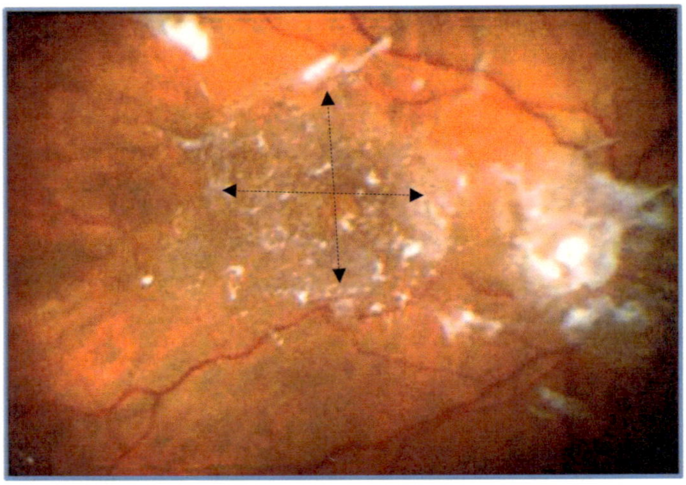

Figure 19.
The macular hole area contrasted can be defined and measured.

the classification of MH with distinguishing of 4 stages was developed on its basis. This classification is widely used at the present time. However, as far as the aim of this study is concerned, this classification has a significant disadvantage since it deals exclusively with the macular area. It does not address other elements of the disease pathogenesis (changes in the VB, vitreoretinal interface) outside the macular area [41, 42].

Currently, a new anatomical classification of MH ha has been created based on optical coherence tomography data [3, 43]. Research showed the sufficient efficiency of this classification in terms of typical OCT features at different stages of MH [6, 18, 26, 44], which in general determined the choice of this classification in the present study.

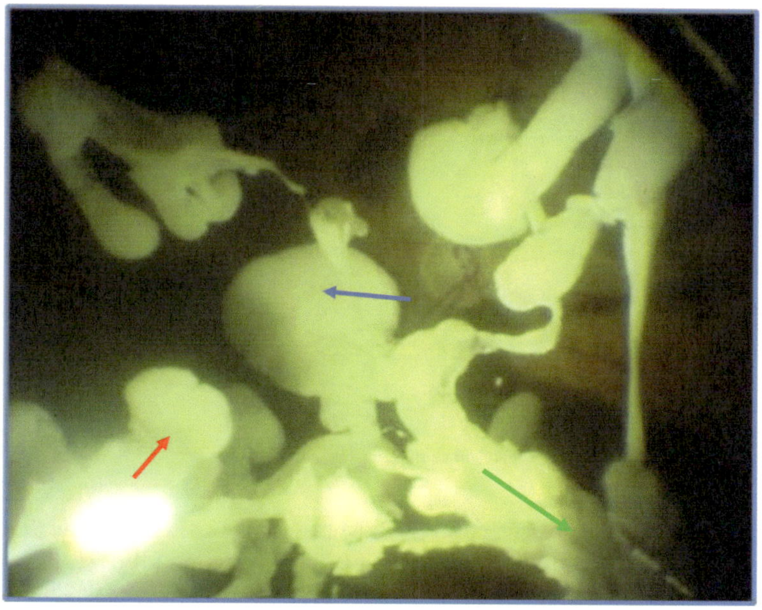

Figure 20.
Visualization of changed intravitreal structures. Elongation of the part of cisterns in the anteroposterior direction (red arrow), complete destruction of the part of the cisterns (green arrow) exit of the contrast agent outside the cavity (blue arrow), big MH, III group patients.

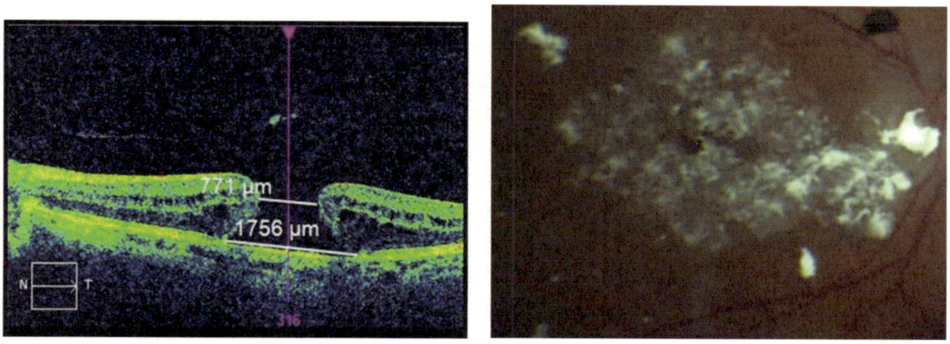

(a) (b)

Figure 21.
a. OCT patient pre-operation (patient A). b. Contrasting by Vitreocontrast. Vitreous body layer visualization in macular hole zone (patient A).

The second point determines the general aspects of MH pathogenesis from the standpoint of anatomical topographic changes in the vitreous. In this regard, it should be emphasized that the trigger for the MH development is the type of the abnormal PVD, which results in the adhesion of a vitreous cortical layer in the macular projection zone. This layer has a similar topography, area, configuration in all cases irrespective of the macular hole size. In small-diameter macular holes (as the initial stage of the pathological process), this layer has no pronounced adhesion to the underlying retinal ILM and in most cases can be removed from its surface. This fact accounts for the positive anatomical effect in small diameter MH in almost 90% of cases without performing retinal ILM peeling [12, 14, 43, 45]. Later, as the pathological proliferative process develops, the

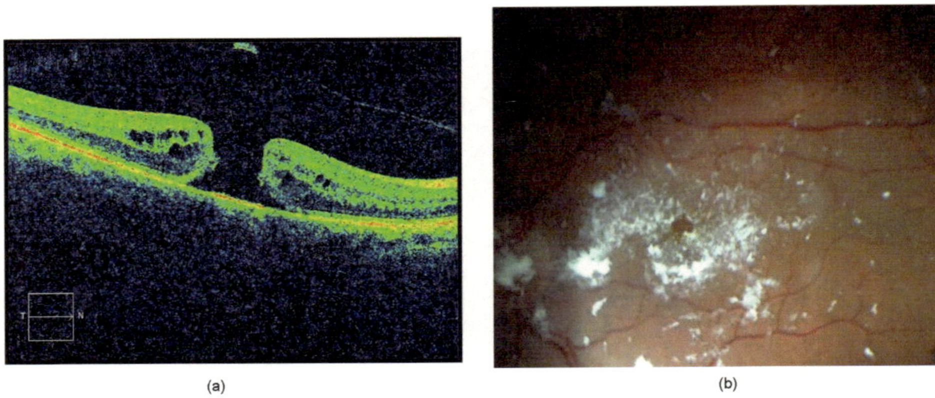

Figure 22.
a. OCT Patient B. b. Vitreous body visualisation in macular hole zone patient B.

adhesion between the vitreous layer and the ILM increases and, apparently, the process is aggravated by the contractile abilities of the ERM in formation [46, 47]. This leads to the intensification of tangential tractions and the gradual growth of MH. This thesis was confirmed by a dense cortical layer that we discovered in the large-diameter MH group of patients. In the vast majority of cases, this layer is fixed to the retinal ILM. Thus, the leading role in the MH pathogenesis belongs to the changes in the ILM of the macular area that is the development of the vitreous layer adhesion in this region. In case of PVD, it leads to its abnormal development, and the residual vitreous cortical layer stays in the macular area on the ILM surface. As the pathological process develops, the degree of the cortical layer adhesion to the retinal ILM and the contractility and tangential traction increase, which leads to an increase in the size of the hole. It should be emphasized that in all the patients, regardless of MH size, anatomical topographic changes in the vitreous were identical and were expressed primarily in the development of destruction characterized by the elongation of equatorial and retrociliary cisterns and the exit of the contrast agent from cistern cavities and its settling in the macular projection zone. It is also important to note that the destruction of the vitreous was present in small-diameter MH, i.e., at the early stages of the disease, which may indicate that changes in the vitreous occur before the development of visible (ophthalmoscopic or OCT) or clinical manifestations. Changes in the topographic anatomy of intravitreal structures have no significant differences at different stages of idiopathic macular holes, hence do not significantly influence the progression of the pathological process. The third point is related to the results of our comparative analytical assessment of the clinical diagnostic efficiency of MH treatment according to the developed techniques of VB visualization and the traditional classification. Our analysis proved to the fundamentally higher level of anatomical and morphological diagnosis of the various stages of MH by the developed techniques of VB visualization (on the basis of the original Vitreocontrastography method). In our opinion, this is associated with the following general drawbacks in the traditional classification [3, 15, 45, 48]:

- according to a number of authors, the leading role in the development of MH belongs to changes in the vitreous, but even indirect data (including B-scanning) are not taken into account when making these classifications;
- in current classification, PVD is assessed only on the basis of OCT data, which is limited exclusively to the macular area;

- the main substrate for the development of the abnormal PVD is vitreous cortical layers with a tight adhesion to the retinal ILM. However, the existing classification does not allow assessing of the characteristic features (configuration, area, number, degree of adhesion to the ILM) of these cortical layers, which, according to some authors, are the main pathogenetic risk factor for the development of MH;

- there are virtually no data characterizing the occurrence and localization of vitreoschisis zones associated with vitreous lamination;

- the visualized band of the hyperreflective image is interpreted as HGM and PVD according to the classification, despite the principal impossibility of this method to visualize transparent structures and differentiate vitreous cortical layers;

- the development of pathological process on the retinal ILM surface around MH is generally considered to be based on the formation of the ERM that has tangential traction effect on the retinal ILM; however, ERM anatomical topographic characteristics are not provided in the classification.

Thus, the traditional classification of MH [1, 49] does not fully reflect the basic characteristics of the pathological process (volume, topography, degree of changes in the retinal tissue) and, most importantly, practically does not assess the changes in the VB, which can trigger this disease. The stated disadvantages are certainly related to the limitations of OCT data in terms of coverage, ability to visualize transparent structures, and dependence on technical capabilities of the equipment used. Practical application of the developed VB visualization technique (based on the original vitreocontrastography method) provided the following fundamentally new possibilities for anatomical and morphological evaluation of VRI under MH:

- visualization of changes in the vitreous structures involved in the pathological process;

- staining of vitreous cortical layers to control intraoperatively induced PVD;

- visualization of vitreous cortical layers adhered to the retinal ILM with the possibility to determine the exact size of vitreoschisis zone in any of the meridians;

- possibility to remove the visualized vitreous layer in order to determine not only the topographic anatomy but also to make histological preparations for light or electron microscopy or immunohistochemical studies;

- possibility to assess the number of vitreous fibers adhered to ILM surface after removing a vitreous layer and staining of the ILM surface;

- possibility to assess the necessity of ILM peeling.

The fourth point defines a number of MH classificational anatomic morphological signs (CAMS) from the standpoint of the vitreoretinal surgery improvement (**Table 1**).

The data presented in **Table 1** make it possible to formulate the following main directions of MH surgical treatment improvement provided by the VB visualization technique on the basis of the original vitreocontastography method:

№ п/п	Classificational anatomic morphological sign	MH size (according to IVTG classification (2013), [4, 22]		
		Small (≤250 μм)	Medium (>250–≤ 400 μм)	Big (>400 μм)
1.	Removal of vitreous cisterns in anterior posterior direction	+	++	+++
2.	Disruption of the integrity of the VB cisterns wall and the exit of the contrast composition beyond the stained cavities.	+	++	+++
3.	VB destruction (violation of the integrity)	+	++	+++
4.	The degree of VB adhesion on the ILM surface	+	+++	+++
5.	The degree of VB adhesion in the macular area	+	+++	+++

Note: "–"—the sign is absent, "+"—the sign is insignificantly expressed; "++"—the sign is moderately expressed, "+++"—the sign is clearly expressed.

Table 1.
Classification of MH anatomical morphological signs developed on the basis of the original technique of VB visualization.

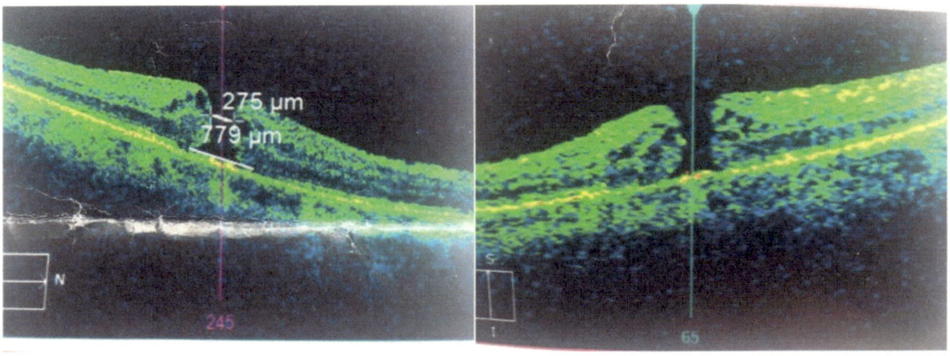

Figure 23.
OCT data (preoperational examination), patient Z.

- in the case of a small-diameter MH and the complete removal of cortical layers from the vitreous surface, it is possible to keep the ILM (patient 1); in the case of medium-diameter MH, the removal of IML can be performed either by the classical method that is a circular maculorrhexis with capturing of the entire ILM area with cortical layers adhered to it or by removing of the ILM with the formation of petals strictly along the contrast agent position keeping the ILM fixation along the hole edge and using any modification of the inverted flap (patient 2);

- in the case of a large-diameter MH and a bilayer vitreoschisis zone (or ERM), it is advisable to perform layer-by-layer removal with staining of each layer (CAMS - 3,4,5);

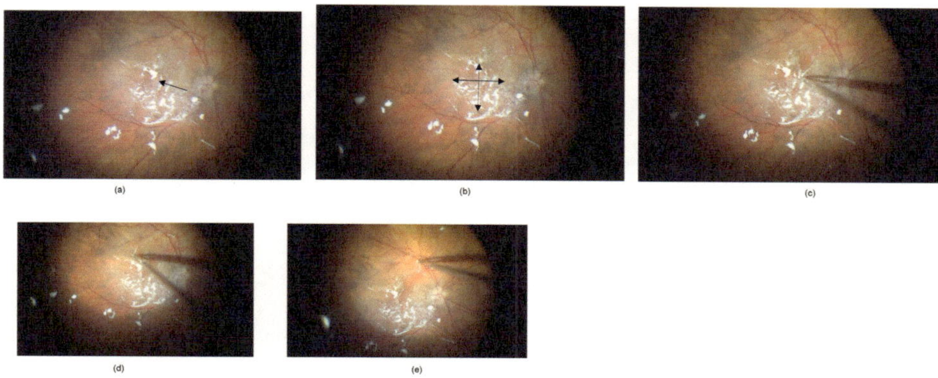

Figure 24.
a. Vitreous layer after the PVD induction, on the retinal surface in the macular area a vitreous layer with clear borders can be seen (patient Z. b. Abnormal PVD. On the retinal surface, a vitreous layer was visualized after complete intraoperative PVD induction (patient Z.). c. Removal of the cortical layer by forceps (patient Z). d–e. Removal of the cortical layer (patient Z.).

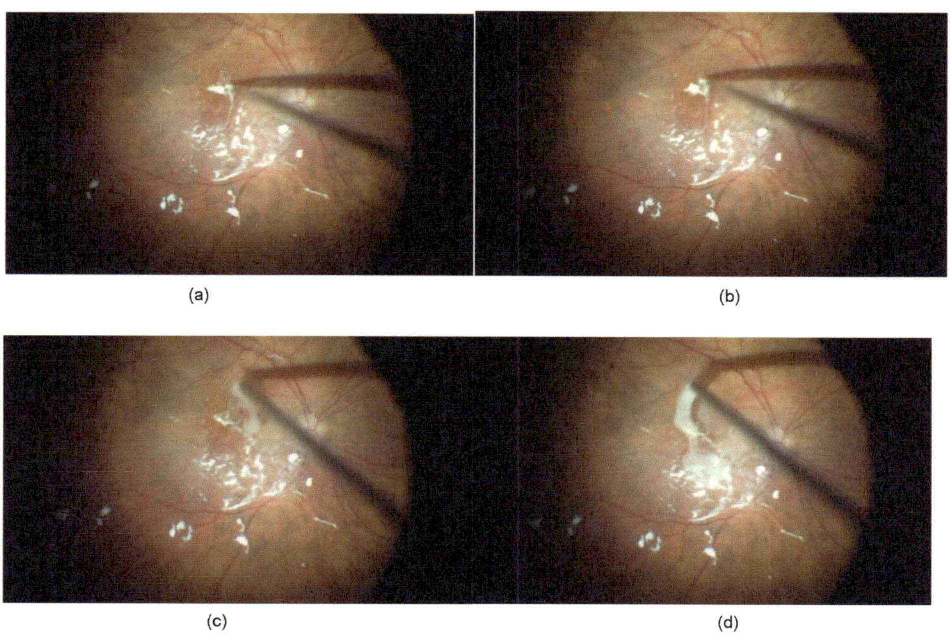

Figure 25.
(a and b) Vitreous layer was fixed to the edges of the MH (patients Z.). (c and d) Highlighting of retinal ILM after the removal of the vitreous cortical layer around the MH (patient Z.).

- in the case of large-diameter MH, it is advisable to perform maximum complete removal of the upper vitreous cortical layer keeping this layer fixed to the MH edges with subsequent staining of the underlying tissues. ILM with the vitreous layer is removed along the edge (or the area) of the stained ILM with the zone of the vitreous cortical layer adhered to it corresponding to the vitreoschisis zone (patient 3).

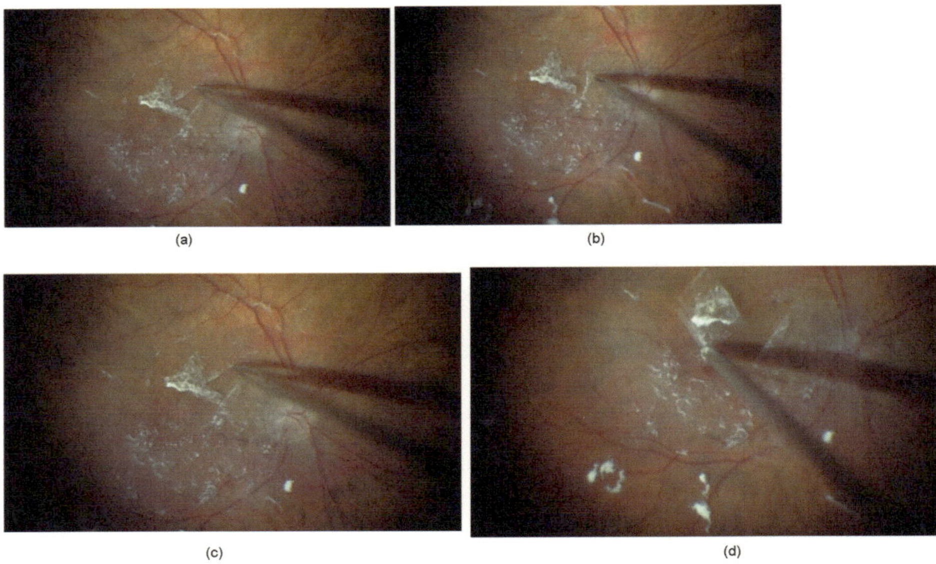

Figure 26.
(a and b) Removal of retinal ILM (patient z) (c) On ILM surface there was no vitreous layer (patient Z) (d) covering of the MH by the inverted ILM flap (patient Z).

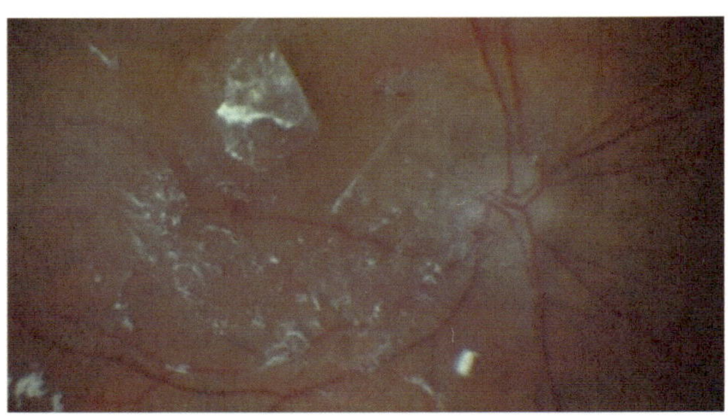

Figure 27.
The flap stayed in the normal position during working with its fragments by the vitreotome (patient Z.).

Thus, application of the developed technique of VB visualization (based on the original vitreocontrastography method) in patients with MH provides a principally new approach to clinical and diagnostic examination that is based on the development of basic classification anatomical morphological signs (visualization of structures and cortical layers (including on retina) of VB, the degree of VB adhesion, etc.) and characterized by principal advantages in comparison with traditional classifications of MR that in general makes it possible to significantly increase the clinical efficiency of vitreoretinal surgical procedures.

The points mentioned above were illustrated by the following clinical example.

Clinical case: patient Z., 64 years old, diagnosis medium diameter MH OS, at admission MCVA – 0.1, after the surgery MCVA – 0.3. The main stages of the diagnosis and treatment are presented in **Figures 23–27**.

5. Conclusion

Vitreoretinal pathology occupies a special place in the structure of eye diseases since these are the most complex and prevalent nosological forms that in many cases require highly qualified surgical treatment, and modern concepts of vitreoretinal surgery involve targeted, selective impact on the structures of the vitreoretinal interface. It should be also noted that the process of vitreoretinal intervention itself is constantly being improved in order to increase the clinical effeciency of surgical treatment both in the postoperative period and with regard to long-term results. The following main areas of improvement in vitrectomy can be conventionally identified as:

- the "technical" one aimed at developing and optimizing equipment for vitreoretinal surgical interventions;
- the "medicamental" one aimed at drug "support" for vitreoretinal surgery; the "diagnostic" one aimed at improving preoperative and intraoperative diagnosis

Currently, the following modern diagnostic methods that make it possible to visualize various vitreoretinal structures have been tested to the greatest extent. These are ultrasound examination (USE), optical coherence tomography (OCT), confocal laser scanning ophthalmoscopy (CLSO), and chromovitrectomy (CV). The use of water-soluble dyes and suspensions is considered the most relevant for the evaluation of intravitreal and preretinal structures within the framework of CV method. At the same time, despite the wide introduction of various staining agents for VB and retinal structures by CV technique into clinical practice, the selection of an optimal staining agent is still a topical issue due to specific requirements for vital dyes in terms of the visualization level as well as safety characteristics imposed on products that come into contact with the internal components of the eye for a long time.

However, in literature, there are only some sporadic studies that allow determining the size of intravitreal structures under normal, age-related, and pathological conditions of the vitreous and to define the comprehensive approach to the surgical treatment of vitreoretinal pathology depending on the morpho-functional condition. Thus, the problem of VB imaging needs further consideration both conceptually and along individual specific lines.

The abovementioned provisions served as a basis for the present study performed with the purpose of scientific substantiation, experimental and morphological development, and evaluation of the clinical efficiency of the complex technique of VB imaging for diagnosis and surgical treatment of vitreoretinal disorders.

The method of the study was based on three main conditions:

1. Complex approach to the assessment of the effeciency of the new VB imaging technique based on the study of anatomo-topographic, morpho-functional, clinical, sanitary-chemical, toxicological parameters as well as the patient's "quality of life."

2. Adequate and tested methods of collecting the required volume of clinical material (a total of 143 patients (143 eyes) and 6t autopsied eyes were examined).

3. Stage-wise approach (three stages) and the study consistency.

During the first stage of the study, the imaging efficiency and safety and various agents for chromo-vitrectomy were assessed on the basis of clinical and *in vitro*, *ex vivo* comparative assessment of various staining agents for the imaging technique of the vitreous body—, Kenalog-40, and original Vitreocontrastography method based on the use of Vitreocontrast suspension. Results of anatomical and morphological evaluation showed that Vitreocontrast due to its properties that are determined by its physical and chemical characteristics had a significantly higher level of visualization compared with Kenalog-40 as it stained not only all intravitreal structures but also the revealed PVD areas. At the same time, the researchers found that during PVD some cortical layers could completely detach from the retinal surface, while others having a higher degree of fixation to the retinal surface could laminate, thus forming an abnormal PVD. In this case, Vitreocontrast suspension had a sufficient degree of adhesion and allowed for the visualization of this condition.

Besides, it is important to emphasize that according to the studies, the Vitreocontrast suspension fully complied with the sanitary and chemical (pH 7.25 + 0.02 pH units (with the permissible value of 7.20–7.60 pH units). pH) and toxicological (according to the results of toxicity index (100 ± 10)% with the permissible values of 70–120%) indicators, the results of morphological evaluation (cyto- and phototoxicity *in vitro*), as well as the parameters of solubility (27 days), as well as parameters of adhesion resistance and biological inertness.

It is important to mention that in our opinion, the use of the new staining agent (Vitreocontrast) cannot be viewed from the point of chromovitrectomy improvement. The above principal advantages of Vitreocontrast suspension reasonably allowed us to substantiate a new, original technique of VB contrast staining that we called Vitreocontrastography (VRCG). The proposed term was adapted to vitreoretinal pathology based on the techniques widely used in medical practice (radiography, tomography, etc.) allowing for the determination of both qualitative and quantitative parameters of the organ under examination. The practical expediency of Vitreocontrastography technique application is explained by the following main advantages:

- high level of adhesion, due to which the intensity of staining of intravitreal structures does not change over time;
- possibility to stain not only all intravitreal structures but also the stripped cortex areas in PVD;
- possibility to determine middle-sized intravitreal structures;
- possibility to identify various anatomical variants of the arrangement of intravitreal canals;
- possibility to identify VB defects (hernias) as a pathogenetic risk factor for retinal detachment;
- required safety characteristics for products that come into contact with the internal structures of the eye for a long time in sanitary-chemical and toxicological (cyto- and phototoxicity) parameters, indicators of sterility, solubility, and biological inertness.

DOI: http://dx.doi.org/10.5772/intechopen.109264

During the second stage of the current work, our efforts were dedicated to the development (in the *ex vivo* experiment) of the next algorithm (step by step) of macro and microscopic experimental morphological study of the anatomical topographic characteristics of isolated vitreous structures from the point of view of normal anatomy [28].

5.1 Macroscopic examination by the technique of preparation with staining of structures

1. Evaluation of anatomical topographic changes of vitreoretinal interface (by PVD to evaluate its view, whether it is true or abnormal).

2. Staining and evaluation of the topographic anatomy of intravitreal structures (canals, bursae, and cisterns), to evaluate the degree of VB destruction.

3. Evaluation of the topographic anatomy of the anterior cortex and vitreolenticular interface.

5.2 Microscopic examination by light (electronic) microscopy of each isolated VB structure

1. Isolated preparation of vitreous structures and layers.

2. Fixation by the original method with the use of a special substrate.

3. Evaluation of microscopic changes by light (electronic) microscopy.

5.3 Making an individual map of VB macromicroscopic topographic anatomy

This algorithm is characterized by the ability to distinguish any VB structure in isolation and to distinguish each cortical layer with the possibility to study its anatomo-topographic features and relations with the underlying tissues (retinal ILM, ciliary body, lens capsule).

The size of intravitreal structures was determined during the study (average size of retrociliary cisterns was 10–12 mm, equatorial cisterns were 15–17 mm, petal-like cisterns were 8–10 mm). Besides, it was revealed for the first time that the anterior cortical layers consistently line the pars plana, the posterior surface of the lens, the ciliary zone fibers and can laminate. Closer to the posterior surface of the lens, a tendency for gradual thinning and lamination of the detected VB layers came into being. For the first time, a separate anatomical structure in the Berger's space projection zone was revealed, making us suggest the possibility of the existence of a retrolenticular bursa not previously described in literature, its anterior multilamellar wall was tightly fixed to the posterior lens capsule and inseparable from it mechanically. It is also important to mention that in the course of the preparation during the formation and cutting off retinal petals, cortex delamination was detected, which could serve as an adaptive mechanism to prevent retinal detachment. It was revealed by modern diagnostic techniques and interpreted as PVD. In addition, after the separation of cortical layers, a defect was formed in the area of the preoptic cistern or premacular bursa, with the subsequent separation of the posterior pole sclera section from the cortical layers and the development of vitreous herniation. In such a case, the VB structure was disturbed, Vitreocontrast suspension stains altered and elongated VB cisterns, and exited through the cortex defect. We noted that when the intraocular pressure increased, the cortex rupture occurred in the defect area with emptying of intravitreal structures and subsequent contraction of the cortical layers. This mechanism can serve as one of the links in the pathogenesis of regmatogenic retinal detachment.

Scientific substantiation of the complex technique of vitreous body imaging (CTVBI, original Vitreocontrastography method in combination with the developed step-by-step algorithm of macroscopic and microscopic examination) for the diagnosis and the surgical treatment of vitreoretinal pathology was based on the efficiency criteria that were developed using the following four groups of imaging methodological principles tested in literature:

1. Basic principles of information imaging in technical systems that made the basis of the following efficiency criteria—penetrating capacity, resolution, breadth of coverage, ability to apply digital data analysis, stability, subjectivity.

2. Main principles of intravital imaging in clinical anatomy that made the basis of the following criteria: possibility to determine the size of intravitreal structures, anatomic variants of the arrangement of intravitreal structures, prediction of pathological processes in retina from the viewpoint of defects in VB, and identification of disorders within an individual vitreous layer.

3. Main principles of morphological investigations in ophthalmology that made the basis for the following efficiency criteria: imaging efficiency in decreased transparency of optical media of the eye with a consideration of VB transparency in hard-to-reach localization or the minimal size of pathological changes as well as in the identification of normal and abnormal morpho-functional state of VB.

4. Main principles of creating the systems of vitreoretinal interface imaging tested in clinical practice including: versatility, staging, structured and stable conduction, realistic, controllable and segmentation of the obtained image with the possibility of pathological process modeling.

Comparative analytical evaluation of the developed technique with the approved methods of VB imaging according to the first three groups of efficiency criteria was performed in scores from 0 (no efficiency) to 3 (high efficiency). The results of the analytical evaluation revealed that the mean score of complex technique of VB imaging (CTVBI) was 2.8; CV -1.9; OCT - 1.4; ultrasound - 1.3 and CLSO - 1.2, respectively. Thus, the data obtained indicate the undoubted advantages of CTVBI where the level of VB imaging efficiency is 93% of the required one.

It is also important to note that our proposed system of the complex technique fully complies with the following basic principles of vitreoretinal interface imaging systems tested in clinical practice.

Universality principle was implemented in the possibility of imaging (based on the vitreocontrastography method) both in experimental (on donor eyes) and in real (intraoperatively during vitrectomy) conditions.

Principle of staging was characterized by our step-by-step technique of VB preparation.

Structuredness principle providing VB macroscopic and microscopic analysis from the position of the system of interconnected structures that in general allowed for the analysis of the internal structure and activating and regulating mechanisms.

Stability principle was characterized by the pronounced stability of the vitreocontrastography to adhesion throughout the surgical intervention.

Realism and controllability principles reflected the possibility of applying the developed VB imaging system in real time and in the required for each specific case duration and volume that is especially important in the process of surgical intervention.

Obtained image segmentation principle was characterized by the possibility of the isolated identification of each of the VB layers and structural elements (cisterns, canals).

Pathological process modeling principal lied in the effectiveness of the developed imaging system in detecting VB defects (hernias) as a pathogenetic risk factor of retinal detachment development.

The studies of the third stage of the work addressed the evaluation of clinical and diagnostic efficiency of the developed complex technology of VB imaging in MH.

The following anatomo-morphological classification criteria were determined for the diagnosis of MH of different sizes (143 patients, 143 eyes): elongation of VB cisterns in anteroposterior direction, disruption of the wall integrity of VB cisterns and exit of the staining composition beyond stained cavities, destruction (disruption of structural integrity) of VB, degree of VB adhesion to the ILM surface, degree of VB layer adhesion in the macular zone.

Our analysis testified to a fundamentally higher level of anatomical and morphological diagnosis of different stages of MH using the developed VB imaging technique that, in our opinion, was associated with the following general drawbacks of the traditional classification:

- according to a number of authors, the leading role in the development of MH belongs to VB changes; however, even indirect data (including B-scan) were not taken into account while developing this classification;

- in the current classification, PVD is evaluated only by OCT data that is restricted exclusively to the macular area;

- the main substrates of the development of abnormal PVD are VB cortical layers that are tightly adhered to the retinal ILM. However, the current classification does not allow the evaluation of the characteristic signs of such cortical layers (configuration, area, their number, the level of adhesion to ILM). And according to a number of authors, these cortical layers constitute the main pathogenic risk factor for MH development;

- there are practically no data characterizing the occurrence and localization of vitreoschisis zones associated with the lamination of the vitreous;

- the visualized band of the hyperreflective image is interpreted as PHM and PVD by the classification despite the principal impossibility of this method to visualize transparent structures and differentiate between vitreous cortical layers;

- according to the generally accepted views, the development of the pathological process on the retinal ILM surface around the MH is based on the formation of ERM that has a tangential traction effect on the retinal ILM, but the ERM anatomo-topographic characteristics are not provided for in the classification. Summarizing the above clinical data, it should be noted that in the present study the classification anatomo-morphological criteria established on the basis of the developed technique of vitreous body imaging allowed (taking into account the presented clinical examples) us to formulate a number of general and specific practical recommendations for the improvement of surgical treatment.

Thus, on the basis of the studies performed, theoretical provisions were developed. Accumulatively, they ensured an increase in clinical efficiency of vitreoretinal surgical intervention based on the application of the proposed complex system of VB imaging.

The practical application of the developed system of VB imaging is possible in the following areas:

- the research one—for macroscopic and microscopic (histological) examination of all the vitreous structures;

- the diagnostic one—for intravital imaging of the state and morpho-functional changes of VB;

- the surgical one—to increase the level of imaging during vitrectomy that ensures the high quality of surgical intervention.

6. Key take-aways

1. The results of experimental and morphological (*in vitro*, *ex vivo*) and clinical studies ensured the development of a comprehensive vitreoretinal imaging technique for the diagnosis and surgical treatment of various types of vitreoretinal pathology based on the use of original techniques ("Vitreocontrastography", macro and microscopic vitreous body algorithm) as well as basic principles of vitreoretinal interface visualization (universality, stage-by-stage approach, structuredness, stability of carrying out, realism, manageability, and segmentation of received images with a possibility to model pathological process.

2. The developed complex technique of VB imaging is characterized, in comparison with traditional methods (ultrasound examination, optical coherence tomography, confocal laser scanning ophthalmoscopy, and chromovitrectomy), by significantly higher level of imaging efficiency according to three-point criteria developed in accordance with basic principles of intravital imaging in clinical anatomy (mean score – 3.0 0.5; 1.0; 0.25 and 1.5, respectively) and morphological studies in ophthalmology (mean scores of 3.0; 1.25; 0.75; 1.0 and 1.8, respectively).

3. The results of the complex (clinical, *in vitro*, *ex vivo*) comparative assessment of various staining techniques of vitreous body (MembraneBlue®Dual,

Kenalog-40 (Triamcinolone acetonide), the original Vitreocontrastography technique) testify to the principal advantages of Vitreocontrastography associated with a high (93% of that required according to the developed criteria) level of imaging efficiency confirmed (according to digital colorimetry) by the highest (22.87 ± 6.67) value of mean Euclidean distance CIELAB), as well as compliance with sanitary and chemical (pH 7.25+0.02 units) values. pH (with an admissible value of 7.20–7.60 pH units), toxicological (by the results of the toxicity index evaluation (100 ± 10)% with admissible values of 70–120%) and morphological evaluation), solubility (27 days) parameters, resistance to adhesion and biological inertness.

4. An algorithm for macro- and microscopic experimental and morphological examination of the vitreous body was developed (in *ex vivo* experiment) that made it possible to determine the size of intravitreal structures (average size of retrociliary cisterns was 10–12 mm, equatorial—15–17 mm, petal—8–10 mm), the existence of a new structure (retrolenticular bursa), the mutual arrangement of the posterior zonules and anterior cortical layers and the three variants of PVD in terms of retinal detachment pathogenesis.

5. Application of the developed technique of vitreous body imaging in patients with macular holes (MH) of various sizes provides a principally new approach to clinical and diagnostic examination based on the development (depending on the stage of the pathological process) of basic classificational anatomical and morphological features (elongation of the vitreous cisterns in anteroposterior direction, violation of the integrity of the vitreous cistern wall and probability of staining composition exit beyond the stained cavities, the level of the vitreous adhesion on the inner limiting membrane surface, etc). and characterized by advantages in comparison with traditional MH classifications that allows for the significant increase in the level of vitreoretinal surgery clinical efficiency.

7. Practical recommendations

1. In order to improve surgical intervention for various types of vitreoretinal disorders, it is advisable to use the developed technique VB imaging based on the original Vitreocontrastography method providing (in general terms) the following advantages:

    - imaging of the changes in the vitreous structures involved in the pathological process;

    - staining of VB cortical layers to control induced PVD intraoperationally;

    - imaging of VB cortical layers adhered to retinal ILM with a possibility to determine the exact sizes of the vitreoschisis in any of the meridians;

    - the possibility to remove the visualized VB layer not only to determine the topographic anatomy but also to prepare histological preparations for light or electronic microscopy or immunohistochemical studies;

- the possibility to assess the number of VB fibers adhered to ILM surface after VB layer removal and ILM surface staining.

2. Vitreoretinal surgical intervention (based on the developed technique) in patients with macular holes of different diameters should be performed taking into account the following recommendations:

    - In cases of the complete removal of VB cortical layers from ILM surface and the presence of small-diameter MH, it is possible to refrain from ILM removal or maculorhexis temporal side only (**Figures 28–32**)

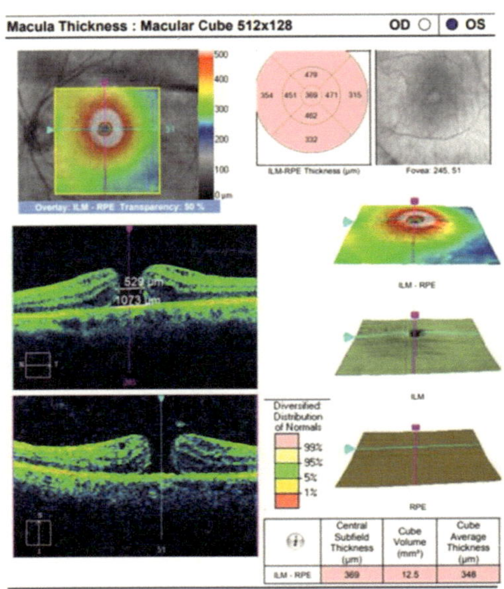

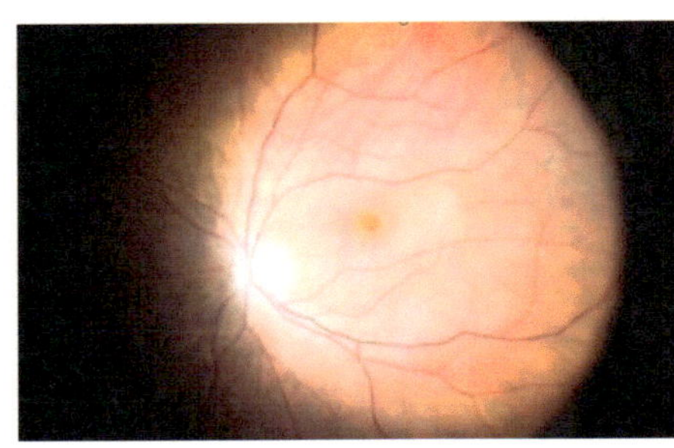

ILM removal in the presence of a middle-sized MH can be done using the classical technique, i.e., circular maculorexis with the catchment of the entire ILM zone including the vitreous cortex adhered to it and the ILM removal with the formation of petals strictly according to the area of the staining agent location keeping the ILM fixation along the edge of the hole and with the inverted flap of any modification; in case of a bilayer vitreous zone in the presence of MH, a layer-by-layer removal with staining of each layer is advisable; in the presence of large-diameter MH, the maximum complete removal of the upper vitreous cortical layer is highly advisable (if possible) followed by staining of underlying tissues and preserving the fixation of this layer to the edges of the MH; In cases of the removal of the ILM with the cortical layer is performed according to the edge of the stained ILM with cortical layers adhered to it. The adhered zone corresponds to the vitreoschisis (**Figures 33–39**).

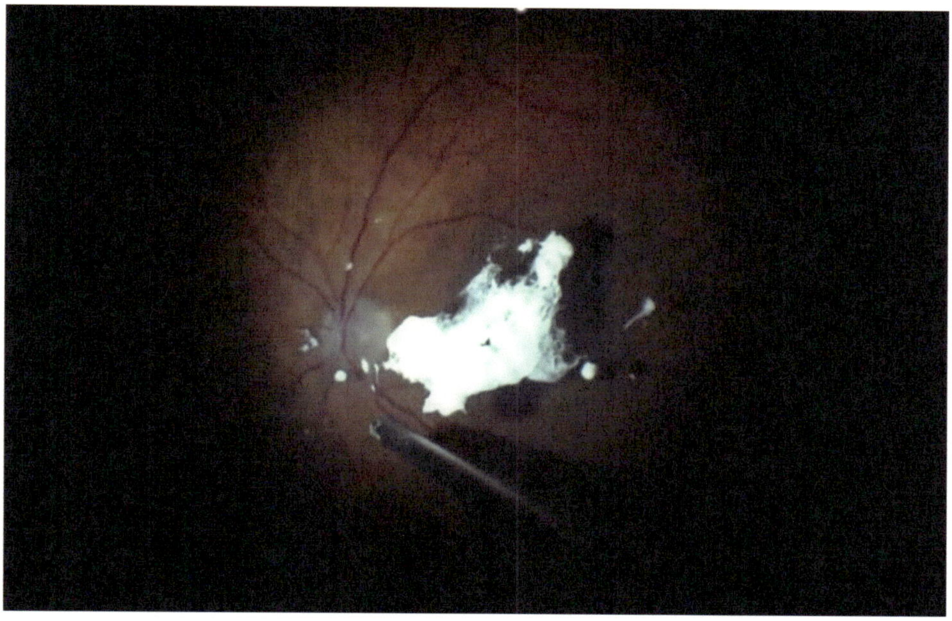

Figure 28.
Cortical layers contrasting with Vitreocontrast suspension. Posterior vitreous detachment induction.

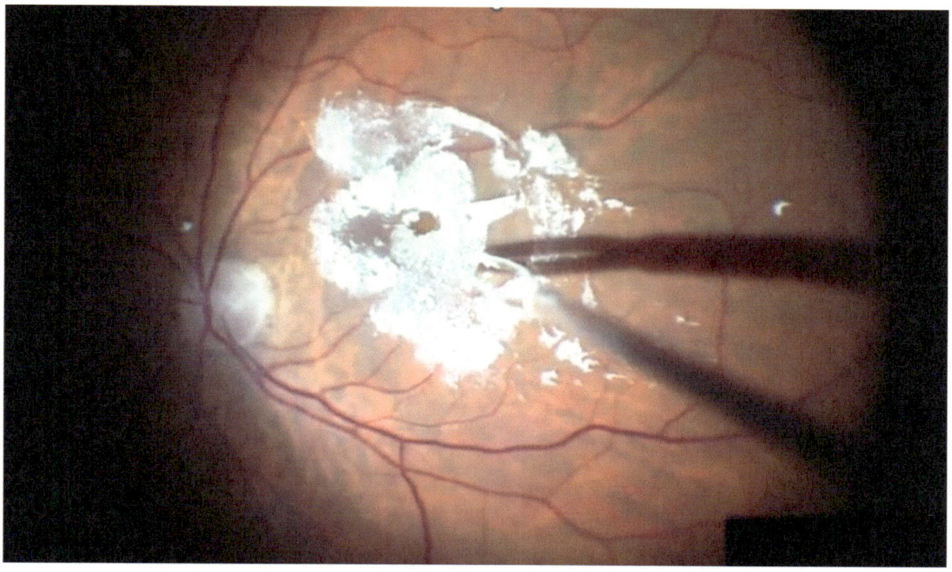

Figure 29.
ILM contrasting with remaining vitreous body on the surface.

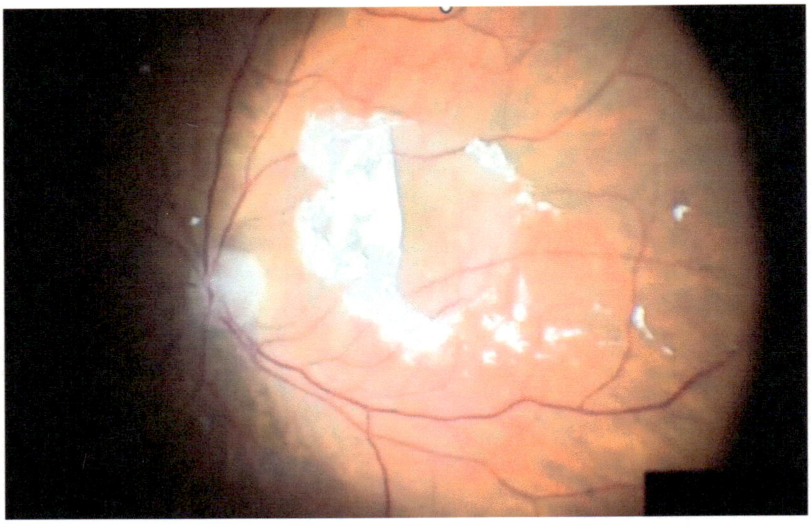

Figure 30.
ILM pilling in the contrasted layer area, temporal side only, laying the lap on the projection of the macular hole. The layer is held in normal position due to Vitreocontrast particles adhesion.

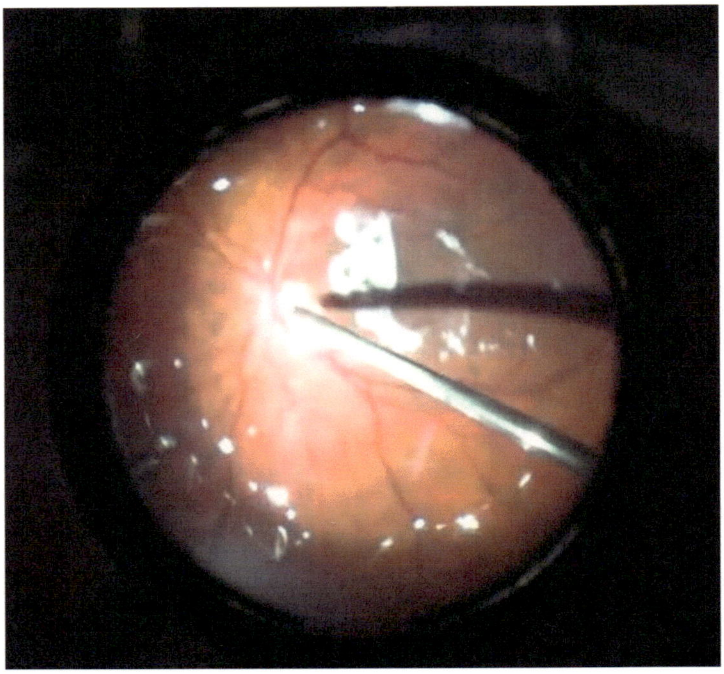

Figure 31.
Vitreal tamponade by the air.

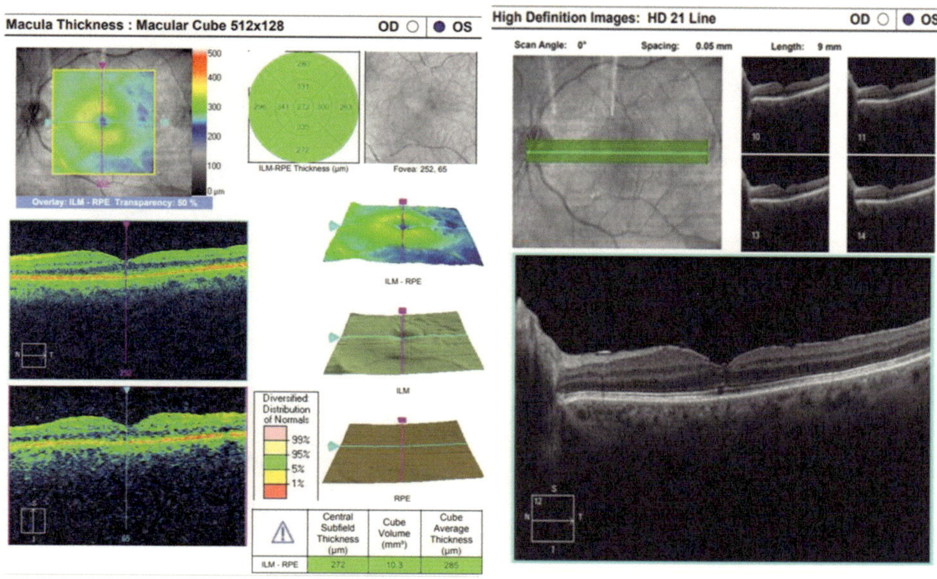

Figure 32.
OCT image of the patient (7 days after surgery).

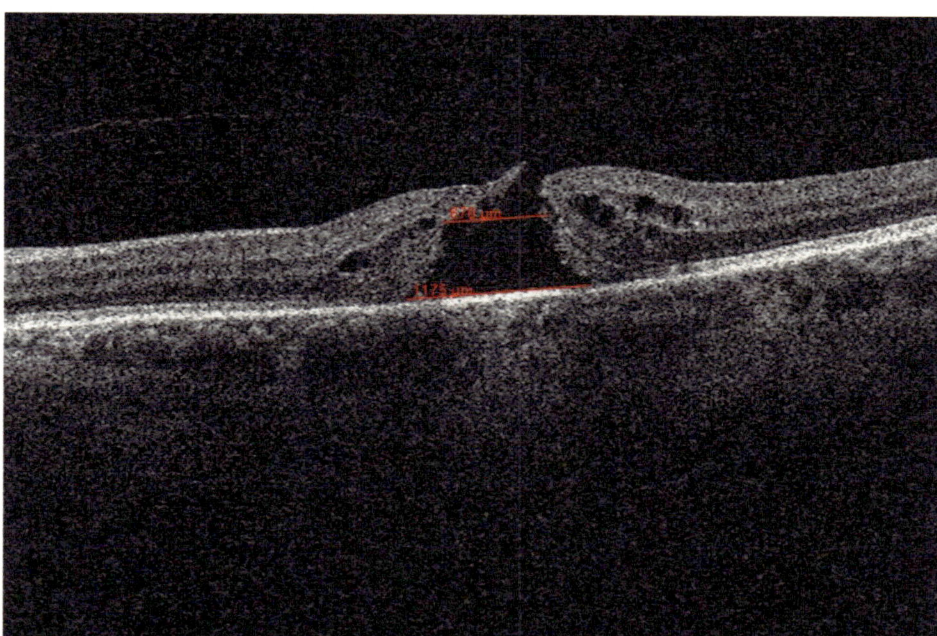

Figure 33.
Posterior vitreous detachment induction with Vitreocontrast suspension.

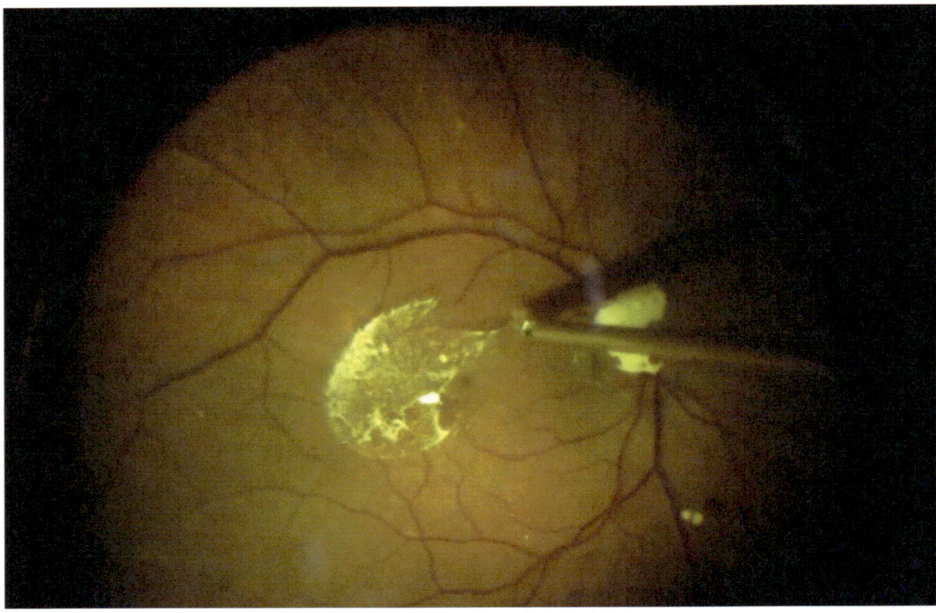

Figure 34.
Posterior vitreous detachment induction with Vitreocontrast suspension.

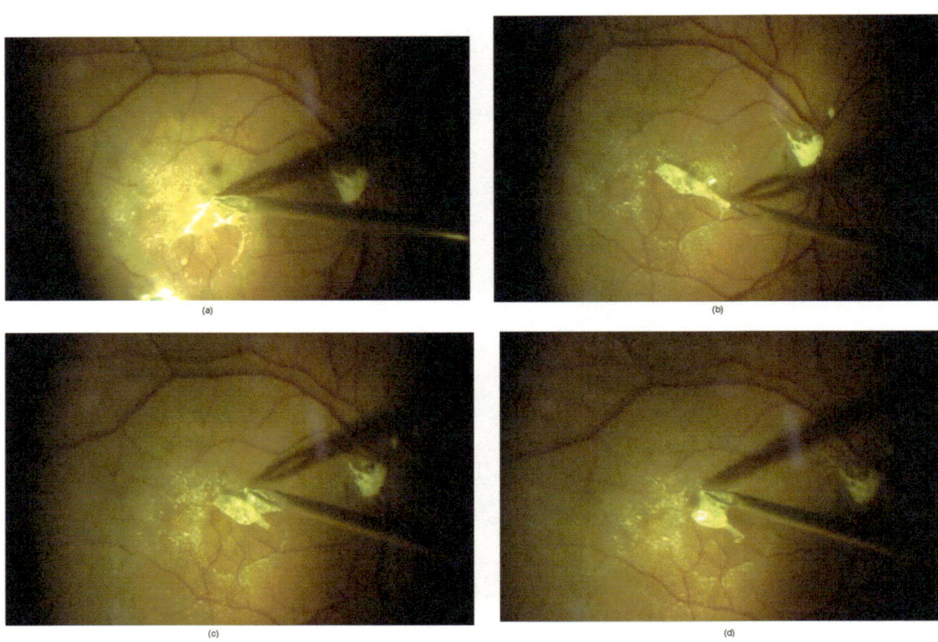

Figure 35.
ILM flaps forming (a–d).

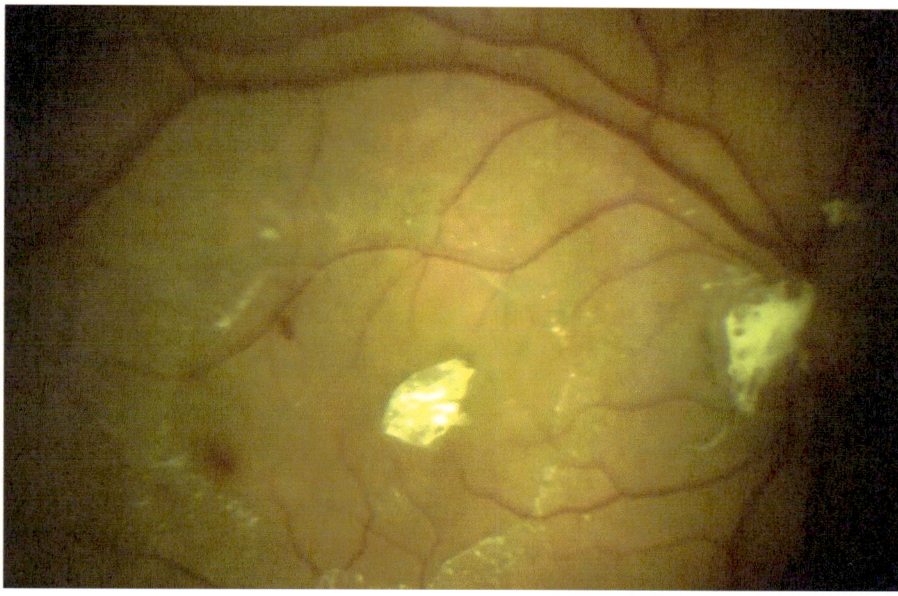

Figure 36.
The reposition of inverted ILM flaps in the macular hole projection. ILM flaps held in the normal position due to Vitreocontrast properties.

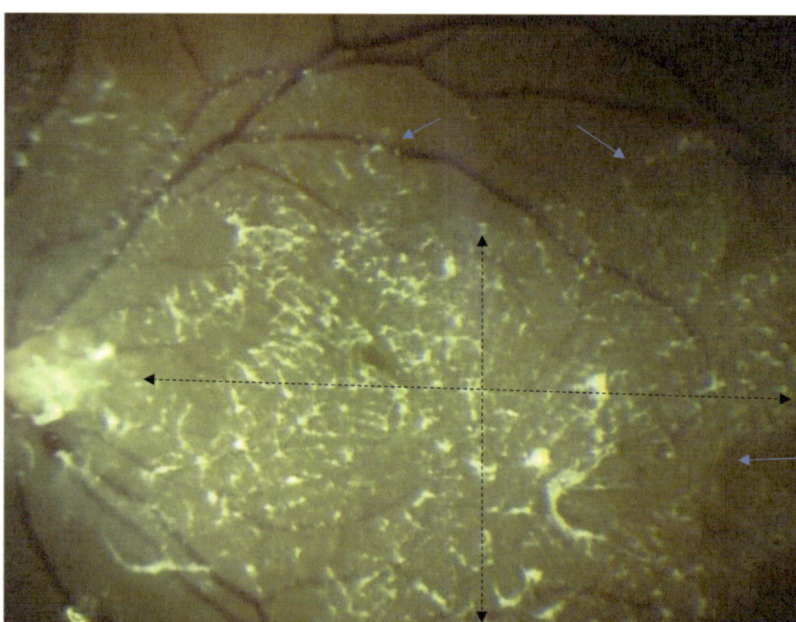

Figure 37.
Cortical layer contrasting on the ILM surface. Cortical layer tightly bound to ILM had clear boundaries (blue arrows) and occupies a certain area that can be measured (black arrows).

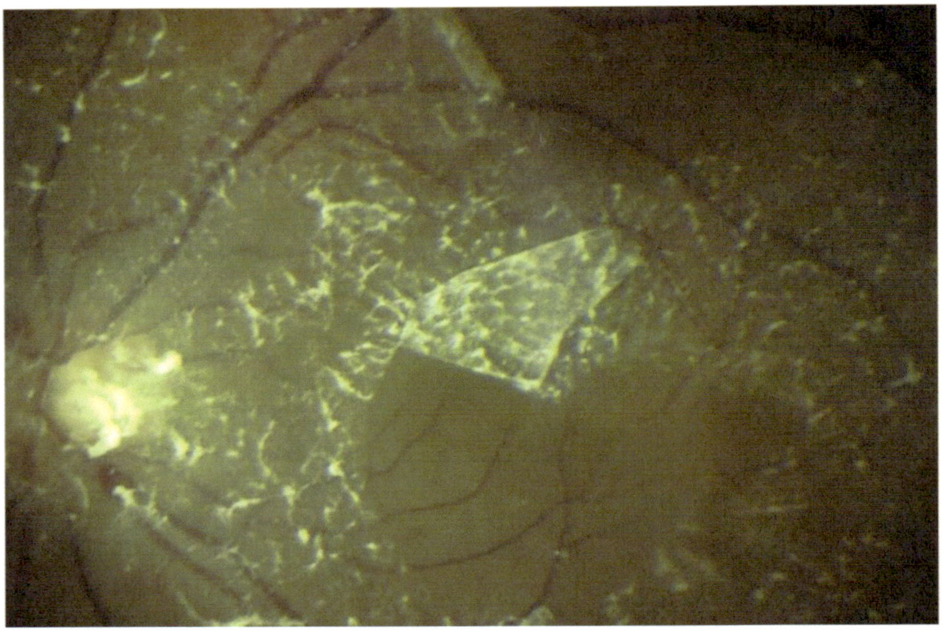

Figure 38.
ILM flaps formation.

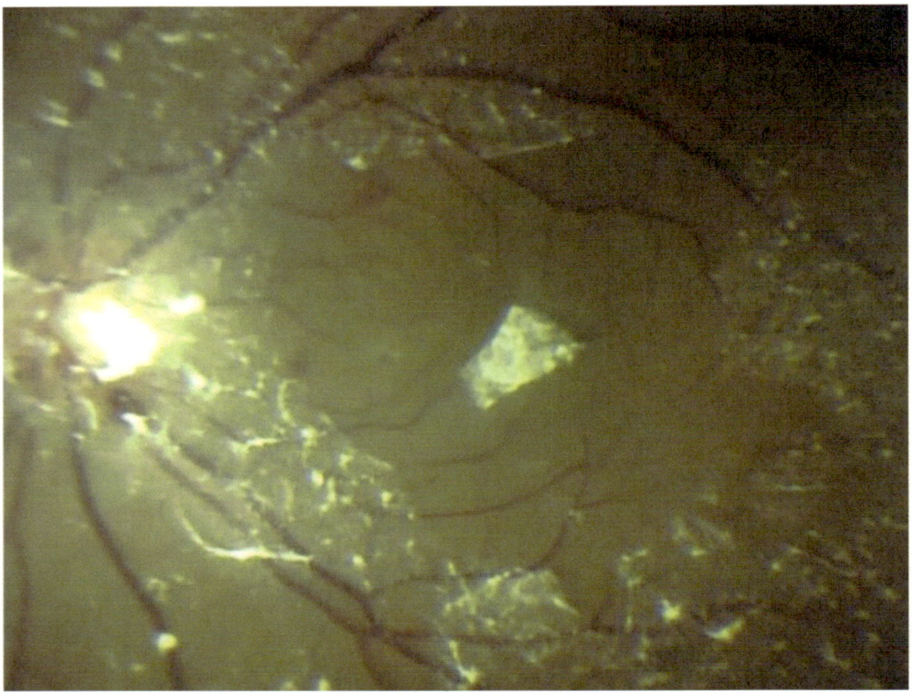

Figure 39.
Macular hole blocked by the inverted flap. ILM removed in the contrasted zone area, in this case ILM removed area corresponded with vitreoschisis zone after abnormal posterior vitreous detachment progress.

Author details

Natalia Kislitsyna[1] and Sergei Novikov[2]*

1 Fyodorov's Eye Microsurgery Complex, Moscow, Russia

2 SEP Ltd Eye Microsurgery, Moscow, Russia

*Address all correspondence to: snovikov@yandex.ru

References

[1] Duker JS et al. The International Vitreomacular Traction Study Group classification of vitreomacular adhesion, traction and macular hole. Ophthalmology. 2013;**120**(12):2611-2619

[2] Sebag J. The vitreoretinal interface and its role in the pathogenesis of vitreomaculopathies. Der Ophthalmologe. 2015;**112**(1):10-19

[3] Gass JDM. Reappraisal of biomicroscopic classification of stages of development of a macular hole. American Journal of Ophthalmology. 1995;**119**(6):752-759

[4] Kislitsyna NM, Novikov SV, Kolesnik SV, Veselkova MP, Dibirova S. Anatomic-topographic features of the anterior cortical layers of the vitreous body Fyodorov's eye microsurgery Complex, Moscow, Russia. EC Ophthalmology. 2019;**10**(12):1-10

[5] Lang Y, Zemel E, Miller B, et al. Retinal toxicity of intravitreal kenalog in albino rabbits. Retina. 2007;**27**(6):778-788

[6] Kislitsyna NM, Kolesnik SV, Novikov SV, et al. [Anatomical and topographic features of the posterior vitreous detachment in various vitreoretinal diseases] Anatomo-topograficheskie osobennosti zadney otsloyki steklovidnogo tela pri razlichnoy vitreoretinal'noy patologii //Sovremennye tekhnologii v oftal'mologii. Современные технологии в офтальмологии. 2017;**1**:123-126

[7] Worst JGF. A SEM-correlation of the anatomy of the vitreous body: Making visible the invisible. Ophthalmologica. 1986;**64**(1):117-127

[8] Mein CE, Flynn HW. Recognition and removal of the posterior cortical vitreous during vitreoretinal surgery for impending macular hole. American Journal of Ophthalmology. 1991;**111**:611-613

[9] Gupta P et al. Vitreoschisis in macular diseases. The British Journal of Ophthalmology. 2011;**95**(3):376-380

[10] Rodrigues EB. Chromovitrectomy: A new field in vitreoretinal surgery. Graefe's Archive for Clinical and Experimental Ophthalmology. 2005;**243**(4):291-293

[11] Kislitsyna NM, Kolesnik SV, Novikov SV, Kolesnik AI, Veselkova MP. Modern possibilities for the vireoretinal interface contrasting (Experimental Study). Ophthalmology in Russia. 2018;**15**(2S):231-238. DOI: 10.18008/1816-5095-2018-2S-231-238

[12] Peyman GA, Cheema R, Conway MD. Triamcinolone acetonide as an aid to visualization of the vitreous and the posterior hyaloid during pars plana vitrectomy. Retina. 2000;**20**:554-555

[13] Kislitsyna N, Novikov SV, Belikova SV. [The use of a new vital dye for the visualization of vitreous structures (experimental study)] Primeneni kontrastnogo veshchestva dlya vizualizatsii struktur steklovidnogo tela (eksperimental'noe issledovanie). Obshchestvo oftal'mologov Rossii FGU MNTK. 2010;**1**(1):55

[14] Simon RB. Chromodissection of the Vitreoretinal interface. Retinal Physician. 2009;**4**:16-21

[15] Kislitsyna NM et al. [Clinical and morphological study of the influence of

"Vitreocontrast" suspension on rabbit eye tissues] Kliniko-morfologicheskoe issledovanie vliyaniya suspenzii. Oftal'mokhirurgiya. 2011;**4**:59-64

[16] Machemer R, Sugita G, Tano Y. Treatment of intraocular proliferations with intravitreal steroids. Transactions of the American Ophthalmological Society. 1979;**77**:171-180

[17] Machemer R. Proliferative vitreoretinopathy (PVR): A personal account of its pathogenesis and treatment. Investigative Ophthalmology & Visual Science. 1988;**29**:1771-1783

[18] Graham RO, Peyman GA. Intravitreal injection of dexamethasone. Treatment of experimentally induced endophthalmitis. Archieves in Ophthalmology. 1974;**92**:149-154

[19] Kampougeris G, Cheema R, McPherson R, Gorman C. Safety of Triamcinolone acetonide- assisted pars plana vitrectomy in macular hole surgery. Eye. 2007;**21**:591-594

[20] Furino C, Micelli FT, Boscia F. Triamcinolone-assisted pars plana vitrectomy for proliferative vitreoretinopathy. Retina. 2003;**23**:771-776

[21] Horio N, Horiguchi M, Yamamoto N. Triamcinolone acetonide-assisted the internal limiting membrane peeling during idiopathic macular hole surgery, Arch. Ophthalmologica. 2005;**123**:96-99

[22] Matsumoto H, Yamanaka I, Hisatomi T. Triamcinolone acetonide-assisted pars plana vitrectomy improves residual posterior vitreous hyaloids removal: Ultrastructural analisis of the inner limitimg membrane. Retina. 2007;**27**:174-179

[23] Enaida H, Hata Y, Ueno A, et al. Possible benefits of triamcinolone-assisted pars plana vitrectomy for retinal diseases. Retina. 2003;**23**:764-770

[24] Narayanan R, Mungcal JK, Kenney MK, Seigel GM, Kuppermann BD. Toxicity of triamcinolone acetonide on retinal neurosensory and pigment epithelial cells. Investment in Ophthalmological Visual Science. 2006;**47**(2):722-728

[25] Albini T, Abd-El-Barr M, Carvounis PE, Iyer MN, Lakhanpal RR, Pennesi ME, et al. Long-term retinal toxicity of intravitreal commercially available preserved triamcinolone acetonide (Kenalog) in rabbit eyes. Investigative Ophthalmology. 2007;**48**:390-395

[26] Dyer D, Callanan D, Bochow T, Abraham P, Lambert HM, Lee SY, et al. Clinical evaluation of the safety and efficacy of preservative-free triamcinolone (triesence(r) [triamcinolone acetonide injectable suspension] 40 mg/ml) for visualization during pars plana vitrectomy. Retina. 2009;**29**(1):38-45

[27] Kislitsyna N, Novikov S. Anatomic and topographic vitreous and vitreoretinal interface features during chromovitrectomy of A, B, C stages of proliferative diabetic vitreoretinopathy (P. Kroll's Classification of Proliferative Diabetic Vitreoretinopathy, 2007): Fyodorov's Eye Micro. In: Giudice MGL, editor. Diabetic Eye Disease—From Therapeutic Pipeline to the Real World. London: IntechOpen; 2022

[28] Kislitsyna NM, Shatskih SM, Dibirova DM, Sultanova MP, Veselkova SV. Macromicroscopic method for vitreous body anatomy studying. Ophthalmology in Russia. 2022;**19**(1):123-132. DOI: 10.18008/1816-5095-2022-1-123-132

[29] See the Invisible, Achieve the Impossible: Anatomical Features of Vitreous and Vitreomacular Interface in Idiopathic Macular Holes of Large Diameter Posted by N.M. Kislitsina, S.V. Novikov, A.I. Kolesnik and S.V. Kolesnik on Apr 26, 2018 in 2018 EVRS Congress – Prague, EDITED FILMS PRAGUE | Comments Off on See the Invisible, Achieve the Impossible: Anatomical Features of Vitreous and Vitreomacular Interface in Idiopathic Macular Holes of Large Diameter. https://www.evrs.eu/see-the-invisible-achieve-the-impossible-anatomical-features-of-vitreous-and-vitreomacular-interface-in-idiopathic-macular-holes-of-large-diameter/

[30] Michalewski J et al. Evolution from a macular pseudohole to lamellar macular hole. Clinical & Experimental Ophthalmology. 2011;**249**:175-178

[31] Kislitsyna N, Novikov SV, Belikova SV. [The use of a new vital dye for the visualization of vitreous structures (experimental study)] Primenenie novogo kontrastnogo veshchestva dlya vizualizatsii struktur steklovidnogo tela (eksperimental'noe issledovanie). Obshchestvo oftal'mologov Rossii FGU MNTK. 2010;**1**(1):55

[32] Kislitsyna NM et al. [Clinical and morphological study of the influence of "Vitreocontrast" suspension on rabbit eye tissues] Kliniko-morfologicheskoe issledovanie vliyaniya suspenzii «Vitreokontrast» na tkani glaza krolikov. Oftal'mokhirurgiya. 2011;**4**:59-64

[33] Samoĭlov AN, Khaibrakhmanov TR, Fazleeva GA, Samoylova PA. Idiopathic macular hole: History and status quo review. Vestnik Oftalmologii. 2017;**133**(6):131-137

[34] Sebag J. Morphology and ultrastructure of human vitreous fibers. Investigative Ophthalmology & Visual Science. 1989;**30**(12):1867-1871

[35] Russell SR. What we know (and do not know) about vitreoretinal adhesion. Retina. 2012;**32**:181-186

[36] Restori M. Imaging the vitreous: Optical coherence tomography and ultrasound imaging. Eye. 2008;**22**(10):1251-1256

[37] Ando F et al. Anatomic and visual outcomes after indocyanine green-assisted peeling of the retinal internal limiting membrane in idiopathic macular hole surgery. American Journal of Ophthalmology. 2004;**137**(4):609-614

[38] Narayanan R et al. Toxicity of triamcinolone acetonide on retinal neurosensory and pigment epithelial cells. Investigative Ophthalmology & Visual Science. 2006;**47**(2):722-728

[39] Kimura H. Triamcinolone acetonide-assisted peeling of the internal limiting membrane. American Journal of Ophthalmology. 2004;**137**(1):172-173

[40] Lee SW et al. Vitreous surgery for impending macular hole. Retina. 2011;**31**(5):909-914

[41] Shah GK et al. Triamcinolone-assisted internal limiting membrane peeling. Retina. 2005;**25**:972-975

[42] Nigam N et al. Spectral domain optical coherence tomography for imaging ERM, retinal edema, and vitreomacular interface. Retina. 2010;**30**(2):246-253

[43] Michalewska Z et al. Temporal inverted internal limiting membrane flap technique versus classic inverted internal limiting membrane flap technique: A comparative study. Retina. 2015;**35**(9):1844-1850

[44] Kislitsyna NM, Novikov SV, Kolesnik SV, Kolesnik AI, Veselkova MP. Anatomic and topographic vitreous and vitreoretinal interface features in proliferative diabetic vitreoretinopathy. Ophthalmology in Russia. 2020;**17**(2):249-257. DOI:10.18008/1816-5095-2020-2-249-257

[45] Johnson MW. Posterior vitreous detachment: Evolution and complications of its early stages. American Journal of Ophthalmology. 2010;**149**(3):371-382

[46] Horio N. Triamcinolone acetonide-assisted the internal limiting membrane peeling during idiopathic macular hole surgery. Archives of Ophthalmology. 2005;**123**:96-99

[47] Abdelkader E. Internal limiting membrane peeling in vitreo-retinal surgery. Survey of Ophthalmology. 2008;**53**(4):368-396

[48] Sebag J. To see the invisible: The quest of imaging vitreous. Developments in Ophthalmology. 2008;**42**:5-28

[49] Schechet S. The effect of internal limiting membrane peeling on idiopathic epiretinal membrane surgery, with a review of literature. Retina. 2017;**37**(5):873-880

Chapter 3

Internal Limiting Membrane Peeling in Idiopathic Epiretinal Membrane

Luciana de Sá Quirino Makarczyk

Abstract

The primary management for epiretinal membrane (ERM) is membrane peel after pars plana vitrectomy. However, the rates of postoperative recurrence of epiretinal membrane reported range from 10 to 21%. Internal limiting membrane (ILM) peeling combined with ERM removal has been introduced in an attempt to diminish this recurrence. Some studies showed that this method largely prevented the recurrence compared with those without ILM peeling. Conversely, other studies demonstrated that combined ERM and ILM peeling did not provide a lower recurrence rate. Since the ILM is formed by the basal lamina of Muller cells, removal of this structure must be pondered due to possible mechanical and functional damage to those important cells. In this chapter, current data on this topic are covered.

Keywords: epiretinal membrane peeling, internal limiting membrane, epiretinal membrane recurrence, idiopathic epiretinal membrane, epiretinal membrane (ERM)

1. Introduction

Epiretinal membrane is a prevalent disease [1, 2]. Studies that incorporated ocular coherence tomography (OCT) for detection found a higher prevalence of this pathology, ranging from 3.4 [3] to 34.1% [4].

Most epiretinal membrane (ERM) is idiopathic and increasing age is the most important risk factor, with most patients presenting over 50 years and a peak prevalence in the 7th decade [5, 6]. There is great variability in the reported prevalence of ERM among different racial groups, although studies using similar methodologies reported a higher prevalence in Asians [7, 8].

Vitrectomy with membrane peeling remains the mainstay of treatment for symptomatic ERMs. First, a three ports pars plana vitrectomy is performed and then the ERM is peeled. Dyes are often used to better visualize the ERM and the internal limiting membrane (ILM).

2. Epiretinal membrane

Idiopathic ERMs occur when there are no associated ocular pathologies. Secondary ERMs are considered those associated with an ocular pathology and account for about 30% of ERMs [8].

Regardless of its etiology, an epiretinal membrane is formed by an innermost single or multilayer of cells and an outermost noncellular layer, which is in contact with the ILM. The cellular layer constituents include retinal glial cells, hyalocytes, retinal pigment epithelial cells, and fibroblasts, and these cells originate myofibroblasts through transdifferentiation [9–11]. The main component of the outermost layer is different types of extracellular collagen divided into native vitreous collagen, reminiscent on the retinal surface after posterior vitreous detachment (PVD), and newly formed collagen, synthesized and secreted by the cellular layer [12, 13].

Since a PVD is present in the majority of cases [14, 15] it has been suggested its participation during idiopathic ERM formation. After PVD, it is theorized that reminiscent of hyalocytes on the retinal surface starts a process of metaplasia and ends up forming the ERM [16].

Another etiology proposed, although less accepted, is the migration of retinal glial cells to the retinal surface through defects on ILM after a PVD [17].

Classification based on clinical findings proposed by Gass [18] is still widely used. Along with developments in OCT (optical coherence tomography), several classifications based on this technology have been proposed based on the identification of associated retinal anatomic changes [19–23].

Based on new OCT findings, including ectopic inner foveal layers, a recent grading scheme had been proposed [24]. Stage 1 was defined as the presence of an ERM, seen as a hyperreflective line above the inner retina, with negligible retinal anatomic changes. Stage 2 was defined as the presence of ERM causing loss of foveal depression and stretching of the outer nuclear layer. Stage 3 was defined as the presence of an ERM with continuous ectopic inner foveal layers added to stage 2 findings. Stage 4 was defined as the presence of stage 3 findings added to the disorganization of retinal layers.

3. Internal limiting membrane

The ILM is composed of an innermost structure formed by a meshwork of collagen fibers, glycosaminoglycans, laminin, and fibronectin called cuticular layer, and an outmost structure, facing the retina surface, formed by the footplates of Müller cells [25, 26]. The internal limiting membrane has a smooth vitreal side and an irregular retinal side where folds are in apposition to Muller cells footplates [27].

Muller cells are the main glial cell of the retina. They give structural stability to the fovea and have an important role in metabolic functions, such as regulating the balance of relevant ions, removing metabolic waste, and providing trophic substances to neurons [28]. The inner processes of Muller cells, formed by its footplates (**Figure 1**), participate in the outmost structure of ILM [25]. The outer processes of Muller cells surround the somata of photoreceptor cells and together constitute the external limiting membrane (ELM) (**Figure 1**).

Muller cells are differentiated into two groups according to their fovea location: Müller cell cone and outer processes of the Müller cells of the foveal walls [29, 30]. The Muller cell cone acts as a plug binding together the receptor cells in the foveola,

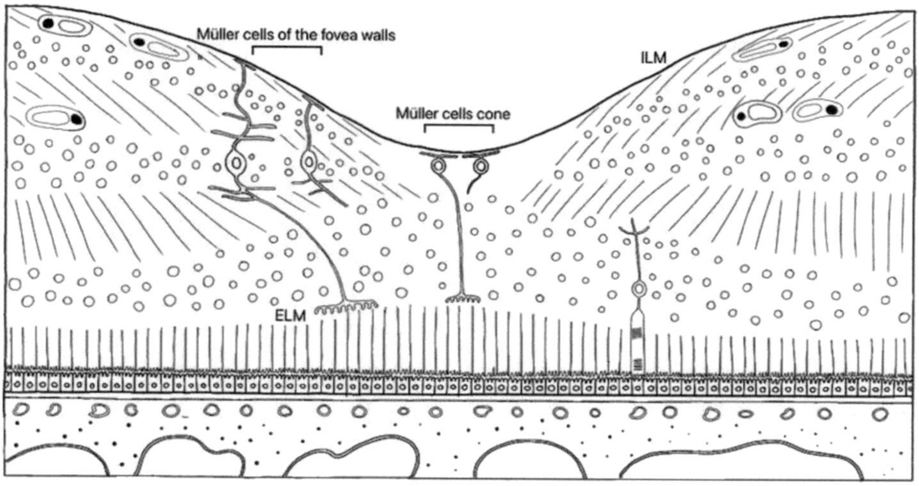

Figure 1.
Muller cells of foveal walls, Muller cells cone, external limiting membrane (ELM), and internal limiting membrane (ILM). Schematic drawing by Luciana S.Q. Makarczyk.

increasing resistance against mechanical stress, since the radiating nerve fibers would be highly susceptible to disruption in this region [31]. It has been suggested that the Muller cells of the foveal wall give stability to the outer layers of the fovea and parafovea [32, 33].

Muller cells of the foveal walls display a z-shaped pattern as a result of the centrifugal displacement of the inner retina and the centripetal displacement of the outer retina and photoreceptors. Muller cells' vertical processes run from the ILM to the inner nuclear layer (INL), then diagonally within Henle's fiber layer (HFL) and, once more, vertically to the outer limiting membrane (OLM). The morphology of this type of Müller cell may absorb mechanical tension according to a physical model study [34]. This model considered those cells as the main determinants of force transmission and suggested their importance in the structural stability of the parafovea by increasing retinal compliance to mechanical stress.

The thickness of the ILM within 400 μm from the foveal center ranges from 0.050 to 0.2 μm. From 400 to 600 μm from the center of the fovea, its thickness varies from 0.08 to 1.0 μm. At a distance of 600 to 900 μm from the foveal center, ILM showed a thickness from 1.4 to 2.4 μm. Between 900 and 1050 μm from the foveal center, ILM reaches 4.0 μm of thickness. At the disc, its thickness ranges from 0.07 to 0.1 μm and it is thicker in the posterior pole than the equator [27, 35].

Analyses of ILM stiffness matched thickness findings according to geographical distribution, meaning that higher stiffness values were found in the posterior pole compared with the mid-peripheral quadrants [27].

Biomechanical analyses of the ILM showed that it provides a protective function to the retina. Removal of the ILM showed to reduce the mean strength of the central retina by 53.6% [36].

Several diseases affecting the vitreomacular interface could be attributed to foveal mechanical instability: vitreous adhesion, a higher thickness and stiffness of the ILM at the macular area added to a known absence of cellular connections between the cells of the Müller cell cone and the outer processes of the Müller cells of the foveal walls [30, 37].

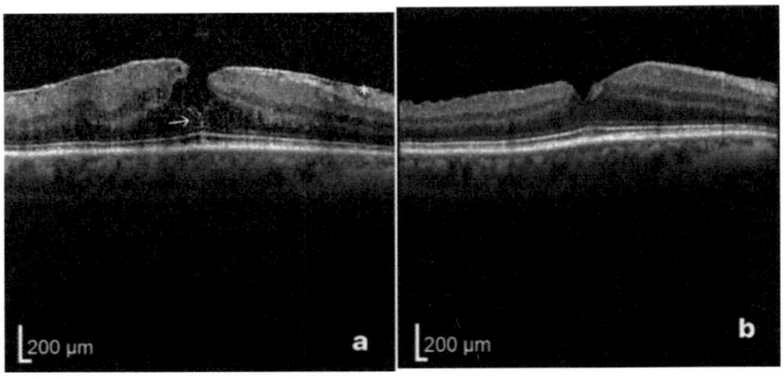

Figure 2.
Epiretinal membrane causing tractional lamellar hole. a. Before surgery. Ectopic inner foveal layer (asterisks). Stretched Muller cell cone processes (arrow). b. Two months after ERM and ILM peeling and absorption of C3F8 gas - Luciana S.Q. Makarczyk, MD, PhD.

3.1 Ectopic inner foveal layers

Ectopic inner foveal layers have been defined by Govetto et al. [37, 38] as displacement of retina architecture with gliosis and proliferation of Muller cells, characterized on OCT as a continuous, homogenous, hypo or hyper-reflective band, extending from the inner nuclear layer and inner plexiform layer across the foveal region (**Figure 2**). This ectopic layer does not possess contractile characteristics.

4. Epiretinal membrane and internal limiting membrane peeling

The aim of surgery is to remove tractions caused by ERM and ectopic inner foveal layers. Three-port pars plana vitrectomy followed by an ERM peeling, using 23-, 25-, or 26-gauge instruments is the standard of care. The use of smaller gauges allows for a faster surgery recovery [39].

Since the separation of the ILM has been shown to be compatible with a good visual function [40–42], intentional removal of the ILM has been performed in order to increase macula elasticity, which could be beneficial for treating several macular disorders, such as macular holes, chronic diabetic macular edema, vitreomacular traction, and myopic foveschisis [28, 29]. Removal of the macular ILM has been demonstrated to greatly improve the anatomical success rate of the surgical treatment of macular holes [43, 44].

The ILM is suspected to provide a scaffold for cellular proliferation and its active peeling has become a common practice during ERM removal. Simultaneous ILM peel is a frequent occurrence during ERM surgery when there is a complete ERM macula adhesion on OCT [45].

Postoperative recurrence of epiretinal membrane range from 10 to 21%. Specimens of recurrent ERM evaluated by electron microscopic demonstrate mainly myofibroblasts, but also fibrocytes, retinal pigment cells, fragments of ILM, and new collagen [45, 46]. Also, some studies had demonstrated remnants of ERM or cell remnants on ILM vitreous surface specimens [47–49].

Thus, ILM peeling combined with ERM removal has been performed in an attempt to remove cells from the retina surface that would serve as potential sites for ERM reproliferation [50].

Chromovitrectomy is frequently used as an adjuvant to facilitate ILM identification. It involves the use of dyes intended to improve ERM and ILM visibility. Trypan blue (TB), brilliant blue G (BBG), and indocyanine green (ICG) are the most frequently used dyes.

Trypan blue stains mainly the ERM while BBG stains mainly the ILM. ICG is an excellent dye for ILM stain, although it has significant evidence of retina and optic nerve toxicity [51, 52].

Despite its toxicity evidence, ICG is still used since it has been described to facilitate ILM peeling by adding an ILM stiffening effect through a collagen IV cross-linking [53] and also having a higher ILM staining property than BBG [54].

A thicker and stiffer ILM facilitates surgical removal and according to previously described, a region within a foveal distance of roughly 1000 μm would be ideal for starting the peeling. Also, in this region, a better stain during chromovitrectomy is expected [27].

The use of BBG has been proven helpful in better visualizing ILM and decreasing ERM fragments, which may be the source of recurrent ERMs [55].

5. Updated data on maintaining ILM versus ILM peeling in ERM treatment

Even more than 10 years after additional ILM peeling has been introduced, there is still a discussion of the best surgical approach for ERM treatment in order to prevent its recurrence.

Some studies showed that ILM peeling prevented ERM recurrence [48, 56, 57]. According to those studies, groups that had ILM peeling had no recurrence of ERM, while in groups where double peeling was not performed, the recurrence reached 17,6%.

On contrary, some other studies showed that patients who had ERM peeling without removing the ILM had an even better anatomical and visual outcome [58–60].

Ahn et al. [60] compared the OCT postoperative status and visual acuity after ERM removal with or without additional ILM peeling. They found that patients who had epiretinal membrane surgery with additional ILM peeling showed worse visual acuity and most severe cone outer segment tips and inner and outer segment junction line defects. Those photoreceptors defects were gradually restored at 12 months postoperatively. A possible reason for this finding is that by removing the ILM, the footplates of Muller cells are also being removed, leading to mechanical and functional damage to those important cells.

There is a supposition that ILM peeling spares the ganglion cells and is limited to the Müller cell footplates. Some studies have suggested that injury to Müller cells was due to direct and indirect traumas, caused by surgical instruments and traction during membrane removal, respectively [61–63].

Deltour et al. [64], in a retrospective study, demonstrated that active peeling induces more numerous and deeper microscotomas than spontaneous peeling. Later, a prospective, randomized, controlled, single-blind, multicentered trial with two parallel arms investigated differences between active ILM peeling and passive ILM peeling, and showed similar findings [65].

A recent meta-analysis of randomized and controlled trials showed no statistically significant difference in final visual acuity and recurrence rate of ERM when ILM peeling was performed. As for the central macular thickness (CMT), it was thicker within 6 months postoperatively in those patients who had additional ILM peeling.

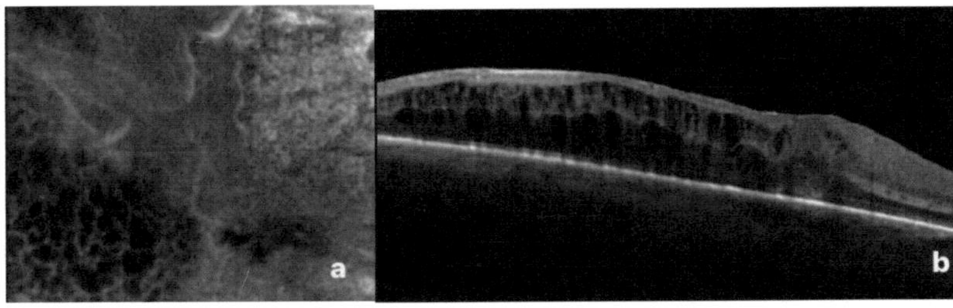

Figure 3.
DONFL after double peeling for stage 4 ERM. a. Enface OCT showing numerous dark areas corresponding to retinal cavitations. b. B scan OCT showing increased foveal thickness due to hyporeflective spaces—images shared by Michelle Gantois, MD.

A possible reason for a thicker CMT in a combined ERM and ILM peeling is that it could induce retinal edema. Also, this meta-analysis data showed that ILM peeling seemed to result in more complications, including intraoperative retinal breaks and nonarteritic anterior ischemic optic neuropathy [66].

Distinct spectral domain optical coherence tomography (SD-OCT) findings on the inner retina have been associated with ILM peeling. Swelling of the arcuate fiber layer (SANFL) is an earlier pathology that is characterized on B scan OCT as hyperreflective images and on infrared as hyperfluorescent arcuate areas. SANFL is followed by dissociated optic nerve fiber layer defect (DONFL) [67]. DONFL (**Figure 3**) presents on SD-OCT as irregular depressions in the nerve fiber layer due to thinning of the ganglion cell layer [67, 68] and more visible with shorter wavelength illumination [69, 70]. It is thought to be due to trauma to Muller cells after the ILM is peeled, disconnecting their attached foot plates [62, 70, 71], and exposing the retinal nerve fiber layers. Trauma to Muller footplates would possibly result in changes in the bundling of the nerve fiber layer and also a volume reduction in the ganglion cell layer where the Muller cell bodies are located [72].

It also had been reported that (DONFL) would also cause a reduction in central retinal sensitivity and paracentral scotomas. Terasaki et al. also reported a delayed recovery of the b-wave amplitude of the focal macula electroretinogram after ILM peeling during macular hole surgery [73].

It is still unclear the cause of DONFL development, but it has been also associated with surgical trauma during ILM peeling [74].

6. Conclusion

The surgical procedures for removing ERM are well-established and safe. However, there is still not enough data to affirm if an additional ILM peeling is always an important surgical step or would be better to be performed only in selected ERM cases.

There are proven morphological and functional retina modifications with an additional ILM peeling, although is not known whether those changes could cause progressive retinal damage in the medium or long term.

In my own experience, recurrence rates of ERM are not common, even when ILM is not removed. And since ILM peeling can lead to complications, in my point of view, it is not essential, unless when associated with macular holes. In addition, ILM removal could also be needed when epiretinal proliferation is present under the

ERM. Evaluation of ILM status after removal of ERM is also important to decide if it is worth to removed.

Intraoperative optical coherence tomography is an emerging technology that has been evolving and improving in reproducibility and motion artifacts. Soon it will help guide decision-making in the surgical approach for treating ERM, including better visualization of debris left on the retina surface that needs to be removed, as well as when ILM should not be left in place.

Author details

Luciana de Sá Quirino Makarczyk
Hospital Oftalmológico de Brasília, Brasília, Brazil

*Address all correspondence to: luciana.quirino@alumni.utoronto.ca

References

[1] Xiao W, Chen X, Yan W, Zhu Z, He M. Prevalence and risk factors of epiretinal membranes: A systematic review and meta-analysis of population-based studies. BMJ Open. 2017;7(9):e014644

[2] Kim B, Choi A, Park JH, Jeon S. Prevalence of epiretinal membrane in the phakic eyes based on spectral-domain optical coherence tomography. PLoS One. 2021;**16**(1):e0245063

[3] Duan XR, Liang YB, Friedman DS, Sun LP, Wei WB, Wang JJ, et al. Prevalence and associations of epiretinal membranes in a rural Chinese adult population: The Handan eye study. Investigative Ophthalmology & Visual Science. 2009;**50**(5):2018-2023

[4] Meuer SM, Myers CE, Klein BE, Swift MK, Huang Y, Gangaputra S, et al. The epidemiology of vitreoretinal interface abnormalities as detected by spectral-domain optical coherence tomography: The beaver dam eye study. Ophthalmology. 2015;**122**(4):787-795

[5] Mitchell P, Smith W, Chey T, Wang JJ, Chang A. Prevalence and associations of epiretinal membranes. The Blue Mountains eye study, Australia. Ophthalmology. 1997;**104**(6):1033-1040

[6] Klein R, Klein BE, Wang Q, Moss SE. The epidemiology of epiretinal membranes. Transactions of the American Ophthalmological Society. 1994;**92**:403-425

[7] Cheung N, Tan SP, Lee SY, et al. Prevalence and risk factors for epiretinal membrane: The Singapore epidemiology of eye disease study. The British Journal of Ophthalmology. 2017;**101**(3):371-376

[8] Kawasaki R, Wang JJ, Mitchell P, et al. Racial difference in the prevalence of epiretinal membrane between Caucasians and Asians. The British Journal of Ophthalmology. 2008;**92**(10):1320-1324

[9] Bu SC, Kuijer R, Li XR, Hooymans JM, Los LI. Idiopathic epiretinal membrane. Retina. 2014;**34**(12):2317-2335

[10] Vinores SA, Campochiaro PA, Conway BP. Ultrastructural and electron-immunocytochemical characterization of cells in epiretinal membranes. Investigative Ophthalmology & Visual Science. 1990;**31**(1):14-28

[11] Smiddy WE, Maguire AM, Green WR, et al. Idiopathic epiretinal membranes. Ultrastructural characteristics and clinicopathologic correlation. Ophthalmology. 1989;**96**(6):811-820

[12] Schumann RG, Gandorfer A, Eibl KH, Henrich PB, Kampik A, Haritoglou C. Sequential epiretinal membrane removal with internal limiting membrane peeling in brilliant blue G-assisted macular surgery. The British Journal of Ophthalmology. 2010;**94**(10):1369-1372

[13] Kritzenberger M, Junglas B, Framme C, et al. Different colla- gen types define two types of idiopathic epiretinal mem- branes. Histopathology. 2011;**58**(6):953-965

[14] Hirokawa H, Jalkh AE, Takahashi M, Takahashi M, Trempe CL, Schepens CL. Role of the vitreous in idiopathic preretinal macular fibrosis. American Journal of Ophthalmology. 1986;**101**(2):166-169

[15] Wiznia RA. Posterior vitreous detachment and idiopathic preretinal

macular gliosis. American Journal of Ophthalmology. 1986;**102**(2):196-198

[16] Sebag J. The vitreoretinal interface and its role in the pathogenesis of vitreomaculopathies. Der Ophthalmologe. 2015;**112**(1):10-19

[17] Foos RY. Vitreoretinal juncture - simple epiretinal membranes. Albrecht von Graefes Archiv für Klinische und Experimentelle Ophthalmologie. 1974;**189**(4):231-250

[18] Gass JDM. Macular dysfunction caused by epiretinal membrane contraction. In: Stereoscopic Atlas of Macular Diseases: Diagnosis and Treatment. 4th ed. Vol. 2. St Louis, MO: Mosby; 1997. pp. 938-950

[19] Kim JH, Kim YM, Chung EJ, Lee SY, Koh HJ. Structural and functional predictors of visual outcome of epiretinal membrane surgery. American Journal of Ophthalmology. 2012;**153**(1):103-110

[20] Shimozono M, Oishi A, Hata M, et al. The significance of cone outer segment tips as a prognostic factor in epiretinal membrane surgery. American Journal of Ophthalmology. 2012;**153**(4):698-704

[21] Itoh Y, Inoue M, Rii T, Hirota K, Hirakata A. Correlation between foveal cone outer segment tips line and visual recovery after epiretinal membrane surgery. Investigative Ophthalmology & Visual Science. 2013;**54**(12):7302-7308

[22] Watanabe K, Tsunoda K, Mizuno Y, Akiyama K, Noda T. Outer retinal morphology and visual function in patients with idiopathic epiretinal membrane. JAMA Ophthalmology. 2013;**131**(2):172-177

[23] Tsunoda K, Watanabe K, Akiyama K, Usui T, Noda T. Highly reflective foveal region in optical coherence tomography in eyes with vitreomacular traction or epiretinal membrane. Ophthalmology. 2012;**119**(3):581-587

[24] Govetto A, Lalane RA, Sarraf D, Figueroa MS, Hubschman J-P. Insights into epiretinal membranes evolution: Presence of continuous ectopic inner foveal layers and a new optical coherence tomography staging scheme. Investigative Ophthalmology & Visual Science. 2017;**58**(8):6002

[25] Fine BS. Limiting membranes of the sensory retina and pigment epithelium: An electron microscopic study. Archives of Ophthalmology. 1961;**66**(6):847-860

[26] Wollensak G, Spoerl E. Biomechanical characteristics of retina. Retina. 2004;**24**:967-970

[27] Henrich P, B, Monnier CA, Halfter W, Haritoglou C, Strauss RW, Lim RYH, et al. Nanoscale topographic and biomechanical studies of the human internal limiting membrane. Investigative Ophthalmology & Visual Science. 2012;**53**(6):2561-2570

[28] Willbold E, Layer PG. Müller glia cells and their possible roles during retina differentiation in vivo and in vitro. Histology and Histopathology. 1998;**13**(2):531-552

[29] Yamada E. Some structural features of the fovea centralis in the human retina. Archives of Ophthalmology. 1969;**82**:151-159

[30] Syrbe S, Kuhrt H, Gärtner U, Habermann G, Wiedemann P, Bringmann A, et al. Müller glial cells of the primate foveola: An electron microscopical study. Experimental Eye Research. 2018;**167**:110-117

[31] Gass JDM. Müller cell cone, an overlooked part of the anatomy of the

fovea Centralis: Hypotheses concerning its role in the pathogenesis of macular hole and Foveomacular Retinoschisis. Archives of Ophthalmology. 1999;**117**(6):821-823

[32] Bringmann A, Syrbe S, Gorner K, Kacza J, Francke M, Wiedemann P, et al. The primate fovea: Structure, function and development. Progress in Retinal and Eye Research. 2018;**66**:49-84

[33] Bringmann A, Unterlauft JD, Wiedemann R, Barth T, Rehak M, Wiedemann P. Two different populations of Müller cells stabilize the structure of the fovea: An optical coherence tomography study. International Ophthalmology. 2020;**40**(11):2931-2948

[34] Govetto A, Hubschman JP, Sarraf D, Figueroa MS, Bottoni F, dell'Omo R, et al. The role of Müller cells in tractional macular disorders: An optical coherence tomography study and physical model of mechanical force transmission. The British Journal of Ophthalmology. 2020;**104**(4):466-472

[35] Matsumoto B, Blanks JC, Ryan SJ. Topographic variations in the rabbit and primate internal limiting membrane. Investigative Ophthalmology & Visual Science. 1984;**25**(1):71-82

[36] Wollensak G, Spoerl E, Grosse G, Wirbelauer C. Biomechanical significance of the human internal limiting lamina. Retina. 2006;**26**(8):965-968

[37] Bringmann A, Unterlauft JD, Wiedemann R, Rehak M, Wiedemann P. Morphology of partial-thickness macular defects: Presumed roles of Müller cells and tissue layer interfaces of low mechanical stability. International Journal of Retina and Vitreous. 2020;**6**(6):28

[38] Govetto A, Lalane RA 3rd, Sarraf D, Figueroa MS, Hubschman JP. Insights into Epiretinal membranes: Presence of ectopic inner foveal layers and a new optical coherence tomography staging scheme. American Journal of Ophthalmology. Mar 2017;**175**:99-113

[39] Mitsui K, Kogo J, Takeda H, Shiono A, Sasaki H, Munemasa Y, et al. Comparative study of 27-gauge vs 25-gauge vitrectomy for epiretinal membrane. Eye (London, England). Apr 2016;**30**(4):538-544

[40] Morris R, Kuhn F, Witherspoon CD. Hemorrhagic macular cysts. Ophthalmology. 1994;**101**(1):1

[41] Morris R, Kuhn F, Witherspoon CD, Mester V, Dooner J. Hemorrhagic macular cysts in Terson's syndrome and its implications for macular surgery. Developments in Ophthalmology. 1997;**29**:44-54

[42] Kuhn F, Morris R, Witherspoon CD, Mester V. Terson syndrome: Results of vitrectomy and the significance of vitreous hemorrhage in patients with subarachnoid hemorrhage. Ophthalmology. 1998;**105**(3):472-477

[43] Lois N, Burr J, Norrie J, et al. Internal limiting membrane peeling versus no peeling for idiopathic full-thickness macular hole: A pragmatic randomized controlled trial. Investigative Ophthalmology and Visual Science. 2011;**52**(3):1586-1592

[44] Mester V, Kuhn F. Internal limiting membrane removal in the management of full-thickness macular holes. American Journal of Ophthalmology. 2000;**129**(6):769-777

[45] Tranos P, Wickham L, Dervenis N, Vakalis A, Asteriades S, Stavrakas P. The role of membrane inner retina adherence

in predicting simultaneous internal limiting membrane peeling during idiopathic epiretinal membrane surgery. Eye (London, England). 2017;**31**(4):636-642

[46] Maguire AM, Smiddy WE, Nanda SK, Michels RG, de la Cruz Z, Green WR. Clinicopathologic correlation of recurrent epiretinal membranes after previous surgical removal. Retina. 1990;**10**(3):213-222

[47] Kwok AKH, Lai TYY, Li WWY, Woo DCF, Chan NR. Indocyanine green-assisted internal limiting membrane removal in epiretinal membrane surgery: A clinical and histologic study. American Journal of Ophthalmology. 2004;**138**(2):194-199

[48] Kwok AKH, Lai TYY, Yuen KSC. Epiretinal membrane surgery with or without internal limiting membrane peeling. Clinical and Experimental Ophthalmology. 2005;**33**(4):379-385

[49] Gibran SK, Flemming B, Stappler T, et al. Peel and peel again. British Journal of Ophthalmology. 2008;**92**(3):373-377

[50] Park DW, Dugel PU, Garda J, et al. Macular pucker removal with and without internal limiting membrane peeling: Pilot study. Ophthalmology. 2003;**110**:62-64

[51] Iriyama A, Uchida S, Yanagi Y. Effects of indocyanine green on retinal ganglion cells. Investigative Ophthalmology & Visual Science. 2004;**45**:943-947

[52] Ando F, Yasui O, Hirose H, Ohba N. Optic nerve atrophy after vitrectomy with indocyanine green-assisted internal limiting membrane peeling in diffuse diabetic macular edema. Adverse effect of ICG-assisted ILM peeling. Graefe's Archive for Clinical and Experimental Ophthalmology. 2004;**242**:995-999

[53] Wollensak G, Spoerl E, Wirbelauer C, Pham DT. Influence of indocyanine green staining on the biomechanical strength of porcine internal limiting membrane. Ophthalmologica. 2004;**218**:278-282

[54] Henrich PB, Priglinger SG, Haritoglou C, Josifova T, Ferreira PR, Strauss RW, et al. Quantification of contrast Recognizability during brilliant blue G– And Indocyanine Green–assisted Chromovitrectomy. Investigative Ophthalmology & Visual Science. 2011;**52**(7):4345-4349

[55] Hikichi T, Kubo N, Tabata M. Epiretinal membrane fragments: The origin of recurrent membranes after epiretinal membrane peeling. Canadian Journal of Ophthalmology. 2022;S0008-4182(22)00125-9. DOI: 10.1016/j.jcjo.2022.04.006. Epub ahead of print. PMID: 35718024

[56] Storch MW, Khattab MH, Lauermann P, et al. Macular pucker surgery with and without delamination of the internal limiting membrane-a prospective randomized study. Der Ophthalmologe. 2019;**116**:1038-1045

[57] Bovey EH, Uffer S, Achache F. Surgery for epimacular membrane: Impact of retinal internal limiting membrane removal on functional outcome. Retina. 2004;**24**(5):728-735

[58] Uemura A, Kanda S, Sakamoto Y, Kita H. Visual field defects after uneventful vitrectomy for epiretinal membrane with indocyanine green-assisted internal limiting membrane peeling. American Journal of Ophthalmology. 2003;**136**:252-257

[59] Lee JW, Kim IT. Outcomes of idiopathic macular epiretinal membrane removal with and without internal limiting membrane peeling: A comparative study. Japanese Journal of Ophthalmology. 2010;**54**:129-134

[60] Ahn SJ, Ahn J, Woo SJ, Park KH. Photoreceptor change and visual outcome after idiopathic epiretinal membrane removal with or without additional internal limiting membrane peeling. Retina. 2014;**34**:172-181

[61] Pichi F, Lembo A, Morara M, Veronese M, Nucci P, Ciardella AP. Early and late inner retinal changes after inner limiting membrane peeling. International Journal of Ophthalmology. 2014;**34**:437-446

[62] Tadayoni R, Paques M, Massin P, Mouki-Benani S, Mikol J, Gaudric A. Dissociated optic nerve fiber layer appearance of the fundus after idiopathic epiretinal membrane removal. Ophthalmology. 2001;**108**:2279-2283

[63] Ehlers JP, Han J, Petkovsek D, Kaiser PK, Singh RP, Srivastava SK. Membrane peeling-induced retinal alterations on intraoperative OCT in Vitreomacular Interface disorders from the PIONEER study. Investigative Ophthalmology & Visual Science. 2015;**56**(12):7324-7330

[64] Deltour JB, Grimbert P, Masse H, Lebreton O, Weber M. Detrimental effects of active internal limiting membrane peeling during Epiretinal membrane surgery: Microperimetric analysis. Retina. 2017;**37**(3):544-552

[65] Ducloyer JB, Ivan J, Poinas A, Lebreton O, Bonissent A, Fossum P, et al. Does internal limiting membrane peeling during epiretinal membrane surgery induce microscotomas on microperimetry? Study protocol for PEELING, a randomized controlled clinical trial. Trials. 2020;**21**(1):500

[66] Sun Y, Zhou R, Zhang B. With or without internal limiting membrane peeling for idiopathic epiretinal membrane: A meta-analysis of randomized controlled trials. Retina. 2021;**41**(8):1644-1651

[67] Mitamura Y, Ohtsuka K. Relationship of dissociated optic nerve fiber layer appearance to internal limiting membrane peeling. Ophthalmology. 2005;**112**:1766-1770

[68] Miura M, Elsner AE, Osako M, Yamada K, Agawa T, Usui M, et al. Spectral imaging of the area of internal limiting membrane peeling. Retina. 2005;**25**:468-472

[69] Saurabh K, Roy R, Mishra S, Garg B, Goel S. Multicolor imaging features of dissociated optic nerve fiber layer after internal limiting membrane peeling. Indian Journal of Ophthalmology. 2018;**66**(12):1853-18540

[70] Spaide RF. Dissociated optic nerve fiber layer appearance after internal limiting membrane removal is inner retinal dimpling. Retina. 2012;**32**:1719-1726

[71] Steel DH, Dinah C, White K, Avery PJ. The relationship between a dissociated optic nerve fibre layer appearance after macular hole surgery and Muller cell debris on peeled internal limiting membrane. Acta Ophthalmologica. 2017;**95**(2):153-157

[72] Baba T, Yamamoto S, Kimoto R, Oshitari T, Sato E. Reduction of thickness of ganglion cell complex after internal limiting membrane peeling during vitrectomy for idiopathic macular hole. Eye. Sep 2012;**26**(9):1173-1180

[73] Terasaki H, Miyake Y, Nomura R, Piao CH, Hori K, Niwa T, et al. Focal macular ERGs in eyes after removal of macular ILM during macular hole

surgery. Investigative Ophthalmology & Visual Science. 2001;**42**:229-234

[74] Runkle AP, Srivastava SK, Yuan A, Kaiser PK, Singh RP, Reese JL, et al. Factors associated with development of dissociated optic nerve fiber Layer appearance In the Pioneer intraoperative optical coherence tomography study. Retina. 2018;**38**(Suppl. 1):S103-S109

Chapter 4

Macular Hole Surgery

Sergio Scalia, Peter Reginald Simcock, Simone Scalia, Daniela Angela Randazzo and Maria Rosaria Sanfilippo

Abstract

Macular hole surgery is one of the most rapidly changing fields in vitreoretinal surgery, the authors discuss the recent acknowledgments and surgical options. Macular holes are classified, and surgical techniques are described in order to have the most successful procedure. Diagnostic tools and surgical instruments improvement allow surgeons to face difficult cases with a variety of surgical options unknown until a few years ago and is mandatory nowadays to approach the different patients with a broad mind.

Keywords: macular hole, vitrectomy, inner limiting membrane, expansile gas, autologous platelet concentrate, human amniotic membrane, retinal graft

1. Introduction

A macular hole (MH) is a full-thickness defect of the neurosensory retina involving the fovea **Figures 1** and **2**. The prevalence of macular holes is estimated at 0.1% in individuals aged 40 years or older and 0.8% in those aged over 74 years. Idiopathic macular holes account for up to 85% of all macular holes. Other causes include blunt trauma, high myopia, macular schisis, macular telangiectasia type 2, wet age-related macular and surgical trauma [1, 2]. Most patients are females over 65 years of age and may also be seen with myopic eyes [3].

2. Pathogenesis of idiopathic MH

The posterior vitreous cortex exhibits anteroposterior and tangential traction forces on the fovea [4]. The role of vitreomacular tractions in the formation of the MH is supported by the reduced incidence of bilateral MH in patients with a posterior vitreous detachment (PVD) in the fellow eye as a PVD significantly reduces the risk of MH formation [5].

3. Clinical presentation

Patients with macular hole usually present with decreased vision, central scotoma and metamorphopsia. Slit-lamp bio-microscopy with 78, 90 D or a fundus contact lens

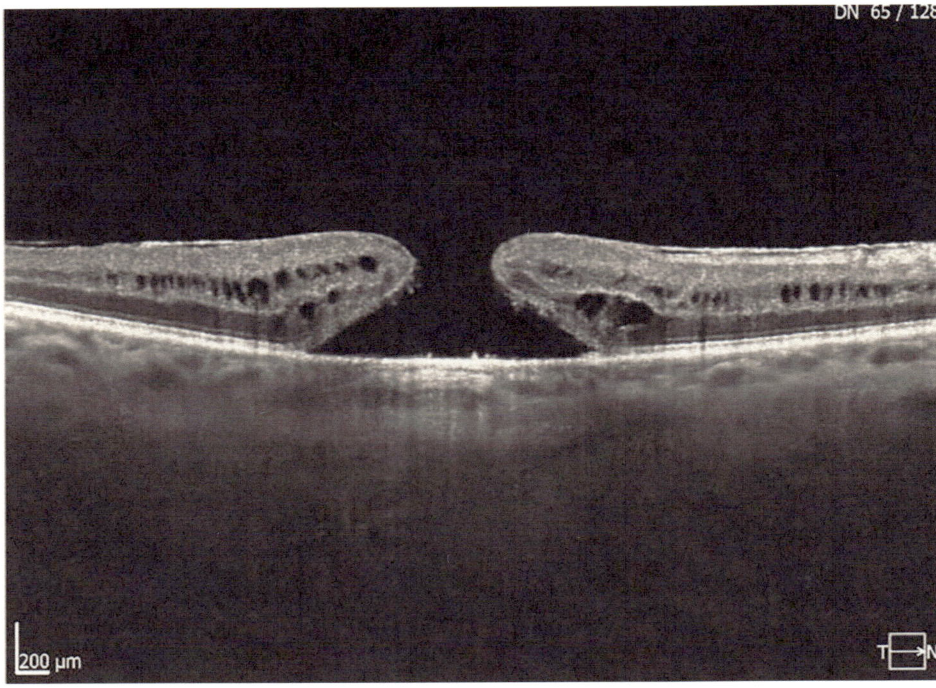

Figure 1.
Full-thickness macular hole OCT cross-sectional image.

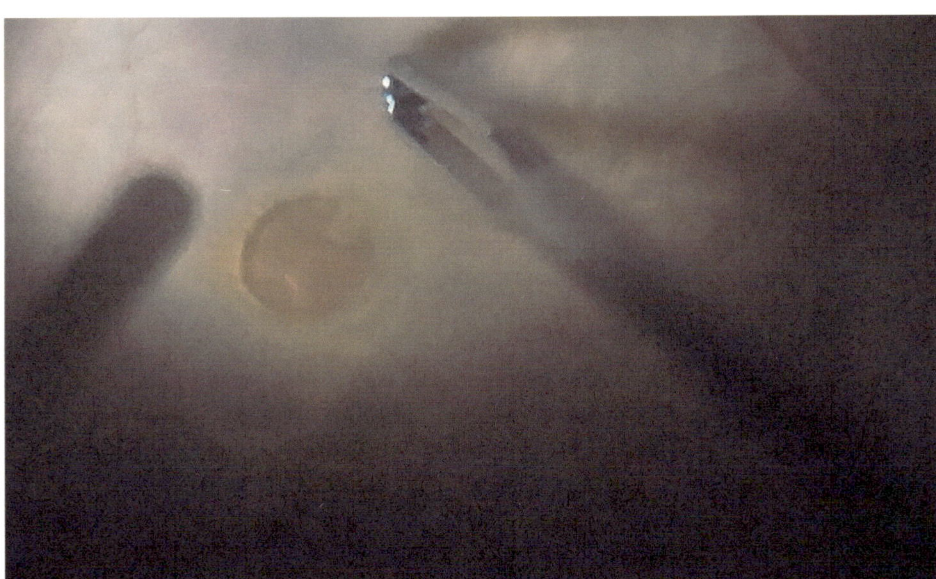

Figure 2.
Intraoperative fundus pictures of a full-thickness macular hole.

is the best way to visualise the hole clinically. The size of macular hole, status of the vitreous, presence of epiretinal membrane (ERM), degenerative changes of the Retinal Pigment Epithelium (RPE), overlying operculum and presence of surrounding cuff of fluid should be reported. Traumatic macular holes can be identified by their ragged and irregular margins and can be easily differentiated from idiopathic macular holes clinically as well as by the history of previous trauma. Full-thickness macular holes can be differentiated from pseudo-holes or lamellar holes by the Watzke-Allen test or laser aiming beam test but these clinical tests have been superseded by the common use of ocular coherence tomography.

4. Investigations

4.1 Ocular coherence tomography

Swept-Source Ocular Coherence Tomography (SS-OCT) gives a high-resolution image of the vitreoretinal interface, neurosensory retina, retinal pigment epithelium and choroid. This investigation identifies surrounding epiretinal membrane, the cuff of subretinal fluid and intraretinal cystic change, vitreo-foveal adhesion, operculum or pseudo-operculum and status of RPE. It also allows accurate calculation of various macular hole indices that have a role in giving a prognosis.

4.2 Macular hole indices

1. Macular Hole height (MHH): Vertical length between RPE and the highest point of the hole

2. Base diameter: Measured at the level of RPE

3. Minimum linear diameter (MLD): Minimum dimension

4. Macular hole inner opening: Distance between innermost layer

5. Tractional hole index (THI): MHH/MLD

6. Macular hole index (MHI): MHH/Base diameter

7. Hole forming factor (HFF): (left arm length of macular hole + right arm length of macular hole)/base diameter

Greater MHI and THI are linked to better post-operative functional results. MHI relates to external limiting membrane (ELM) restoration, while MLD and BD are to anatomical closure (**Figure 3**).

5. Fundus autofluorescence

This test also helps with prognosis. The absence of foveal pigments in macular hole leads to hyper autofluorescence of healthy RPE. Poor autofluorescence from RPE due to pigmentary or other degenerative changes in the RPE is associated with poor visual prognosis.

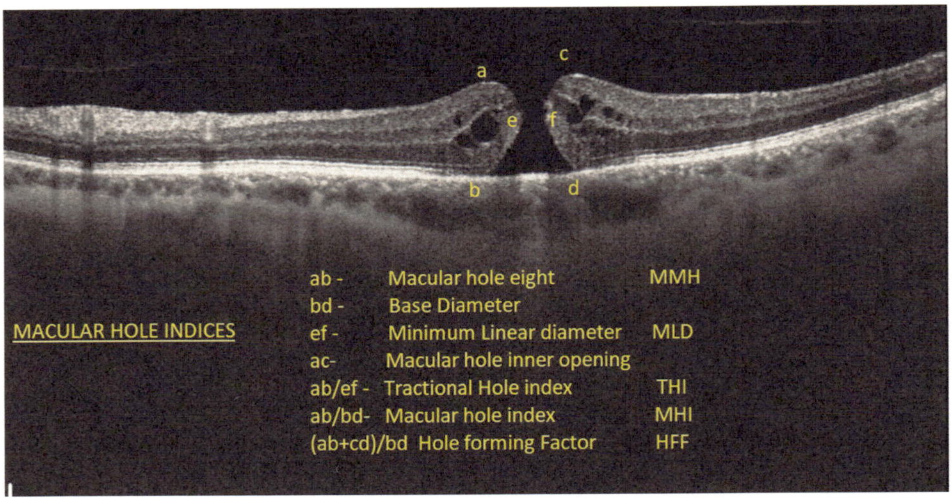

Figure 3.
Preoperative macular hole indices.

5.1 Classification

Idiopathic full-thickness macular holes are produced by traction exerted by the posterior vitreous cortex on the neurosensory retina in the central macular area. Disinsertion of the overlying glial plug may result in the formation of a foveal "cyst." Further traction with removal of the cyst roof produces a free-floating operculum on the posterior vitreous cortex. The neurosensory retina then displaces centrifugally as a full-thickness retinal hole.

Gass described MHs according to clinical evolution:

1. **Stage 1a:** (Impending Hole): 100–200-micron, foveolar detachment- Yellow Spot

2. **Stage 1b:** (Occult Hole): 200–300-micron, foveal detachment- Yellow Ring

3. **Stage 2:** Small full-thickness macular hole less than 400 microns

4. **Stage 3:** Full-thickness macular hole of more than 400 microns with or without an operculum. No Posterior Vitreous Detachment (PVD)

5. **Stage 4:** Full-thickness macular hole with complete PVD.

A new classification introduced by the International Vitreomacular Traction Study Group was facilitated by high-resolution OCT imaging and was defined as: vitreomacular adhesion (VMA), vitreomacular traction (VMT) and macular hole (**Table 1**) [2].

Evidence from a large surgical series of 1483 primary MH repairs reported by Steel et al. [6] treated with vitrectomy, ILM peel, and gas or air tamponade noted that a linear diameter of 500 μm or less was the threshold for successful hole closure. Other studies demonstrated a similar correlation between MH size and successful hole closure, and it was suggested that the definition of large MH's should be changed to

VMA	**Size: focal (<1500 mm) or broad (>1500 mm)**
VMT	Size: focal (<1500 mm) or broad (>1500 mm)
Full-thickness Macular hole	Size: small (250 mm), medium (>250 e < 400 mm), large (>400 mm
Vitreous	Status of vitreous: with or without VMT primary or secondary

Table 1.
International Vitreomacular traction study group classification.

≥500 μm [7–9]. The evolution of holes is variable, with a tendency to progress with time in 74% of cases within 2 years [10]. Small holes may close spontaneously in about 5% of cases and it may be reasonable to closely observe small holes with good vision in case of spontaneous resolution [11].

High myopia is a well-recognised risk factor for unsuccessful MH repair, with an axial length (AL) > 26 mm or refraction higher than −6 Diopters making successful hole closure less likely [12]. Anatomical success is reduced as the degree of myopia increases and ranges from 91.7% (AL: 26–29.9 mm) to 0% in eyes with AL > 30 mm [13].

6. Pharmacologic treatment

The only pharmacologic treatment available to date as an alternative to surgical treatment is Ocriplasmin (OCP). This treatment is approved in cases of symptomatic VMA including VMA with MH less than 400 microns. While Ocriplasmin releases VMT in the majority of eyes, the success rate for macular hole closure remains limited and is in the range of 40–50% in eyes with a small-diameter macular hole but decreases to 15–20% in the medium-sized macular hole [14, 15]. Floaters can still be troublesome after OCP and there is a side effect profile that has resulted in most vitreoretinal surgeons still favouring a formal surgical procedure over pharmacological vitreolysis with OCP.

7. Surgical treatment

7.1 Timing

Jaycock et al. [16] reported a closure rate of 94% among patients having surgery within 1 year of the onset of symptoms. The anatomical success was noted to be reduced to 47% when surgery was postponed more than 12 months. Macular holes operated after 1 year yield poor functional improvement even if - anatomic closure is obtained. Limited visual improvement may be obtained after successful closure of chronic MH and is linked with the MH duration [17]. One possible reason for a failed surgical outcome in chronic MH surgery may be due to a strong adhesion of the photoreceptor layer of the retina to the underlying RPE [18–20].

7.2 Evaluation of outcome of surgery

It is difficult to accurately compare the results of different studies due to the lack of a uniform method for determining the integrity of the outer retinal layers after MH vitrectomy. The rapid development of the OCT has facilitated images with a very high resolution. This has allowed accurate interpretation of the outer retinal layers and the ability to compare them to histological sections of the retina.

The outer retinal layers can be divided into 4 lines or bands [21] and the presence of well-defined bands is associated with good vision. The first band arises from the External Limiting membrane (ELM). The second band is referred to as the inner segment – outer segment (IS-OS) intersection of the photoreceptors. The third band has been described as the COST (cone outer segment tips), intermediate line and more recently the interdigitation zone (IZ). The fourth band corresponds to the RPE. Iwasaki et al. [22] also described a method in which the ELM recovery rate and the EZ recovery rate were evaluated in the treated groups.

Caprani et al. [23] describe the restoration of outer retinal layers from the external limiting membrane (ELM), inner segment/outer segment junction (IS-OS), and cone outer segment tips (COST) to retinal pigment epithelium (RPE) after IMH surgery and its relation to visual acuity. They classified the layers as either present or absent after MH surgery with ILM peeling. They also observed the ELM was the first layer to be restored in the healing process, while the integrity of the ellipsoid zone was present in 53.5% of patients at 3 months and in 73.91% at 6 months.

7.3 Surgical technique

Surgical treatment was pioneered in 1990 by Kelly and Wendel [24] by performing 20 gauge pars plana vitrectomy, PVD induction, intraocular gas tamponade and postoperative face-down positioning. They reported an anatomical closure rate of 58% and 73% and visual improvement in 42% and 55% of cases in two consecutive reports.

Eckardt [25] in 1997, introduced the concept of internal limiting membrane (ILM) peeling in the management of macular holes. Peeling of the internal limiting membrane relieves the tangential traction caused by glial cells and improves the anatomical and visual success rates of macular hole surgery.

A Cochrane review in 2013 [26] showed better visual results, anatomical closure rates and lower re-operation rates in patients who underwent ILM peeling when compared to those who underwent pars plana vitrectomy alone.

7.4 Microincision vitreoretinal surgery (MIVS)

The advent of smaller gauge and better instrumentation, tissue staining during ILM removal, combined phaco-vitrectomy surgery and reduced or no postoperative face-down positioning are all factors that have facilitated surgery and made it technically less challenging as well as being less obtrusive and difficult for the patient.

Shift to small gauge instrumentation in the last 20 years may have resulted in a slightly increased duration of the vitrectomy operation due to the increased cut rates and slight reduction of fluid passage in the eye. MIVS has however caused a significant reduction in complications like entry site retinal breaks and vitreous traction-related retinal damage (**Table 2**).

	PRO	CONS
20G	Instrument stiffness, illumination Easy PVD induction	Scleral wound needs suturing Retinal and entry site breaks
23G	Safer vitreous removal, efficient aspiration for PVD induction	Wounds often require suturing
25G	Sutureless wounds, very controlled vitreous removal	Wounds rarely require suturing Slightly greater flexibility of instruments
27G	Sutureless wounds, safe vitreous base shaving Fast healing	Difficult PVD induction, flexible instruments and less illumination. Longer vitrectomy time, sometimes difficult to grasp the membrane.

Table 2.
Comparison of 20-G, 23-G, and 25-G vitreous cutters and instrumentation.

7.5 Gas tamponade

Filling the vitreous cavity with gas encourages hole closure by preventing fluid from accessing the hole and may facilitate the formation of a glial plug that can contract and help with hole closure. The buoyancy effect of the gas is also thought to play a role by direct pressure on the hole and hence the reason that face-down posturing has been recommended in the postoperative period. Gas mixtures used in different percentages are C3F8, C2F6, SF6 and air. Recent studies have shown that longer-acting gases like C3F8 and C2F6 may not be needed as SF6 and air show similar anatomic results in terms of hole closure and better patient compliance [27, 28]. Silicone oil is rarely used as a tamponade agent and needs a further surgical procedure to remove the oil.

7.6 Postoperative prone posturing

Facedown posturing (FDP) has been recommended because the gas bubble with its surface tension forces may support the apposition of the MH edges and also provide a scaffold for the migration of glial cells and blocking fluid entry into the hole.

The force of the gas bubble is greatest at the apex of the arc of contact to the retinal surface and diminishes from this point [29].

Postoperative face-down positioning night and day for a week was recommended as a critical step for many years to increase the buoyancy force exerted on the posterior pole but studies have subsequently shown that prolonged face-down posturing may not be needed especially for smaller holes. Recent publications report closure rates for small- to medium-size MHs at around 95% in both postured and non-postured groups indicating that prolonged posturing is not necessary for MH closure after surgery. The authors concluded that face-down posturing is not necessary for medium-sized MHs [30–32]. Large holes >400 microns may benefit from prolonged postoperative posturing, but studies still show inconclusive results [33].

Ye et al. [34] in a meta-analysis of five randomised controlled trials compared MH surgeries with ILM peeling with postoperative FDP versus those with non-supine posturing (NSP). The MH closure rate was higher in the FDP group, with a significant difference in the closure rate for MH with size >400 μm, but not for those <400 μm.

Eckardt et al. [35] considered stopping the FDP as soon as the OCT confirmed the closure but in case of non-closure on day 3, it required a second procedure on day 5 or 6 to facilitate hole closure. It has been noted that increased duration between the first and second surgery when there is failed primary repair may result in a worse visual and anatomical outcome [36–38].

Nearly all patients having vitrectomy surgery with a gas bubble will develop cataract. A pilot study by P R Simcock and S Scalia [39] showed that combining lens removal at the time of vitrectomy resulted in greater space for the gas bubble and better tamponade and patients had successful hole closure without having to adopt a prone posture as well as the advantage of not having to return for further cataract surgery.

Chakrabarti et al. [40] described the use of autologous gluconated blood (AGBL) in the macular area for treating MH without the use of intraocular gas or prone positioning. They report no significant side effects and 26 patients with large MH's, obtained 100% closure using an inverted ILM flap and AGBL to encourage macular healing with good functional outcome. The technique involves a preparation of AGBC before the surgery (1 mL of 5% glucose added to 2 mL of autologous blood) then an ILM flap was created and AGBC on top to create a macular plug. This technique allowed the patients to adopt a comfortable position without gas tamponade.

8. Staining

Vital dyes were introduced more than 20 years ago to allow better visualisation and removal of the vitreous and staining and removal of epiretinal membranes and the internal limiting membrane [41, 42].

8.1 Triamcinolone acetonide

Triamcinolone crystalline microparticles are trapped in the vitreous gel facilitating gel removal by improving visualisation and determining if there has been a vitreous separation from the retina. The microparticles also tend to settle on membrane surfaces creating a demarcation between the peeled and remaining membrane.

8.2 Indocyanine green (ICG) and Infracyanine green (IfCG)

ICG green stains the ILM because of its affinity to laminin and collagen type IV within the ILM. ILM peeling was popularised as a result of this stain as it was a technically challenging procedure to perform without the stain. It has however been criticised due to complications associated with cytotoxic and phototoxic effects on the exposed RPE. Infracyanine Green at a concentration of 0.5 mg/ml also allows good visualisation of the ILM but with a better safety profile.

8.3 Trypan blue

Trypan blue 0.2% is also used to stain the ILM or ERM during vitreoretinal surgery and is often injected after a fluid air exchange to increase the staining of the membrane (**Figure 4**).

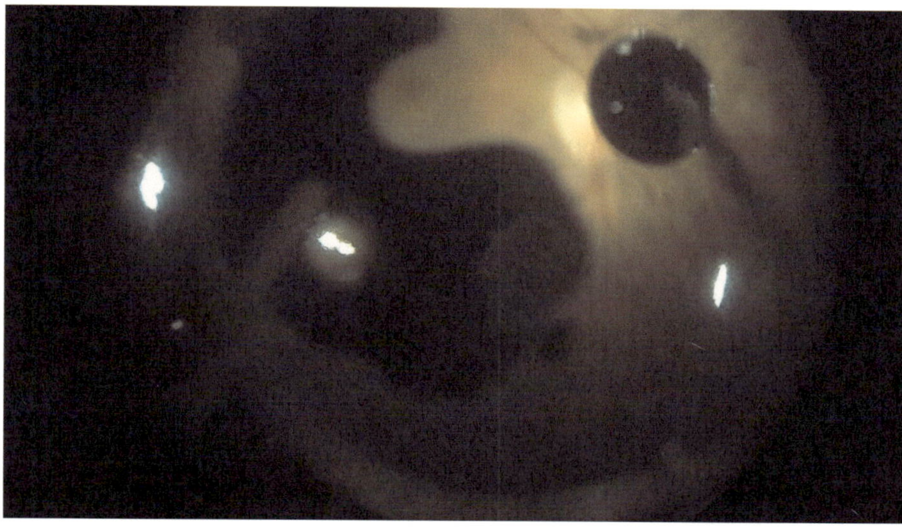

Figure 4.
Trypan blue is injected under the air bubble.

8.4 Brilliant blue G

The brilliant blue stain has been used for selective ILM staining. It was approved in the European Union in 2007 as Brilliant Peel. Brilliant Blue G formulation uses 4% polyethylene glycol (PEG) as a carrier for the dye and prevents the blue stain from diluting in the vitreous cavity. Since the dye is heavier than water it settles at the posterior pole with a standard injection technique.

9. Dye injection techniques

There are different ways to protect the RPE cells during dye injection in MH surgery:

1. gentle injection of the dye (this is the most common way that is used now as Brilliant Blue is very safe to use and not harmful to the RPE)

2. placing substances such as sodium hyaluronate over the MH.

3. perflourocarbons liquids (PFCL),

4. autologous blood

The most common techniques in dye injection are:

1. The “dry method” consists of removing the balanced salt solution (BSS) in the vitreous cavity by a fluid-gas exchange before dye injection. The technique has the advantage of concentrating the dye in the posterior pole, exposing the retinal surface to a higher concentration of dye in the vitreoretinal interface

2. The "wet method" while the surgeon injects the dye in a fluid-filled vitreous cavity. The amount of dye in contact with the retinal surface is lower because it is diluted by the fluid in the vitreous cavity. The wet method is safer and faster but may be less effective in ILM staining, particularly in highly myopic eyes. If a poor stain is encountered, it is often worth re-staining as there may be greater stain uptake on the second attempt.

10. Macular hole closure

A macular hole is said to be closed when there is flattening and reattachment of the hole rim along the whole circumference of the macular hole (**Figures 5** and **6**).

Two types of closure have been defined [43].

- Type 1 closure: No interruption in the foveal retinal tissue above the RPE layer (**Figures 7** and **8**).

- Type 2 Closure: Interruption of inner retinal tissue and central RPE exposure.

Imai et al. [44] gave another OCT-based classification of macular hole closure and divided it into three types:

- Type "U"- Normal foveal contour on OCT

- Type "V"- Steep foveal contour

- Type "W"- Foveal defect of neurosensory retina

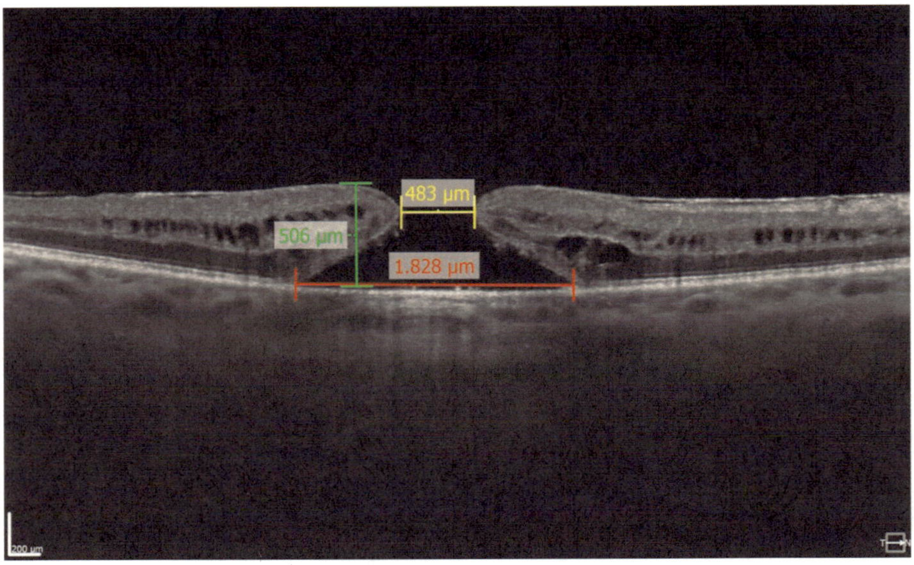

Figure 5.
Full-thickness macular hole preop cross-sectional image and measurements.

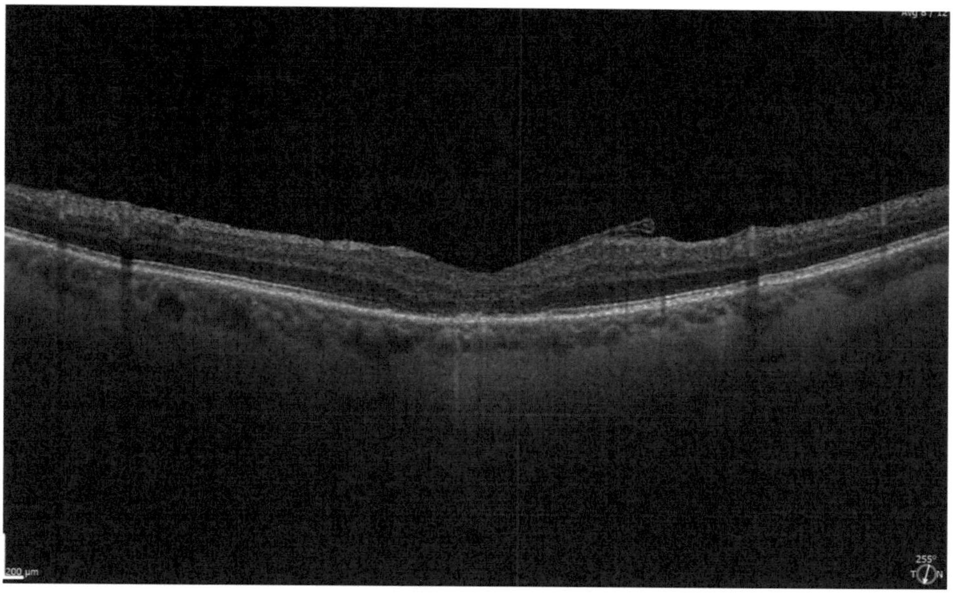

Figure 6.
Macular hole closure after successful vitrectomy, ILM peeling and gas tamponade.

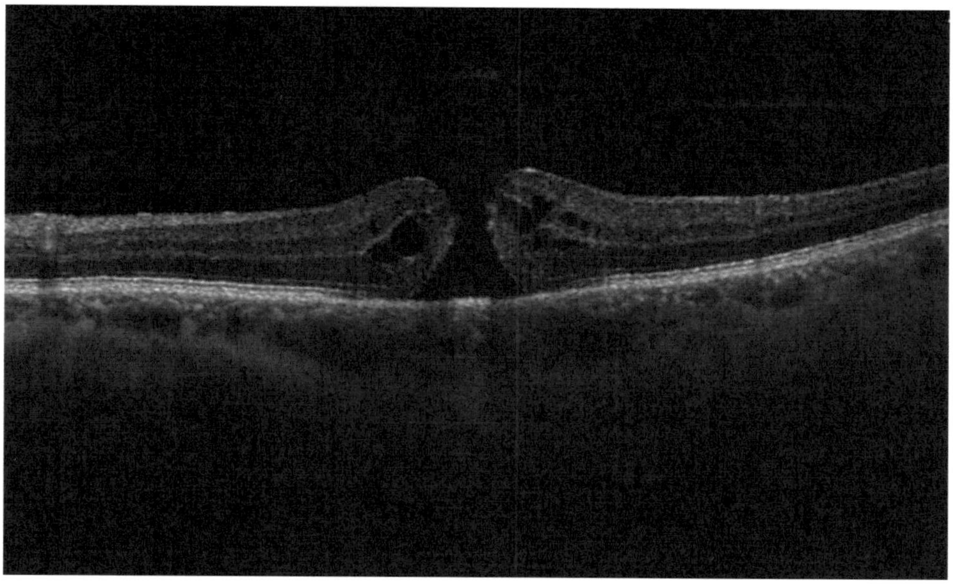

Figure 7.
Full-thickness macular hole with operculum.

The various lines seen in the outer retinal on OCT scanning have been mentioned earlier in this chapter, namely the External limiting membrane (ELM), Inner segment/Outer segment junction (IS/OS junction) or Ellipsoid zone (EZ), Cone outer segment tips (COST) or Interdigitation zone (IZ) and Retinal pigment epithelium (RPE).

Structural changes in the macular region after surgery are correlated to photoreceptor alterations [45–48]. They can be related to the outer retinal bands seen on OCT

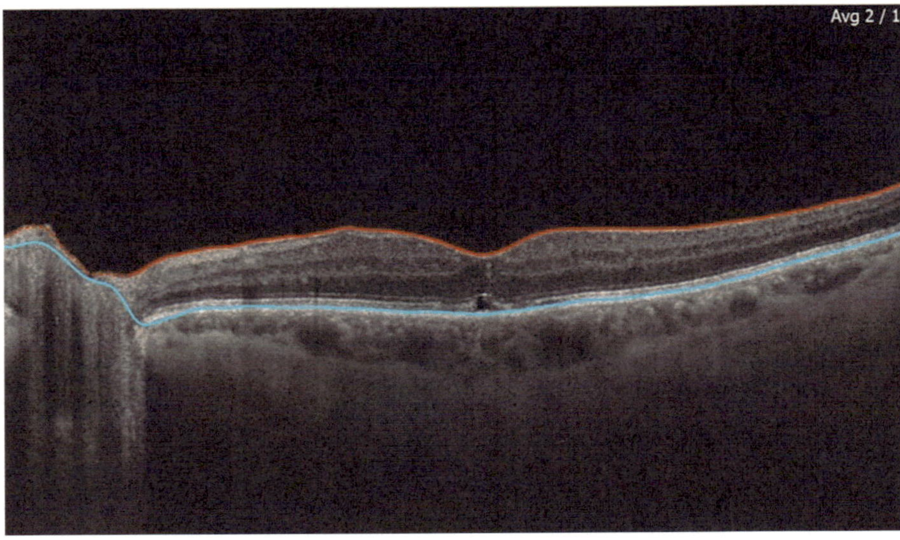

Figure 8.
Macular hole closure after surgical treatment.

scanning. The ELM is the first retinal layer to recover, followed by the IS/OS, and lastly the COST (**Figure 8**).

Min Woo Lee et al. [49] analysed the process of recovery of the ELM, Outer nuclear layer (ONL), and EZ after surgical treatment. They tried to identify the factors affecting changes in visual acuity and those associated with EZ recovery. They divide full-thickness MH healing into the following stages: the first stage occurred when the traction from ILM to the neuroretina was released after surgery resulting in the resolution of intraretinal cysts, this phase occurred when the inner retinal layers grew to the centre of the macular hole and two edges were connected by forming a tissue bridge. At this stage, SRF could still be found on B-scan. Finally, the SRF resolves and photoreceptors begin remodelling, which could lead to restoration of the ellipsoid area (**Figure 9**).

11. Role of the internal limiting membrane

The ILM is the most superficial layer of the retina and is formed by the Muller cell footplates together with a fibrous component. This membrane is 400 nm thick at the retinal periphery, rising to about 1400 nm in the macular region [50]. This structure provides greater mechanical strength than retinal cell layers, being responsible for 50% of retinal stiffness. The rationale for its removal is to relieve all tangential traction around the macular hole and improve hole closure rates [51–53].

During macular hole surgery, central vitrectomy is usually followed by PVD induction by placing the cutter on aspiration mode in the proximity of the optic disk until a Weiss ring is noticed and a wave of circumferential vitreous separation is seen. Vitreous removal with a high-speed cutter to the retinal periphery is then performed. At this stage, any epiretinal membranes (ERM) surrounding the macular hole should be stained and removed up to the borders of the hole. If no ERM is identified, then

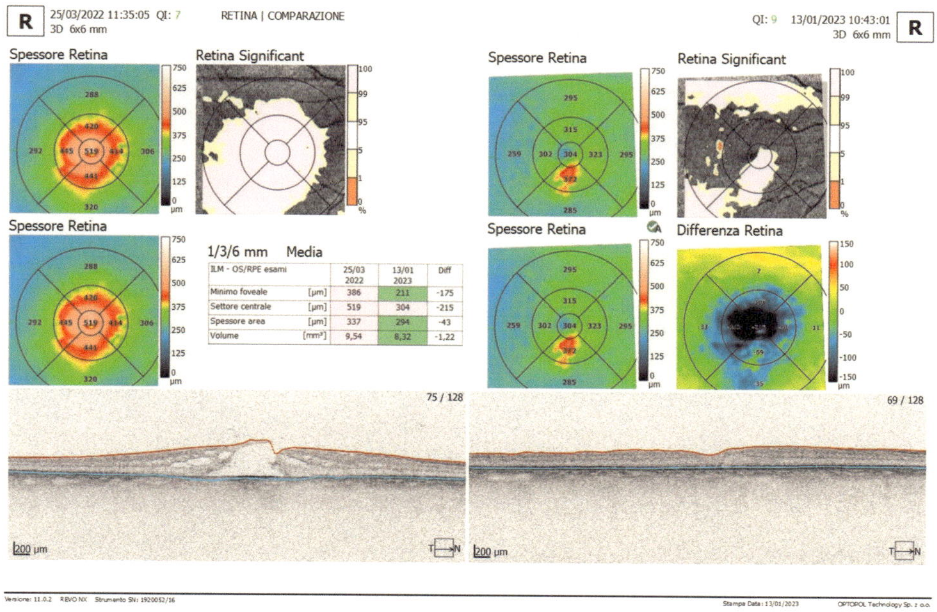

Figure 9.
Macular hole closure: Preoperative optical coherence tomography (OCT) and 10 months postoperative OCT.

most surgeons would routinely remove the ILM. The advent of tissue stains and dedicated surgical instrumentations allows the identification and removal of the inner limiting membrane and this procedure can be described as total peeling (TP) when the ILM around the MH is removed or foveal sparing peeling (FSP).

12. ILM peeling technique

12.1 Initiation

The creation of an ILM flap is a crucial step in ILM peeling. The ideal starting point has been suggested as about 1000 microns above or below the fovea. A small ILM tear is created on the retinal surface by scraping the retinal surface with a diamond-dusted or using picks, bent MVR blades or with dedicated ILM forceps using a pinch and peel technique. Many surgeons utilise custom-designed micro forceps to pinch and lift the ILM and create a small flap to then grasp and customise the direction and shape of the desired flap (**Figure 10**).

12.2 Flap creation

Vitreoretinal forceps and the diamond-dusted membrane scraper are valuable tools for flap creation [54]. The majority of surgeons tend to peel an ILM area of about one disk diameter around the fovea, releasing enough retinal tissue in order to allow macular hole closure (**Figure 11**). A broader area of ILM up to 3 disk diameters may be removed to improve retinal compliance and subsequent retinal closure but it is still unclear regarding the exact dimension of ILM removal needed.

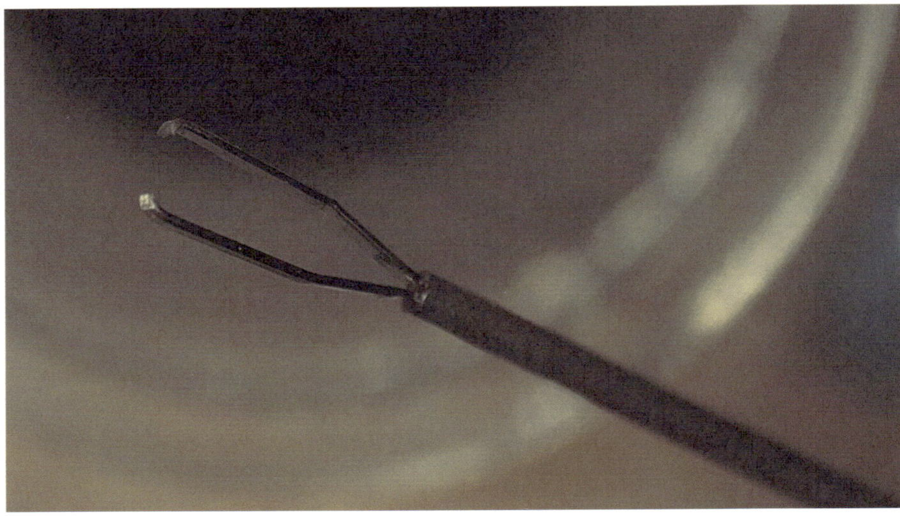

Figure 10.
The finesse SHARKSKIN ILM forceps.

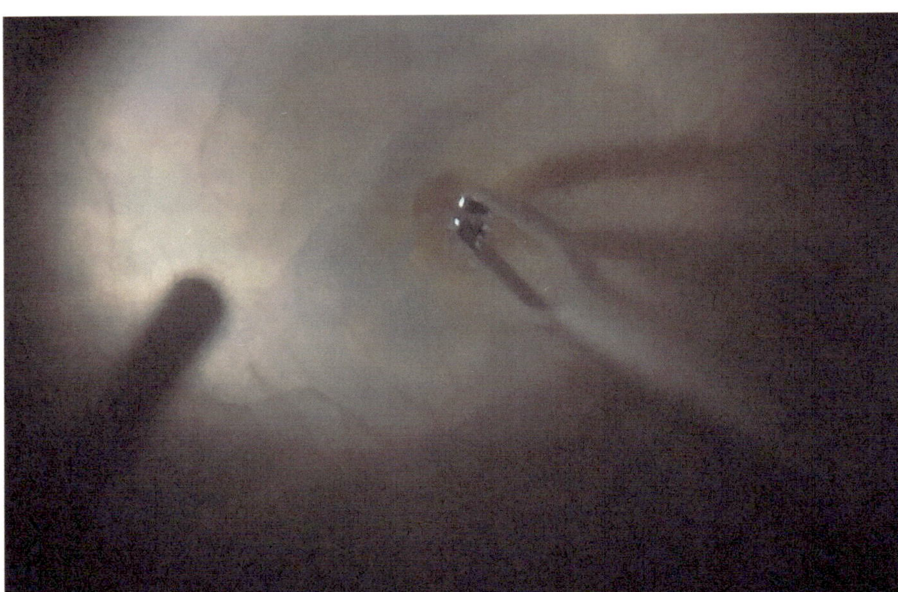

Figure 11.
ILM flap folded over the macular hole.

12.3 Side effects

ILM peeling is one of the most demanding procedures in ophthalmic surgery requiring a high level of manual dexterity. Retinal damage can occur at the initial ILM flap creation point resulting in retinal haemorrhages and nerve fibre layer damage as well as iatrogenic eccentric retinal holes have been reported [55]. A peculiar retinal alteration in the area where the ILM is removed has been described as Disassociated

Optic Nerve Fibre Layer (DONFL) with a characteristic change in inner retinal morphology and appears related to Muller cell end plate damage [56–58].

12.4 ILM peeling variants

12.4.1 Foveal sparing peeling

This technique entails ILM removal but sparing a circular area of 400 microns around the MH rim. In a study by HO [59] foveal sparing resulted in better visual acuity and postoperative anatomy, based on the concept that Muller cells are important for maintaining foveal architecture. Muller cells may improve light transmission to the photoreceptors [60]. In a study by Morescalchi [61], a total of 46 eyes had macular hole surgery and were randomly allocated to complete or foveal-sparing peeling. The latter group demonstrated a greater increase in foveal sensitivity following surgery. Muller cells preservation may therefore provide a better functional outcome after macular hole surgery [62, 63].

12.4.2 ILM abrasion

Mahajan [64] reported a different procedure to reduce trauma during ILM removal by using a diamond-dusted membrane scraper (DDMS) in circumferential and centripetal motions around the MH. This procedure was thought to encourage glial cell activation, losing ILM attachment to the underlying retinal tissue and ultimately encouraging MH closure.

ILM peeling was initially described in 1997 by Eckardt [25]. The rationale for ILM peeling was the removal of residual adherent vitreous cortex remnants, thereby increasing retinal compliance. ILM serves as a scaffold for cellular proliferation, and its removal should encourage MH closure. Peeling the ILM ensures the thorough removal of any tangential tractional components implicated in the development of macular holes. The removal of a potential scaffold for the re-proliferation of myofibroblasts may reduce the possibility of late reopening of surgically closed holes. Furthermore, peeling off the ILM is also believed to stimulate wound healing at the macula, possibly by inducing local expression of growth factors that promote glial repair (**Video 1**, http://bit.ly/433B3XW).

The Cochrane database of systemic reviews concluded in 2013 that there was enough evidence to support the positive effects of ILM peeling for stages 2–4 idiopathic MH's to improve the primary anatomical hole closure rate, although no clear benefit was found for small holes [24].

ILM peeling increases the likelihood of successful macular hole closure, but it has been suggested that the extra manipulation of this membrane at the time of surgery could be harmful to the retina.

Swelling of the arcuate nerve fibre layer after internal limiting membrane peeling was described by Clark [65]. Electrophysiologic studies using focal macular electroretinogram showed a delayed recovery of the b-wave 6 months after macular hole surgery in eyes that underwent ILM peeling compared to those without peeling [66].

Although anatomical closure achieved after complete ILM peeling was associated with improved visual outcomes, the rate of anatomic closure was inversely correlated with the extent of ILM peeling actually achieved. It was suggested that excessive unsuccessful attempts at ILM peeling might enhance anatomic success (possibly through enhanced promotion of glial healing) at the expense of poorer visual outcomes, presumably resulting from damage to inner retinal elements [67].

Inner limiting membrane peeling appears to improve the rate of anatomical closure, but its effect on visual outcome is less predictable and unsuccessful attempts to peel the ILM are associated with poor visual outcome. While ILM peeling may be performed for full-thickness macular holes of any stage, it is more commonly reserved for stage 3 or 4 holes, long-standing holes, those that have failed to close, or those that have re-opened following conventional surgery.

ILM peeling is thought to be beneficial for macular hole closure and in particular for large holes, however, it may also cause side effects on retinal anatomy and functionality. Retinal changes described after ILM peeling included inner retinal dimpling [68], dissociated retinal nerve fibre layer (RNFL), [69] and reduced parafoveal retinal thickness [70].

13. Internal limiting membrane peel extension

ILM peeling has improved surgical success in MH surgery. The ILM can be removed using forceps, diamond dusted scraper or other surgical tools and it has been suggested that at least 2 disc diameter (DD) of ILM should be removed around the fovea. Different surgeons perform this delicate procedure using peel radii from 0.5 to 3 DD. Bae et al. [71] compared peel sizes of 0.75 DD versus 1.5 DD and showed that a larger ILM peel lessens postoperative metamorphopsia. Modi et al. [72] have shown similar results in MH closure rates with 3 mm versus 5 mm peel sizes. No consensus on optimal peel width exists, but case reports of wide peels having success in large MHs have led many surgeons to peel ILM up to the arcades [73].

13.1 Macular holes >400 microns

In macular holes <400 microns conventional ILM peeling provided better functional outcomes compared with the inverted flap technique and should be advocated [74].

FTMH above 400 microns have a reduced rate of success with standard surgery, and other techniques such as ILM flaps and retinal expansion may be preferred for these macular holes [7]. Vitrectomy with the inverted ILM flap technique seems to be effective surgery for large idiopathic and myopic MHs, improving both functional and anatomical outcomes in a study by Rizzo [75] and surgical closure in all patients is reported in a study by Yamashita [76].

The practice of using the ILM on top of a macular hole has many effects, such as a bandage, isolating the retinal hole from the vitreous fluids, as a scaffold stimulating glial tissue proliferation, and will all encourage hole closure. In a study by Michalewska et al. [19] the use of ILM flap increased the rate of MH closure up to 98% for large MHs. This technique has also resulted in a 100% macular hole closure rate in myopic MH's reported in some studies [77, 78].

ILM flaps can be divided into two groups, inverted and non-inverted flaps:

Inverted flaps

- the folded inverted flap
- temporal inverted flap,

- nasal inverted flap (Texas Taco technique)
- superior inverted flap
- the cabbage leaf flap
- SWIFT (superior wide base flap transposition)

These flaps require the presence of ILM still hinged around the hole or near the hole in order to prevent displacement of ILM in the vitreous cavity. Michalewska [79] describes a procedure where the ILM is engaged with ILM forceps and removed almost in its entirely around the macular hole but a tiny residual attachment is left in place. Folded ILM is then packed inside the MH rather than a flap covering it. ILM is massaged into the MH from all sides until it becomes inverted and may be described as an 'ILM plug'. At a microscopic level, the presence of this plug may hamper outer retinal layer healing and prevent visual acuity recovery by interfering with photoreceptor reconstitution [80]. ILM tissue however is also known to work as a scaffold for tissue proliferation, promoting photoreceptors restoration and providing guidance for the correct positioning of the cells [81]. Rossi [82] stated that by using the fill technique, the ILM acts as a filler, glue, and scaffold all at the same time.

Shin [83] first introduced a true flap technique (single-layered flap of the ILM) for covering MH's (larger than 400 μm) with the assistance of perfluoro-n-octane (PFO) in 2014. Perflurocarbon liquid allows ILM flap stabilisation during fluid-air exchange by reducing dislocation or flap loss.

The temporal inverted internal limiting membrane flap was described by Michalewska [79]. The nasal ILM was left in place to protect the tissue from surgical trauma and lessen the occurrence of dissociated optic nerve fibre layer (DONFL).

The opposite approach has also been described and named the "Texas taco" [84]. This procedure involves peeling the nasal ILM and then it is folded temporally to cover the MH.

Ghassemi et al. [85] investigated the results of different ILM flap directions. The techniques used were a hemi circular ILM peel with a temporally hinged inverted flap, a circular ILM peel with a temporally only hinged inverted flap and a circular ILM peel with a superior inverted flap. Similar results were obtained with all flap directions.

Aurora [86] described the Cabbage Leaf Inverted Internal Limiting Membrane Flap technique. Three inverted ILM flaps sealed the hole looking like cabbage leaves. These flaps were connected to the edge of the MH, trimmed and flipped over the MH, one above the other like seen with cabbage leaves.

In cases when the central ILM had already been removed during previous surgery, Tabandeh [87] described the SWIFT flap procedure. An ILM flap is fashioned from superior residual ILM then a narrow strip of residual ILM forms the base of the flap, which is positioned horizontally. The ILM flap is inverted over the macular hole and covers the MH and the retina inferior to the MH **Figures 12** and **13**.

Leisser [88] described a technique where a temporal ILM flap was prepared while the residual ILM around the MH was peeled to the rim of the MH, after which the ILM flap was positioned in an inverted fashion over the MH (**Figures 14** and **15**).

The pedunculated flap technique creates an ILM flap that covers the macular hole from the border of the previous ILM peel. The flap should be large enough to cover the region of the pre-existing ILM peel as well as the macular hole.

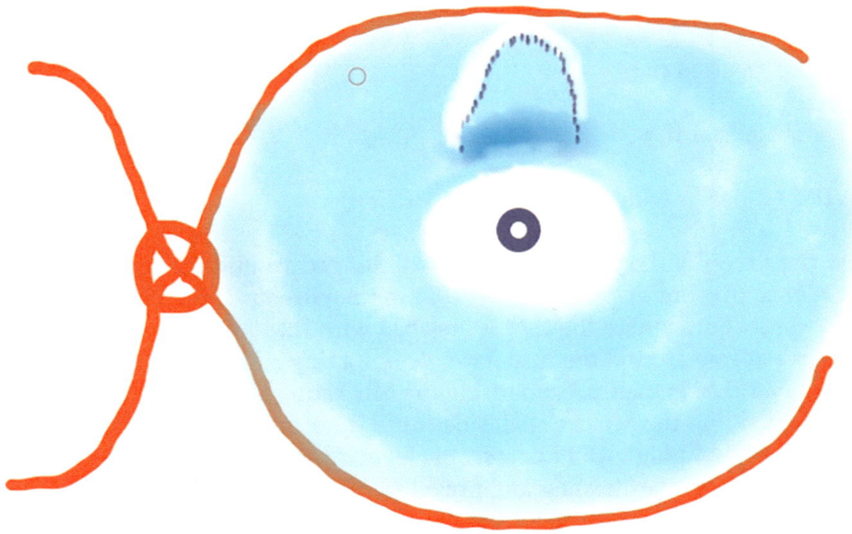

Figure 12.
SWIFT (superior wide-based FLAP transposition) FLAP.

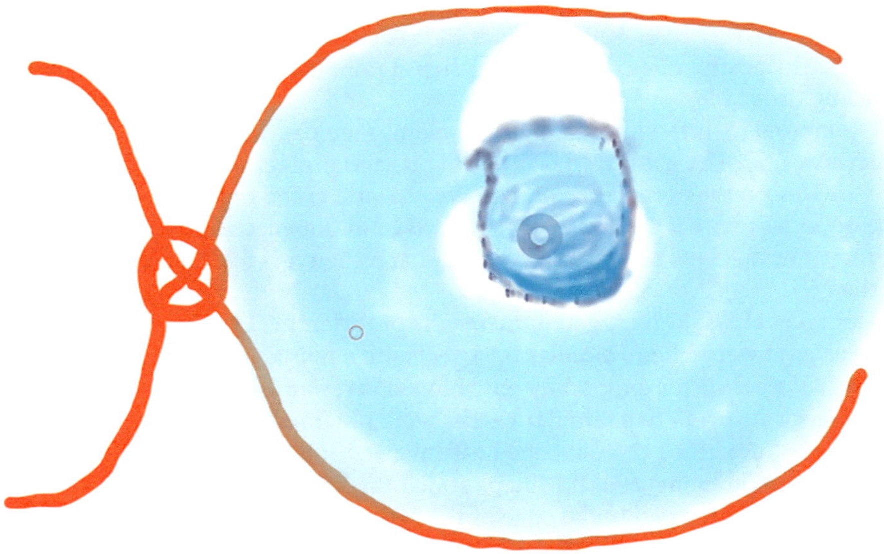

Figure 13.
Macular holes covered with inverted ILM.

Non-inverted flaps

- Pedicle ILM transposition
- Retracting door
- Free flaps

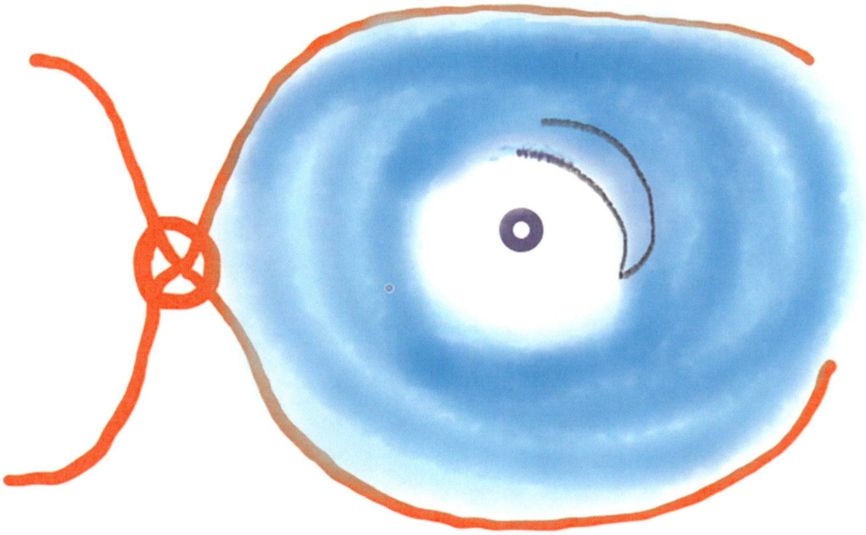

Figure 14.
Temporal residual ILM peduncolated flap.

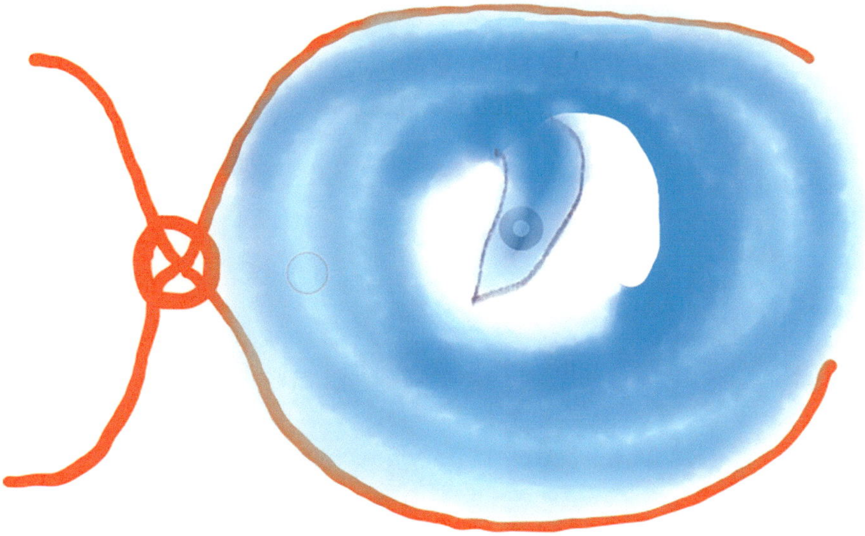

Figure 15.
Macular hole covered.

14. Pedicle ILM transposition

Hu [89] suggested a non-inverted flap provides a more physiological scaffold for healing. The pedicle is created by circular ILM peeling in the macular area but leaving a hinge attached superiorly to pivot the mobilised ILM to cover the hole. This method reduces flap loss during fluid-air exchange observed using free flaps [90].

15. Internal limiting membrane retracting door

Finn [91] performed surgery on myopic MH's using a hinged ILM flap retracted to cover the MH. This procedure addressed the issues of relaxing the stiff ILM in myopic eyes together with providing the scaffold needed for retinal tissue healing (**Figures 16** and **17**).

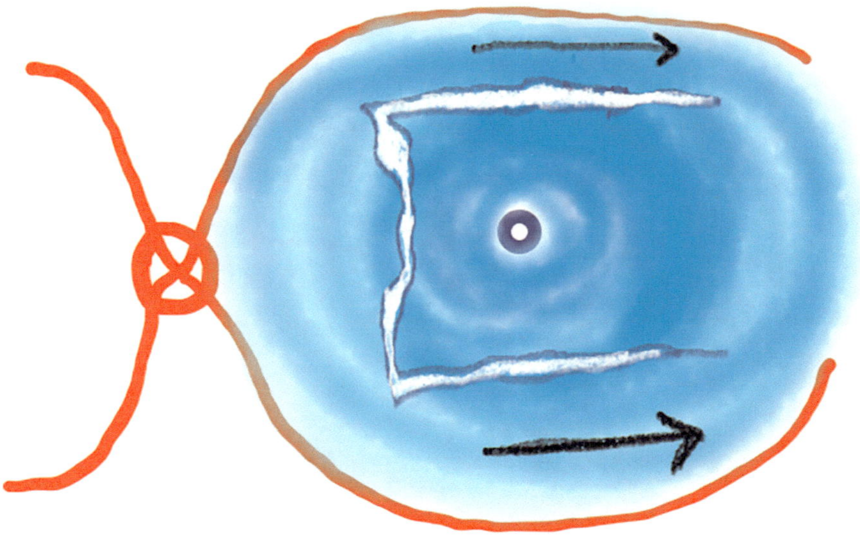

Figure 16.
ILM retracting door flap.

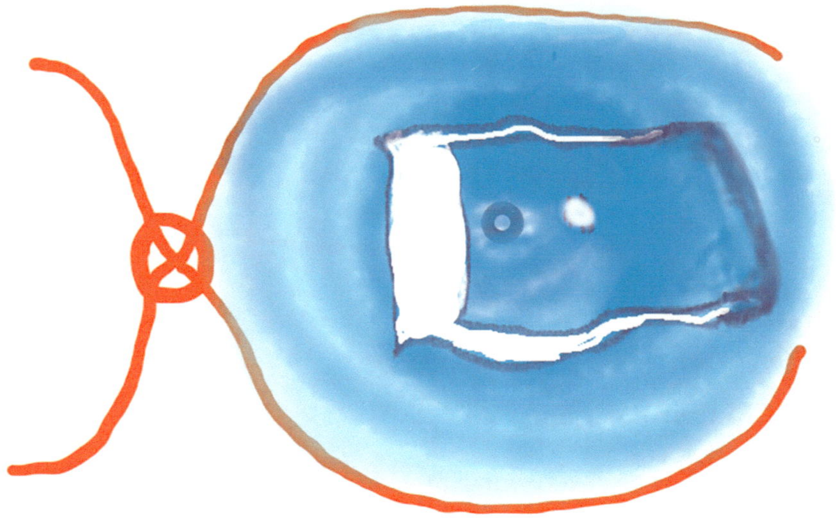

Figure 17.
Macular hole covered with non-inverted ILM.

16. Autologous ILM free flap

Eyes with an extensive ILM peel may benefit from a free ILM flap. Keeping the ILM in place during air-fluid exchange is never easy, but a small amount of heavy liquid or viscoelastic like Viscoat, can stabilise the flap [92, 93]. Patients who have a persistent MH hole following earlier surgery with ILM peeling may benefit from the use of an ILM-free flap [94]. Peripheral peeled ILM is placed on the MH during redo surgery. Successful results may be obtained in the closure of large MHs with this technique, but this procedure may cause damage to the retinal pigment epithelium in the fovea and alterations of the photoreceptor layers [95]. Prolonged exposure of the RPE to the staining fluids and stained ILM may also cause chemical damage to the RPE, as detected by De Novelli [96].

17. Lens capsule flap transplantation (LCFT)

When there is no ILM available, the lens capsule may be used as an alternative tool to encourage MH closure in refractory cases [97]. The procedure entails staining the anterior (AC) or posterior capsule (PC). In phakic patients, combined cataract surgery was performed, and the AC was used, and in pseudophakic patients, the PC. The flap was trimmed and positioned within the hole. Anatomic and functional results are promising but the challenge of flap dislocation remains an issue.

18. Autologous neurosensory retinal transplant (ART)

In 2016, Grewal and Mahmoud introduced the use of an autologous full-thickness retinal free flap for closure of refractory myopic MHs. They applied endolaser and diathermy in a circular pattern around a 2-disc diameter area of the retina and using a bimanual approach with vertical scissors and forceps obtained a retinal free flap. Instillation of perfluoro-noctane heavy liquid over the flap was followed by a direct PFC-silicone oil exchange [98–102].

19. Human amniotic membrane (hAM) transplantation

Rizzo [103] describes the use of a human amniotic membrane (hAM) for MH treatment. A 2 mm disk of hAM grasped by forceps under fluid or perfluorocarbon was transplanted into the subretinal space. It is speculated that the hAM stimulates retinal pigment epithelium (RPE) cells division.

Kuriyan [104] described the use of commercially available human amniograft from Bio-Tissue (Tissue Tech, Miami) using sub- and pre-retinal placement. A dermal punch may be used to trim the tissue for hole placement. The chorion side is supposed to face the retinal pigment epithelium. Once in place inside or on top of the MH, the fluid-air exchange was performed.

20. Autologous platelet concentrate

Gaudric [105] explored the effects of autologous platelet concentrate (APC) in macular hole closure by injecting some APC in the hole at the end of a vitrectomy and obtained an improvement in anatomical closure rate. In a study comparing ILM peeling versus ILM peeling plus platelet-rich plasma (PRP) a significant improvement in anatomic and functional results was reported in eyes that had an application of PRP [106]. Several growth factors and cytokines are released by platelets and platelet-rich plasma has been used in various medical conditions [107]. Autologous PRP has been used in more complex holes such as myopic and refractory MH's with encouraging anatomical and functional results [108]. PRP derived from a patient's peripheral blood requires special tools, which may not be always available. One study found low rates of closure in refractory MHs with autologous blood [109] but a further study found high rates of closure when combining the inverted ILM flap technique with autologous blood for large MHs [110].

21. Subretinal blebs

The concept underlying this technique is that it is thought to increase retinal compliance by releasing the adhesions of photoreceptors to the retinal pigment epithelium (RPE).

The ILM is peeled in the usual manner at the sites of the injection. A small-gauge subretinal cannula (usually 38-41gauge) is used to inject a small volume of fluid under the retina, and usually few blebs are created by injecting BSS into the subretinal space. A confluent perifoveal serous detachment is induced, using a Tano diamond-dusted scraper or a Flex Loop to help massage the sub-retinal fluid until the retina surrounding the macular hole is detached. A fluid-air exchange is performed, and gas or silicone oil is used. This procedure has been shown to be a viable option for the closure of recurrent or persistent holes [20, 111, 112].

Multiple entry sites into the retina may be avoided as suggested by Felfeli [113] using a silicone extrusion cannula to inject fluid through the macular hole. Once the central retina has been detached by refluxing fluid into the macular hole the margins of the hole are once more re-opposed by carefully massaging them and this is followed by a fluid-air exchange and then gas tamponade. In a series of 39 complex cases, this technique resulted in a 95% closure rate. This procedure is especially useful where chorioretinal scarring is present at the macula resulting in extra adhesion of the retinal layers.

22. Retinal relaxing incisions

Charles [114] reported using retinal relaxing incisions in six eyes to release tangential traction and increase retinal elasticity. This procedure does result in damage to the neuroretina and potentially the underlying RPE and visual improvement were limited to 3 cases.

Reiss [115] described 7 patients treated with five radial full-thickness incisions and gas tamponade. Using this procedure, the investigators reported 100% anatomic success in patients with refractory MH's.

The need to perform a deep incision in the retina with no damage to the underlying retinal pigment epithelium and choroid makes this procedure more technically challenging than others and with potentially greater risk.

23. Dragging and peeling

Peng in 2020 described a procedure called ILM dragging and peeling [116]. Two horizontal ILM strips were removed in the upper and lower quadrant of the macula. An upper ILM flap was created and pulled down towards the edge of the MH to try and reduce the size of the hole using the adhesion between the ILM and underlying retina. A similar procedure was performed by creating a lower ILM flap which was pulled upwards, also try and reduce the size of the hole by a similar mechanism. Once these tangential forces were applied to minimise the hole size a standard circular ILM peel was created. This surgical procedure derives from the belief that MH mobility is critical for MH closure and it may be that in some cases peeling alone may not give enough mobility to the retina [117]. The authors did not report significant complications and MH closure rate was 96.2%.

24. Adjuvants with ILM techniques

24.1 Autologous blood

Autologous gluconated blood has been used with inverted ILM flaps as a macular bandage, and one study showed initial surgical success in all patients with MH > 500 without gas tamponade or postoperative positioning [118].

24.2 Heavy fluids

Per-fluro-octane (PFO) has been applied to the MH to stabilise the free or inverted ILM flap in the correct position until the end of the fluid-air exchange [119–121]. PFO could also help flatten the retina whilst the ILM flap is being created by providing a degree of counteraction. Due to its vapour pressure, a small bubble of residual PFO can be removed by evaporation instead of using irrigation, thus reducing the risk of flap displacement [92, 122].

24.3 Viscoelastic

Viscoelastic can facilitate macular hole surgery in a variety of ways. When used before ILM peeling it reduces the toxicity of the dye to the retina. When applied over the ILM flap it can act to reduce the displacement of the flap and keep it in the correct position. It can also act as a binder to stabilise the flap. The functions of adhesive viscoelastic (Viscoat, Alcon) were investigated in a study by Song [123]. Viscoelastic was injected into the MH and then ILM was stained with ICG. The ILM below the hole was removed but the ILM above the hole was used to create an inverted flap. Supplemental viscoelastic was then injected into the surface of the inverted ILM flap prior to the fluid air exchange. This technique resulted in anatomical and functional recovery in highly myopic patients with large MHs.

25. Summary

There are many techniques available for the treatment of macular holes. The authors preferred technique for small to medium-sized macular holes is combined phaco-vitrectomy with 360-degree ILM peel without face down posture but with the patient avoiding lying on his or her back for 1 week. Face-down posturing is reserved for larger holes. With small holes and good vision, a period of observation is an option as these holes can spontaneously improve and so avoid surgery.

With the many techniques available it is possible to postulate a flowchart for patient treatment.

Recent, small Stage 2 MH's may be managed by PPV and gas tamponade although a short period of observation is an option as some can spontaneously improve and avoid surgery.

MH <400 μm with ERM, PPV with ILM peel is suggested.

MH >400 μm or chronic, inverted ILM flap is preferable.

MH >700 μm, primary ART (Autologous neurosensory retinal transplant).

Refractory holes where ILM has been peeled or difficult ILM flap, consider a free ILM flap or hinged ILM flap. If ILM is not available ART, human amniotic membrane graft and lens capsule are all options depending on the availability of tissue and surgical experience (**Figure 18**).

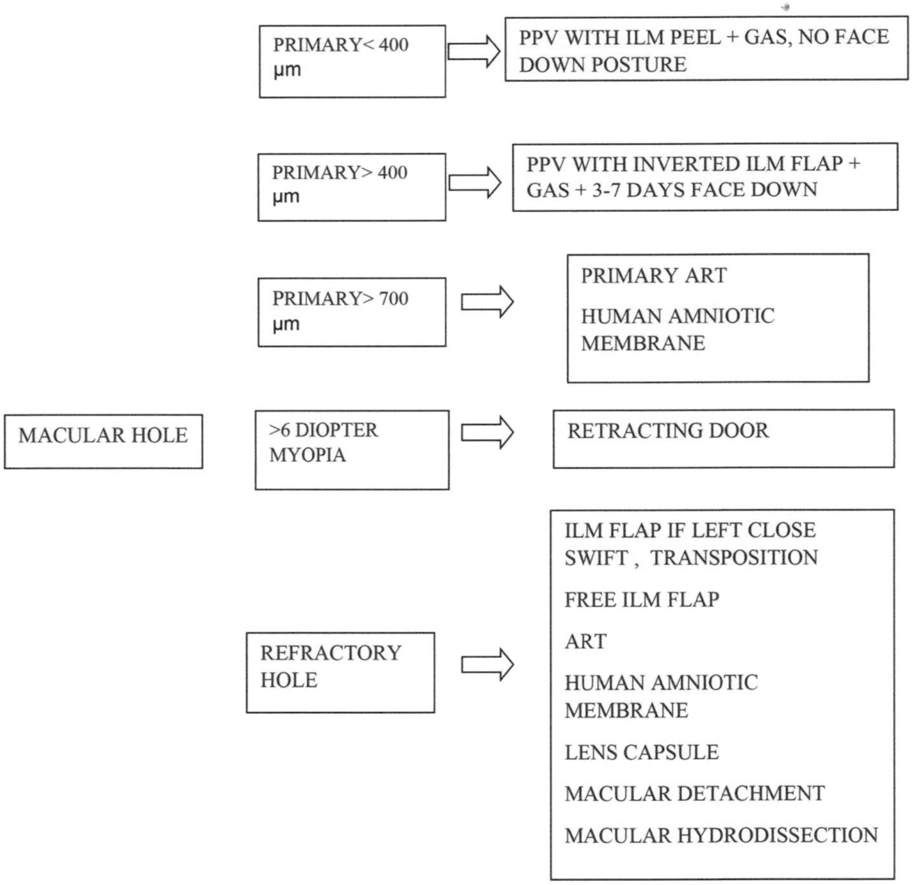

Figure 18.
Macular hole surgery suggested approach.

Author details

Sergio Scalia[1*], Peter Reginald Simcock[2], Simone Scalia[3], Daniela Angela Randazzo[1] and Maria Rosaria Sanfilippo[1]

1 Enna Eye Unit, Enna, Italy

2 West of England Eye Unit, Exeter, UK

3 School of Medicine, University of Catania, Italy

*Address all correspondence to: sergioscalia@yahoo.com

References

[1] Gass JDM. Idiopathic senile macular hole: Its early stages and pathogenesis. Archives of Ophthalmology. 1988; **106**(5):629

[2] Duker JS, Kaiser PK, Binder S, et al. The international Vitreomacular traction study group classification of vitreomacular adhesion, traction, and macular hole. Ophthalmology. 2013; **120**(12):2611-2619. DOI: 10.1016/ j.ophtha.2013.07.042

[3] Ali FS, Stein JD, Blachley TS, Ackley S, Stewart JM. Incidence of and risk factors for developing idiopathic macular hole among a diverse group of patients throughout the United States. JAMA Ophthalmology. 2017;**135**(4): 299-305. DOI: 10.1001/ jamaophthalmol.2016.5870

[4] La Cour M, Friis J. Macular holes: Classification, epidemiology, natural history and treatment. Acta Ophthalmologica Scandinavica. 2002;**80**: 579-587

[5] Bainbridge J, Herbert E, Gregor Z. Macular holes: Vitreoretinal relationships and surgical approaches. Eye (London, England). 2008;**22**: 1301-1309

[6] Steel DH, Donachie PHJ, Aylward GW, Laidlaw DA, Williamson TH, Yorston D. BEAVRS macular hole outcome group. Factors affecting anatomical and visual outcome after macular hole surgery: Findings from a large prospective UK cohort. Eye. 2021;**35**(1):316-325

[7] Ch'ng SW, Patton N, Ahmed M, et al. The Manchester large macular hole study: Is it time to reclassify large macular holes? American Journal of Ophthalmology. 2018;**195**:36-42

[8] Wong R, Howard C, Orobona GD. Retina expansion technique for macular hole apposition report 2. Efficacy, closure rate and risks of a macular detachment technique to close large full-thickness macular holes. Retina. 2018;**38**: 660-663

[9] Yu Y, Liang X, Wang Z, et al. Internal limiting membrane peeling and air tamponade for stage iii and stage iv idiopathic macular hole. Retina. 2020; **40**(1):66-67

[10] Ezra E. Idiopathic full thickness macular hole: Natural history and pathogenesis. The British Journal of Ophthalmology. 2001;**85**(1):102-108. DOI: 10.1136/ bjo.85.1.102

[11] Johnson RN, Gass JD. Idiopathic macular holes. Observations, stages of formation, and implications for surgical intervention. Ophthalmology. 1988; **95**(7):917-924

[12] Wu TT, Kung YH. Comparison of anatomical and visual outcomes of macular hole surgery in patients with high myopia vs. non-high myo- pia: A case-control study using optical coherence tomography. Graefe's Archive for Clinical and Experimental Ophthalmology. 2012;**250**(3):327-331

[13] Suda K, Hangai M, Yoshimura N. Axial length and outcomes of macular hole surgery assessed by spectral-domain optical coherence tomogra- phy. American Journal of Ophthalmology. 2011;**151**(1):118-27.e1

[14] Stalmans P, Benz MS, Gandorfer A, et al. Enzymatic vitreolysis with ocriplasmin for vitreomacular traction and macular holes. The New England Journal of Medicine. 2012;**367**(7): 606-615. DOI: 10.1056/NEJMoa1110823

[15] Singh RP et al. Anatomical and visual outcomes following ocriplasmin treatment for symptomatic vitreomacular traction syndrome. British Journal of Ophthalmology. 2014;**98**: 356-360

[16] Jaycock PD, Bunce C, Xing W, et al. Outcomes of macular hole surgery: Implications for surgical management and clinical governance. Eye (London, England). 2005;**19**(8):849-884

[17] Willis AW, Garcia-Cosio JF. Macular hole surgery. Comparison of longstanding versus recent macular holes. Ophthalmology. 1996;**103**(11): 1811-1814

[18] Lytvynchuk L, Ruban A, Stieger K. Strong adhesion of RPE to photoreceptors explains in part the failure of macular detachment technique for large macular hole closure: iOCT findings. Investigative Ophthalmology & Visual Science. 2020;**61**(9):B0034.41

[19] Yun C, Oh J, Hwang SY, Togloom A, Kim SW, Huh K. Morphologic characteristics of chronic macular hole on optical coherence tomography. Retina. 2012;**32**(10):2077-2084

[20] Meyer CH, Szurman P, Haritoglou C, et al. Application of subretinal fluid to close refractory full thickness macular holes: Treatment strategies and primary outcome: APOSTEL study. Graefe's Archive for Clinical and Experimental Ophthalmology. 2020;**258**(10):2151-2161

[21] Wong IY, Iu LP, Koizumi H, Lai WW. The inner segment/outer segment junction: What have we learnt so far? Current Opinion in Ophthalmology. 2012;**23**(3):210-21822

[22] Iwasaki M, Kinoshita T, Miyamoto H, Imaizumi H. Influence of inverted internal limiting membrane flap technique on the outer retinal layer structures after a large macular hole surgery. Retina. 2019;**39**:1470-1477

[23] Caprani SM, Donati S, Bartalena L. Macular hole surgery: The healing process of outer retinal layers to visual acuity recovery. European Journal of Ophthalmology. 2017;**27**(2):235-239

[24] Kelly NE, Wendel RT. Vitreous surgery for idiopathic macular holes. Results of a pilot study. Archives of Ophthalmology. 1991;**109**(5):654-659. DOI: 10.1001/archopht.1991.010800 50068031

[25] Eckardt C, Eckardt U, Groos S, Luciano L, Reale E. Removal of the internal limiting membrane in macular holes. Clinical and Morphological Findings. Ophthalmologe. 1997;**94**(8): 545-551

[26] Spiteri Cornish K, Lois N, Scott N, Burr J, Cook J, Boachie C, et al. Vitrectomy with internal limiting membrane (ILM) peeling versus vitrectomy with no peeling for idiopathic full-thickness macular hole (FTMH). Cochrane Database of Systematic Reviews. 2013;**2013**(6): CD009306

[27] Hasegawa Y, Hata Y, Mochizuki Y, et al. Equivalent tamponade by room air as compared with SF(6) after macular hole surgery. Graefe's Archive for Clinical and Experimental Ophthalmology. 2009;**247**(11): 1455-1459. DOI: 10.1007/s00417-009-1120-8

[28] Sano M, Inoue M, Itoh Y, et al. Duration of prone positioning after macular hole surgery determined by swept-source optical coherence tomography. Retina. 2017;**37**(8):

1483-1491. DOI: 10.1097/IAE.00000 00000001394

[29] Mohamed S, Lai TYY. Intraocular gas in vitreoretinal surgery. HKJO. 2010; **14**(1):8-13

[30] Yamashita T, Sakamoto T, Yamashita T, et al. Individualized, spectral domain-optical coherence tomography-guided facedown posturing after macular hole surgery: Minimizing treatment burden and maximizing outcome. Retina. 2014;**34**(7):1367-1375. DOI: 10.1097/IAE.0000000000000087

[31] Zhang Y, Chen X, Hong L, et al. Facedown positioning after vitrectomy will not facilitate macular hole closure based on swept-source optical coherence tomography imaging in gas-filled eyes: A prospective. Randomized Comparative Interventional Study. Retina. 2019; **39**(12):2353-2359

[32] Solebo AL, Lange CA, Bunce C, Bainbridge JW. Face-down positioning or posturing after macular hole surgery. Cochrane Database of Systematic Reviews. 2011;**12**:CD008228

[33] Pasu S, Bell L, Zenasni Z, et al. Facedown positioning following surgery for large full-thickness macular hole: A multicenter randomized clinical trial. JAMA Ophthalmology. 2020;**138**(7):725

[34] Ye T, Yu JG, Liao L, Liu L, Xia T, Yang LL. Macular hole surgery recovery with and without face-down posturing: A meta-analysis of randomized controlled trials. BMC Ophthalmology. 2019;**19**(1):265

[35] Eckardt C, Eckert T, Eckardt U, Porkert U, Gesser C. Macular hole surgery with air tamponade and optical coherence tomography-based duration of face-down positioning. Retina. 2008; **28**(8):1087-1096

[36] D'Souza MJ, Chaudhary V, Devenyi R, Kertes PJ, Lam WC. Re-operation of idiopathic full-thickness macular holes after initial surgery with internal limiting membrane peel. The British Journal of Ophthalmology. 2011; **95**(11):1564-1567

[37] Patel R, Gopalakrishnan M, Giridhar A. Timing and outcome of surgery for persistent macular hole. Retina. 2017;**39**:314-318

[38] Moisseiev E, Fabian ID, Moisseiev J, Barak A. Outcomes of repeated pars plana vitrectomy for persistent macular holes. Retina. 2013; **33**:1137-1143

[39] Simcock PR, Scalia S. Phacovitrectomy without prone posture for full thickness macular holes. The British Journal of Ophthalmology. 2001; **85**(11):1316-1319. DOI: 10.1136/ bjo.85.11.1316

[40] Chakrabarti M, Benjamin P, Chakrabarti K, Chakrabarti A. Closing MH with "macular plug" without gas tamponade and postoperative posturing. Retina. 2017;**37**(3):451-459. DOI: 10.1097/IAE.0000000000001206

[41] Nguyen QD, Rodrigues EB, Farah ME, Mieler WF, Do DV. Retinal Pharmacotherapeutics. Dev Ophthalmol. Basel, Karger. 2016;**55**:365-375. DOI: 10.1159/000438963

[42] Al-Halafi AM. Chromovitrectomy: Update. Saudi Journal of Ophthalmology. 2013;**27**(4):271-276. DOI: 10.1016/j.sjopt.2013.10.004 Epub 2013 Oct 17

[43] Kang SW, Ahn K, Ham D-I. Types of macular hole closure and their clinical implications. The British Journal of Ophthalmology. 2003;**87**(8):10159

[44] Imai M, Iijima H, Gotoh T, Tsukahara S. Optical coherence tomography of successfully repaired idiopathic macular holes. American Journal of Ophthalmology. 1999;**128**(5): 621-627

[45] Inoue M, Watanabe Y, Arakawa A, et al. Spectral-domain optical coherence tomography images of inner/outer segment junctions and macular hole surgery outcomes. Graefe's Archive for Clinical and Experimental Ophthalmology. 2009;**247**(3):325-330

[46] Haritoglou IC, Neubauer AS, Reiniger IW, et al. Long-term functional outcome of macular hole surgery correlated to optical coherence tomography measurements. Clinical and Experimental Ophthalmology. 2007; **35**(3):208-213

[47] Mitamura Y, Mitamura-Aizawa S, Katome T, et al. Photoreceptor impairment and restoration on optical coherence tomographic image. Journal of Ophthalmology. 2013;**2013**: 518170

[48] Ooka E, Mitamura Y, Baba T, et al. Foveal microstructure on spectral-domain optical coherence tomographic images and visual function after macular hole surgery. American Journal of Ophthalmology. 2011;**152**(2):283-290

[49] Lee MW, Kim TY, Song YY, et al. Changes in each retinal layer and ellipsoid zone recovery after full-thickness macular hole surgery. Scientific Reports. 2021;**11**:11351

[50] Candiello J, Balasubramani M, Schreiber EM, et al. Biomechanical properties of native basement membranes. The FEBS Journal. 2007; **274**(11):2897-2908. DOI: 10.1111/ j.1742-4658.2007.05823.x

[51] Wollensak G, Spoerl E, Grosse G, Wirbelauer C. Biomechanical significance of the human internal limiting lamina. Retina. 2006;**26**(8): 965-968. DOI: 10.1097/01. iae.0000250001.45661.95

[52] Morescalchi F, Costagliola C, Gambicorti E, Duse S, Romano MR, Semeraro F. Controversies over the role of internal limiting membrane peeling during vitrectomy in macular hole surgery. Survey of Ophthalmology. 2017; **62**(1):58-69. DOI: 10.1016/j.survo phthal.2016.07.003

[53] Smiddy WE, Flynn HW Jr. Pathogenesis of macular holes and therapeutic implications. American Journal of Ophthalmology. 2004;**137**(3): 525-537. DOI: 10.1016/j. ajo.2003.12.011

[54] Steel DH, Dinah C, Habib M, White K. ILM peeling technique influences the degree of a dissociated optic nerve fibre layer appearance after macular hole surgery. Graefe's Archive for Clinical and Experimental Ophthalmology. 2015;**253**(5):691-698. DOI: 10.1007/s00417-014-2734-z

[55] Mason JO III, Feist RM, Michael A, Albert J. Eccentric macular holes after vitrectomy with peeling of epimacular proliferation. Retina. 2007;**27**(1):45-48. DOI: 10.1097/01.iae.0000256661. 56617.69

[56] Rubinstein A, Bates R, Benjamin L, Shaikh A. Iatrogenic eccentric full thickness macular holes following vitrectomy with ILM peeling for idiopathic macular holes. Eye. 2005; **19**(12):1333-1335. DOI: 10.1038/sj. eye.6701771

[57] Miura M, Elsner AE, Osako M, Iwasaki T, Okano T, Usui M. Dissociated optic nerve fiber layer appearance after internal limiting membrane peeling for

idiopathic macular hole. Retina. 2003; **23**(4):561-563. DOI: 10.1097/00006982-200308000-00024

[58] Mitamura Y, Ohtsuka K. Relationship of dissociated optic nerve fiber layer appearance to internal limiting membrane peeling. Ophthalmology. 2005;**112**(10): 1766-1770. DOI: 10.1016/j.ophtha.2005.04.026

[59] Ho TC, Yang CM, Huang JS, Yang CH, Chen MS. Foveola nonpeeling internal limiting membrane surgery to prevent inner retinal damages in early stage 2 idiopathic macula hole. Graefe's Archive for Clinical and Experimental Ophthalmology. 2014;**252**(10): 1553-1560. DOI: 10.1007/s00417-014-2613-7

[60] Franze K, Grosche J, Skatchkov SN, et al. Muller cells are living optical fibers in the vertebrate retina. Proceedings of the National Academy of Sciences of the United States of America. 2007;**104**(20): 8287-8292. DOI: 10.1073/pnas.0611180104

[61] Morescalchi F, Russo A, Bahja H, Gambicorti E, Cancarini A, Costagliola C, et al. Fovea-sparing versus complete internal limiting membrane peeling in vitrectomy for the treatment of macular holes. Retina. 2020;**40**(7): 1306-1314. DOI: 10.1097/IAE.0000000000002612

[62] Hu Z, Qian H, Fransisca S, et al. Minimal internal limiting membrane peeling with ILM flap technique for idiopathic macular holes: A preliminary study. BMC Ophthalmology. 2020;**20**: 228. DOI: 10.1186/s12886-020-0154

[63] Murphy DC, Fostier W, Rees J, Steel DH. Foveal sparing internal limiting membrane peeling for idiopathic macular holes: Effects on anatomical restoration of the fovea and visual function. Retina. 2019;**40**(11): 2127-2133. DOI: 10.1097/IAE.0000000000002724

[64] Mahajan VB, Chin EK, Tarantola RM, et al. Macular hole closure with internal limiting membrane abrasion technique. JAMA Ophthalmology. 2015;**133**(6):635-641. DOI: 10.1001/jamaophthalmol.2015.204

[65] Clark A, Balducci N, Pichi F, et al. Swelling of the arcuate nerve fiber layer after internal limiting membrane peeling. Retina (Philadelphia, Pa.). 2012; **32**(8):1608-1613. DOI: 10.1097/iae.0b013e3182437e86

[66] Terasaki H, Miyake Y, Nomura R, et al. Focal macular ERGs in eyes after removal of macular ILM during macular hole surgery. Investigative Ophthalmology & Visual Science. 2001; **42**(1):229-234

[67] Smiddy WE, Feuer W, Cordahi G. Internal limiting membrane peeling in macular hole surgery. Ophthalmology. 2001;**108**(8):1471-1476 discussion 1477–1478

[68] Spaide RF. Dissociated optic nerve fiber layer appearance after internal limiting membrane removal is inner retinal dimpling. Retina (Philadelphia, Pa). 2012;**32**(9):1719-1726

[69] Hisatomi T, Tachibana T, Notomi S, Nakatake S, Fujiwara K, Murakami Y, et al. Incomplete repair of retinal structure after vitrectomy with internal limiting membrane peeling. Retina (Philadelphia, Pa). 2017;**37**(8):1523-1528

[70] Ohta K, Sato A, Senda N, Fukui E. Comparisons of foveal thickness and slope after macular hole surgery with and without internal limiting membrane

peeling. Clinical Ophthalmology (Auckland, NZ). 2018;**12**:503-510

[71] Bae K, Kang SW, Kim JH, Kim SJ, Kim JM, Yoon JM. Extent of internal limiting membrane peeling and its impact on macular hole surgery outcomes: A randomized trial. American Journal of Ophthalmology. 2016;**169**: 179-188

[72] Modi A, Giridhar A, Gopalakrishnan M. Comparative analysis of outcomes with variable diameter internal limiting membrane peeling in surgery for idiopathic macular hole repair. Retina. 2017;**37**:265-273

[73] Al Sabti K, Kumar N, Azad RV. Extended internal limiting membrane peeling in the management of unusually large macular holes. Ophthalmic Surgery, Lasers & Imaging. 2009;**40**: 185-187

[74] Ventre L, Matteo F, Antonio L, Guglielmo P, Andrea R, Vincenza B, et al. Conventional internal limiting membrane peeling versus inverted flap for small-to-medium idiopathic macular hole: A randomized trial. Retina. 2022; **42**(12):2251-2257

[75] Rizzo S, Tartaro R, Barca F, Caporossi T, Bacherini D, Giansanti F. Internal limiting membrane peeling versus inverted flap technique for treatment of full-thickness macular holes: A comparative study in a large series of patients. Retina. 2018;**38**:S73-S78. DOI: 10.1097/IAE.000000000 0001985

[76] Yamashita T, Sakamoto T, Terasaki H, Iwasaki M, Ogushi Y, Okamoto F, et al. Best surgical technique and outcomes for large macular holes: Retrospective multicentre study in Japan. Acta Ophthalmologica. 2018;**96**: e904-e910. DOI: 10.1111/aos.13795

[77] Hu Z, Lin H, Liang Q, Wu R. Comparing the inverted internal limiting membrane flap with autologous blood technique to internal limiting membrane insertion for the repair of refractory macular hole. International Ophthalmology. 2020;**40**(1):141-149

[78] Michalewska Z, Michalewski J, Dulczewska-Cichecka K, Adelman RA, Nawrocki J. Temporal inverted internal limiting membrane flap technique versus classic inverted internal limiting membrane flap technique: A comparative study. Retina. 2015;**35**(9): 1844-1850. DOI: 10.1097/ IAE.0000000000000555

[79] Michalewska Z, Michalewski J, Adelman RA, Nawrocki J. Inverted internal limiting membrane flap technique for large macular holes. Ophthalmology. 2010;**117**(10):2018-2025

[80] Chen BS, Yang C. Inverted internal limiting membrane insertion for macular hole-associated retinal detachment in high myopia. American Journal of Ophthalmology. 2016;**165**:206-207

[81] Chin EK, Almeida DRP, Sohn EH. Structural and functional changes after macular hole surgery. International Ophthalmology Clinics. 2014;**54**(2): 17-27

[82] Rossi T, Gelso A, Costagliola C, et al. Macular hole closure patterns associated with different internal limiting membrane flap techniques. Graefe's Archive for Clinical and Experimental Ophthalmology. 2017;**255**(6):1073-1078

[83] Shin MK, Park KH, Park SW, Byon IS, Lee JE. Perfluoro-n-octaneassisted single-layered inverted internal limiting membrane flap technique for macular hole surgery. Retina. 2014;**34**(9):1905-1910

[84] Major JJ, Lampen SI, Wykoff CC, Ou WC, Brown DM, Wong TP, et al. The Texas taco technique for internal limiting membrane flap in large full-thickness macular holes: A short-term pilot study. Retina. 2020;**40**(3):552-556

[85] Ghassemi F, Khojasteh H, Khodabande A, Dalvin LA, Mazloumi M, Riazi-Esfahani H, et al. Comparison of three different techniques of inverted internal limiting membrane flap in treatment of large idiopathic full-thickness macular hole. Clinical Ophthalmology. 2019;**13**:2599-2606. DOI: 10.2147/OPTH.S236169

[86] Aurora A, Seth A, Sanduja N. Cabbage leaf inverted flap ILM peeling for macular hole: A novel technique. Ophthalmic Surgery, Lasers & Imaging Retina. 2017;**48**(10):830-832

[87] Tabandeh H, Morozov A, Rezaei KA, Boyer DS. Superior Wide-Base internal limiting membrane flap transposition for macular holes: Flap status and outcomes. Ophthalmology Retina. 2021;**5**(4): 317-323. DOI: 10.1016/j.oret.2020.12.003

[88] Leisser C, Ruiss M, Pilwachs C, Findl O. ILM peeling with ILM flap transposition vs. classic ILM peeling for small and medium macula holes-a prospective randomized trial. Spektrum Augenheilkd. 2022;**37**:1-6. DOI: 10.1007/s00717-022-00515-y Epub ahead of print

[89] Hu Z, Ye X, Lv X, Liang K, Zhang W, Chen X, et al. Non-inverted pedicle internal limiting membrane transposition for large macular holes. Eye. 2018;**32**(9):1512-1518

[90] Gekka T, Watanabe A, Ohkuma Y, Arai K, Watanabe T, Tsuzuki A, et al. Pedicle internal limiting membrane transposition flap technique for refractory macular hole. Ophthalmic Surgery, Lasers & Imaging Retina. 2015; **46**(10):1045-1046

[91] Finn AP, Mahmoud TH. Internal limiting membrane retracting door for myopic macular holes. Retina. 2019;**39** (Suppl 1):S92-S94. DOI: 10.1097/IAE.0000000000001787

[92] Shin MK, Park KH, Park SW, Byon IS, Lee JE. Perfluoro-n-octane-assisted single-layered inverted internal limiting membrane flap technique for macular hole surgery. Retina Philadelphia PA. 2014;**34**(9):1905-1910. DOI: 10.1097/IAE.0000000000000339

[93] Lai C-C, Wu A-L, Chou H-D, et al. Sub-perfluoro-noctane injection of ocular viscoelastic device assisted inverted internal limiting membrane flap for macular hole retinal detachment surgery: A novel technique. BMC Ophthalmology. 2020;**20**(1):116. DOI: 10.1186/s12886-020-01393-1

[94] Morizane Y, Shiraga F, Kimura S, et al. Autologous transplantation of the internal limiting membrane for refractory macular holes. American Journal of Ophthalmology. 2014;**157**(4): 861-869 e1. DOI: 10.1016/j.ajo.2013.12.028

[95] Lee SM, Kwon HJ, Park SW, Lee JE, Byon IS. Microstructural changes in the fovea following autologous internal limiting membrane transplantation surgery for large macular holes. Acta Ophthalmologica. 2018;**96**(3):e406-e408. DOI: 10.1111/aos.13504

[96] De Novelli FJ, Preti RC, Monteiro MLR, Pelayes DE, Nóbrega MJ, Takahashi WY. Autologous internal limiting membrane fragment transplantation for large, chronic, and refractory macular holes. Ophthalmic Research. 2016;**55**(1):45-52. DOI: 10.1159/000440767

[97] Chen SN, Yang CM. Lens capsular flap transplantation in the management of refractory macular hole from multiple aetiologies. Retina. 2016;**36**(1): 163-170. DOI: 10.1097/IAE.0000000000000674

[98] Grewal DS, Mahmoud TH. Autologous neurosensory retinal free flap for closure of refractory myopic macular holes. JAMA Ophthalmology. 2016;**134**(2):229-230. DOI: 10.1001/jamaophthalmol. 2015.5237

[99] Grewal DS, Charles S, Parolini B, Kadonosono K, Mahmoud TH. Autologous retinal transplant for refractory macular holes: Multicenter international collaborative study group. Ophthalmology. 2019;**126**(10): 1399-1408. DOI: 10.1016/j.ophtha. 2019.01.027

[100] Ding C, Li S, Zeng J. Autologous neurosensory retinal transplantation for unclosed and large macular holes. Ophthalmic Research. 2019;**61**(2):88-93. DOI: 10.1159/000487952

[101] Chang Y-C, Liu P-K, Kao T-E, et al. Management of refractory large macular hole with autologous neurosensory retinal free flap transplantation. Retina Phila PA. 2020;**40**(11):2134-2139. DOI: 10.1097/IAE.0000000000002734

[102] Tanaka S, Inoue M, Inoue T, et al. Autologous retinal transplantation as a primary treatment for large chronic macular holes. Retina Phila PA. 2020; **40**(10):1938-1945. DOI: 10.1097/IAE.0000000000002693

[103] Rizzo S, Caporossi T, Tartaro R, et al. A human amniotic membrane plug to promote retinal breaks repair and recurrent macular hole closure. Retina Phila PA. 2019;**39**(Suppl 1):S95-S103. DOI: 10.1097/IAE.0000000000002320

[104] Kuriyan AE, Hariprasad SM, Fraser CE. Approaches to refractory or large macular holes. Ophthalmic Surgery, Lasers & Imaging Retina. 2020; **51**(7):375-382

[105] Gaudric A, Massin P, Paques M, et al. Autologous platelet concentrate for the treatment of fullthickness macular holes. Graefe's Archive for Clinical and Experimental Ophthalmology. 1995; **233**(9):549-554. DOI: 10.1007/BF00404704

[106] Shpak AA, Shkvorchenko DO, Krupina EA. Surgical treatment of macular holes with and without the use of autologous platelet-rich plasma. International Ophthalmology. 2021; **41**(3):1043-1052. DOI: 10.1007/s10792-020-01662-4

[107] Foster TE, Puskas BL, Mandelbaum BR, Gerhardt MB, Rodeo SA. Platelet-rich plasma: From basic science to clinical applications. The American Journal of Sports Medicine. 2009;**37**(11):2259-2272

[108] Figueroa MS, Govetto A, de Arriba-Palomero P. Short-term results of platelet-rich plasma as adjuvant to 23-G vitrectomy in the treatment of high myopic macular holes. European Journal of Ophthalmology. 2016;**26**(5):491-496

[109] Purtskhvanidze K, Frühsorger B, Bartsch S, Hedderich J, Roider J, Treumer F. Persistent full-thickness idiopathic macular hole: Anatomical and functional outcome of revitrectomy with autologous platelet concentrate or autologous whole blood. Ophthalmologica. 2018;**239**(1):19-26

[110] Lyu W-J, Ji L-B, Xiao Y, Fan Y-B, Cai X-H. Treatment of refractory giant macular hole by vitrectomy with internal limiting membrane transplantation and

autologous blood. International Journal of Ophthalmology. 2018;**11**(5):818

[111] Meyer CH, Borny R, Horchi N. Subretinal fluid application to close a refractory full thickness macular hole. International Journal of Retina and Vitreous. 2017;**3**:44. DOI: 10.1186/s40942-017-0094-7

[112] Oliver A, Wojcik EJ. Macular detachment for treatment of persistent macular hole. Ophthalmic Surgery, Lasers & Imaging. 2011;**42**(6):516-518. DOI: 10.3928/15428877-20110825-01

[113] Felfeli T, Mandelcorn ED. MACULAR hole hydrodissection: Surgical technique for the treatment of persistent, chronic, and large macular holes. Retina. 2019;**39**(4):743-752

[114] Charles S, Randolph JC, Neekhra A, Salisbury CD, Littlejohn N, Calzada JI. Arcuate retinotomy for the repair of large macular holes. Ophthalmic Surgery, Lasers & Imaging Retina. 2013;**44**(1):69-72. DOI: 10.3928/23258160-20121221-15

[115] Reis R, Ferreira N, Meireles A. Management of Stage IV macular holes: When standard surgery fails. Case Reports in Ophthalmology. 2012;**3**(2):240-250. DOI: 10.1159/000342007 Epub 2012 Aug 8

[116] Peng J, Zhang LH, Chen CL, Liu JJ, Zhu XY, Zhao PQ. Internal limiting membrane dragging and peeling: A modified technique for macular holes closure surgery. International Journal of Ophthalmology. 2020;**13**(5):755-760. DOI: 10.18240/ijo.2020.05.09

[117] Alpatov S, Shchuko A, Malyshev V. A new method of treating macular holes. European Journal of Ophthalmology. 2007;**17**(2):246-252. DOI: 10.1177/112067210701700215

[118] Lai CC, Chen YP, Wang NK, Chuang LH, Liu L, Chen KJ, et al. Vitrectomy with internal limiting membrane repositioning and autologous blood for macular hole retinal detachment in highly myopic eyes. Ophthalmology. 2015;**122**(9):1889-1898

[119] Park SW, Pak KY, Park KH, Kim KH, Byon IS, Lee JE. Perfluoro-n-octane assisted free internal limiting membrane flap technique for recurrent macular hole. Retina. 2015;**35**(12):2652-2656

[120] Pak KY, Park JY, Park SW, Byon IS, Lee JE. Efficacy of the perfluoro-N-octane-assisted single-layered inverted internal limiting membrane flap technique for large macular holes. Ophthalmologica. 2017;**238**(3):133-138

[121] Ozdek S, Baskaran P, Karabas L, Neves PP. A modified perfluoro-n-octane-assisted autologous internal limiting membrane transplant for failed macular hole reintervention: A case series. Ophthalmic Surg lasers imaging. Retina. 2017;**48**(5):416-420

[122] Nishimura A, Kita K, Segawa Y, Shirao Y. Perfluorocarbon liquid assists in stripping the ILM to treat detached retina caused by macular hole. Ophthalmic Surgery and Lasers. 2002;**33**(1):77-78

[123] Song ZM, Li M, Liu JJ, Hu XT, Hu ZX, Chen D. Viscoat assisted inverted internal limiting membrane flap technique for large macular holes associated with high myopia. Journal of Ophthalmology. 2016;**2016**:8283062

Section 2

Vitreous and Ocular Disease: Glaucoma, Ocular Tumors, Inflammation and New Perspective

Chapter 5

Perspective Chapter: Role of the Vitreoretinal Interface Condition in the Development of Glaucoma

Alexey Ermolaev

Abstract

Until now, there are no objective criteria to understand the moment of transition of eyes, anatomically predisposed to primary angle-closed glaucoma, from the risk group to the real form of PACG. IOP on the predisposed eyes may remain normal until advanced age without treatment. The aim of this study is to identify factors that can act as a trigger mechanism that starts such transition and the role of vitreous-retinal interface (VRI) condition in this process. A risk group that included 259 eyes (37–88 years old) predisposed to PACG was formed. The criteria for forming the group were gonioscopy, predictive coefficients Lowe and Chirshikov, provocative Hyams test, and ultrasound examination. Monitoring was carried out for up to 4 years. In the risk group, there were eyes in which the state of predisposition was transformed into a real form of PACG during monitoring. Such a transition was accompanied by the occurrence of PVD, which was not detected at the beginning of the monitoring. In eyes with normal IOP predisposed to PACG, PVD appearance leads to destabilization of the vitreous body position inside the vitreous cavity, possibility for iris-lenticular diaphragm displacement forward, appearance of hydrodynamic blocks and undulating IOP increases, and appearance of the real form of PACG.

Keywords: primary angle-closed glaucoma (PACG), vitreous-retinal interface, posterior vitreous detachment (PVD), predisposition to PACG, Hyams test

1. Introduction

Due to the rapid development of vitreoretinal surgery, the vitreoretinal interface (VRI) is the subject of active discussions among ophthalmologists. However, the question of the VRI role in the hydrodynamics of the eye has been studied not enough. One of the subjects of our interest is the influence of VRI condition on the mechanisms of primary angle-closure glaucoma (PACG) development.

The fact is that the development of PACG can occur only in the eyes, in which there is an anatomical predisposition to this disease. This includes a narrow-angle of the anterior chamber of the eye (ACA), which is formed against the background of a disproportionate ratio of the short axial length of the eye and the excessive thickness of the lens. Usually, such eyes have hypermetropic refraction. The primary manifestation of PACG and intraocular pressure (IOP) increases according to the "closed-angle" type occurs on the background of age-related changes. More often these will be undulating IOP increases but in some cases, acute attacks of PACG may develop.

Although in most cases a predisposition to PACG can be identified at an early age, physicians with extensive clinical experience know that IOP in such eyes can remain normal for an indefinitely long time. However, it is difficult to predict the moment when the primary manifestation of PACG in the predisposed eyes will occur.

In cases where we are dealing with eyes at-risk group of PACG to prevent diseases from developing, at some moment it is necessary to make a laser iridectomy. We need an objective criterion in order to decide when to do it, whether laser iridectomy needs to be done urgently, and when the patient can be left for monitoring at the risk group. We assume that the study of the VRI condition can help in solving this issue.

2. Purposes of the research

- To find the relationship between IOP increases in "closed-angle" type and PACG primary manifestation with VRI condition and PVD appearance;
- To find an objective criterion for the moment of laser iridectomy on the eyes with a predisposition to PACG.

3. Reasons to initiate research

The starting point for the research was the observation of one clinical case with a high predisposition to PACG.

The clinical case: The patient S. 55-year-old; high hypermetropia in both eyes; extremely abnormal anatomical parameters (presented in **Table 1**). The coefficients that determine the predisposition to the development of PACG (see below) in both eyes were extremely unfavorable.

However, despite the very narrow ACA (**Figures 1** and 2), IOP in both eyes remained stable at normal values for long time. The primary manifestation of PACG

Eye	Vision acuity and refraction	Axial length of the eye (mm)	Anterior chamber depth (mm)	Lens thickness (mm)	Prognostic Lowe coefficient* ($N \geq 0.2$)	Axial Chirshikov coefficient** ($N \leq 10.0$)
OD	sph + 7.5D = 0.8	16.0	0.6	5.8	0.06	60
OS	sph + 7.5D = 0.7	16.1	0.6	5.9	0.06	60

**Lowe coefficient (CLowe) [1]—the coefficient of predisposition to PACG is calculated by the formula:*
$CLowe = \left(ACD + \frac{1}{2}LTh\right) : ALE$
Predisposition to PACG is if $CLowe \leq 0.2$.
***Axial Chirshikov coefficient (AShC) [2]—the coefficient of predisposition to PACG is calculated by the formula:*
$AShC = (Lth\ x\ 100) : (ACD\ x\ ALE)$
Predisposition to PACG is if $AshC \geq 10.0$.
ACD, anterior chamber depth; LTh, lens thickness; ALE, axial length of the eye.

Table 1.
Parameters of the patient' S. eyes. 55years old. High predisposition to PACG.

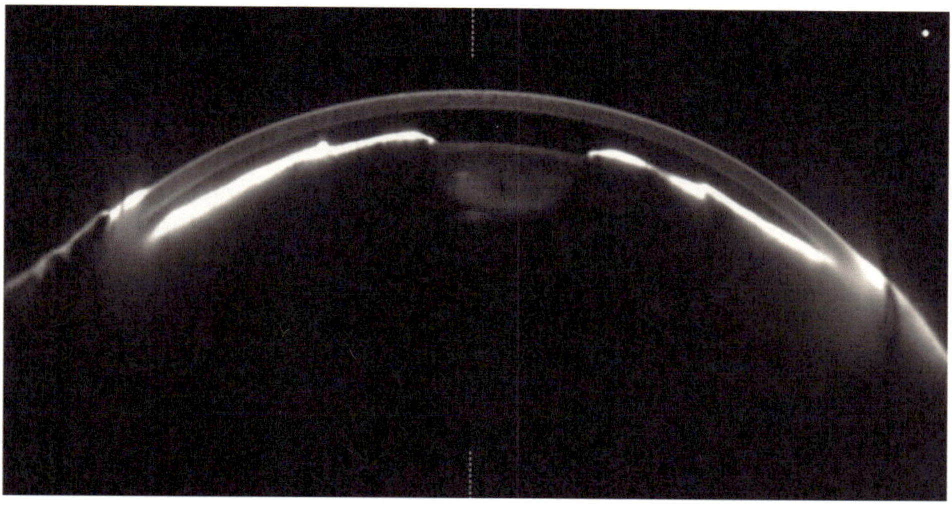

Figure 1.
The anterior chamber angle of the left eye. Patient S., 55 years old, high predisposition to PACG. Extremely narrow anterior chamber angle (Pentacam, author' photo).

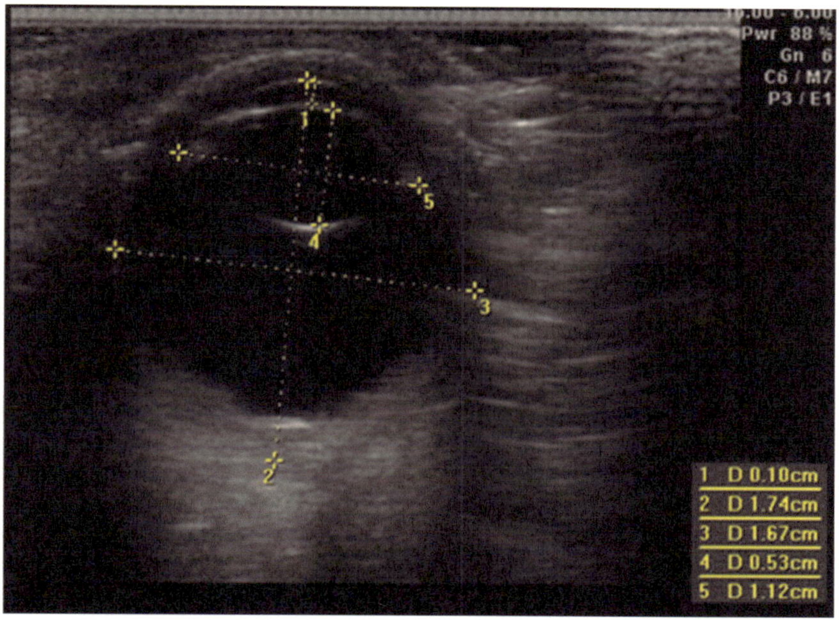

Figure 2.
Patient S., 55 years old. Hypermetropia +7.5 D. Internal dimensions of OD (the OS parameters are the same) (US B-scan, author' photo). There is a combination of the short axial length of the eye with a disproportionately lens thickness, narrow anterior chamber angle.

on OS with undulating IOP increases up to 29 mm Hg was detected only 4 months before the visit to the clinic. At the same time, there were never detected increases of IOP on OD before.

OD: The optic nerve head and visual field are consistent with the norm; OS: The optic nerve head and visual field are consistent with the early stage of glaucoma.

When analyzing this clinical case, the following questions arose:

- How, with such extremely unfavorable anatomical parameters of the eyes, IOP was normal until the age of 55 years old?
- Why did in fellow eyes with identical anatomical parameters the IOP increases were detected on the left eye only, while no hydrodynamic disturbances were detected in the right eye?

When comparing the ultrasound picture of the fellow eyes of patient S., we paid attention to the fact that on OD (IOP was always normal), the vitreous was in close contact with the retina. Unlike this, on the OS, a plane posterior vitreous detachment (PVD) and retrohyaloid space were found (**Figure 3a** and **b**).

We assumed that the reason for PACG primary manifestation on the OS could be the violation of VRI and the appearance of PVD. The presence of retrohyaloid space could be a reason for the destabilization of vitreous body position in the vitreous cavity. This makes it possible for the vitreous body micro-displacement in the sagittal direction. This, in turn, could be a cause for changes in the position of the iris-lens diaphragm (ILD) and its displacement toward the anterior chamber of the eye. As a result of this, there was a narrowing of the ACA, the development of hydrodynamic blocks for the intraocular fluid movement, and IOP increases.

4. Vitreous-retinal interface

The vitreous body is externally bounded by the cortical (hyaloid) membrane, which is a layer 100–200 μm thick, in which the concentration of hyaluronic substances and the density of the fibrillary layer are higher in comparison to other parts of the vitreous [3].

We can talk about two different clinical and anatomical conditions of the posterior hyaloid membrane (PHM)—before and after the development of PVD. Before the PVD appears, PHM is not visible either histologically or clinically, however, after the PVD it can be observed ophthalmoscopically as well as using OCT and ultrasound methods of research [4].

VRI (the contact zone between the retina and PHM) condition is important for the physiology of the eye. The power of the contact of the vitreous with the retina is different: the strongest one is in the area where the optic nerve enters the eyeball ("posterior basis of the vitreous"), in the zone of premacular bursa and in the zone of contact between the vitreous body and retinal vessels [5, 6]. At young age, VRI is most durable but with the age and with some metabolic disorders in vitreous substances, as well as with a progressive increase in the axial size of the eye, the strength of the VRI weakens, which leads to the appearance of PVD.

The functional significance of VRI for the eye is more often considered from the point of view of the retina condition. In our work, we will consider the issue of the VRI role from the point of view of the hydrodynamics of the eye. The subject of the research was the study of VRI in eyes with an anatomical predisposition to the development of PACG.

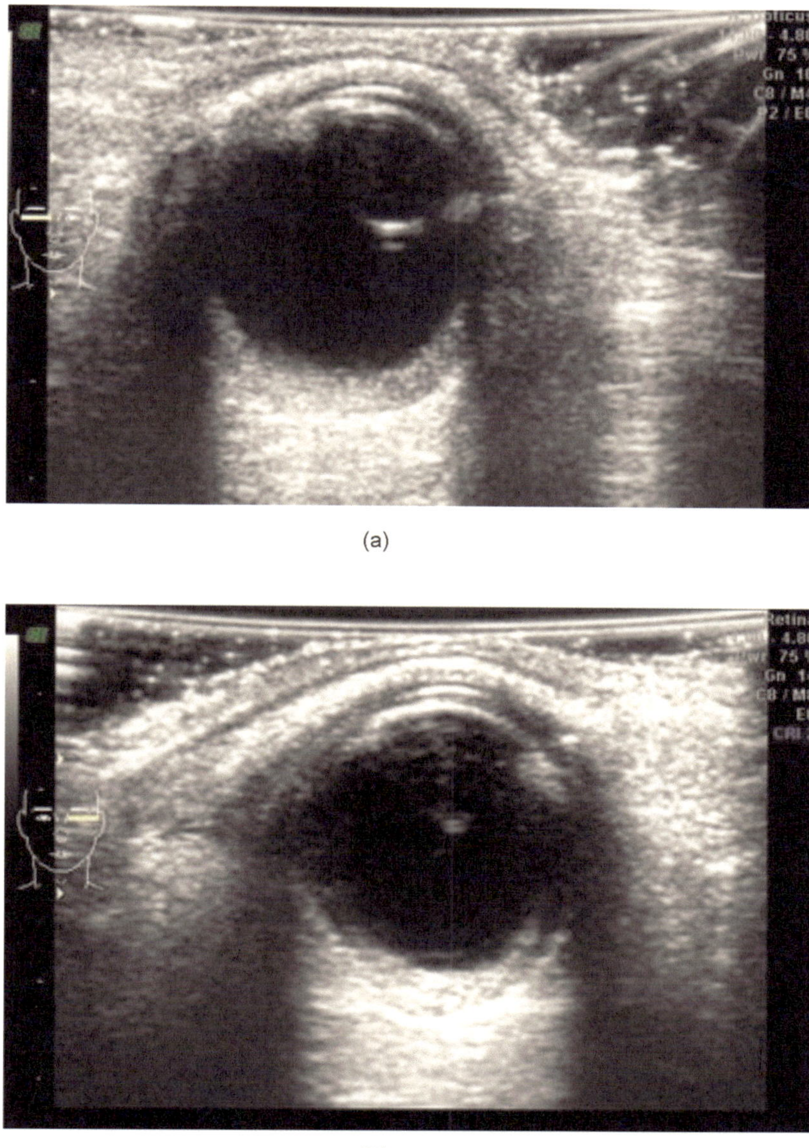

Figure 3.
(a, b) Fellow eyes of patient S., 55 years old (US B-scan, author' photos). (a) OD: the eye is at risk group for the development of PACG, the diagnosis of PACG was not confirmed. IOP is stable within the normal range. PVD is absent. Choroid is thickened. (b) OS: the IOP increases up to 29 mm Hg firstly was detected 4 months ago. Plane PVD. Choroid is thickened. The diagnosis of PACG is confirmed.

5. The hydrodynamic blocks in the eye and the reasons for IOP increases on "angle-closed" type

A special feature of the clinical manifestations of PACG (except the acute attack of glaucoma) is an alternation of IOP increases with periods of IOP normalization (in contrast to primary open-angle glaucoma, in which IOP steadily increases due to outflow ways degradation). In PACG cases, IOP increases occur as a result of the development of hydrodynamic blocks that impede intraocular fluid movement from the zone of secretion in the posterior chamber of the eye to the zone of outflow in the ACA.

There are several blocks, typical for PACG:

- Iris-lenticular block, in which movement of fluid through the space between the anterior surface of the lens and the posterior surface of the iris toward the pupil is disturbed;

- Pupillary block, in which the pupil is obturated by the anterior surface of the lens and fluid movement from posterior chamber into anterior chamber of the eye is disturbed;

- Angular block, in which a critical narrowing of the ACA occurs and the access of fluid to trabecula and uveal-scleral outflow zone is impaired [7, 8].

In eyes with axial myopia weakening of VRI and PVD development occurs at a young age. However, in such eyes, the occurrence of PACG is extremely rare. Even the lens thickness in such eyes is big, there is no anatomical predisposition to the development of hydrodynamic blocks of the "angle-closure" type.

Physicians with extensive clinical experience know that IOP can remain normal indefinitely despite the anatomical predisposition to PACG and the presence of a narrow ACA. However, against the background of age-related changes, once a primary manifestation of PACG is occurring. It is difficult to predict the moment when the primary manifestation of PACG will start. This is very important for tactics of managing patients in risk groups for PACG development. An objective criterion is needed to understand whether it is safe to continue to observe a patient at risk group or whether a laser iridectomy should be performed.

IOP undulated increases are possible only in those cases when there is a fluctuation of ACA width. The reason for such fluctuation may be the appearance of factors leading to the periodic displacement of iris-lenticular diaphragm (ILD) toward the anterior chamber. Normally, ILD is in a stable position, which guarantees a constant width of ACA and normal access of intraocular fluid to the drainage zone of the eye. For this reason, even in situations with very narrow ACA (as it was described in the clinical case), its width remains stable and IOP can remain at a normal level until old age.

There is an opinion that the main factor that leads to displacement of ILD forward and as a result—the PACG development is the involutional increase of lens thickness. However, this cannot fully explain the pathogenesis of the undulating nature of IOP increases, which is so typical for chronic form of PACG. If the development of hydrodynamic blocks occurs only due to the thickening of lens, then IOP increases would have a constant stable lasting nature. In practice, chronic forms of PACG are more common when periods of IOP increase alternate with periods of its normalization.

There is another opinion, that the cause of displacement of ILD forward is increase in the volume (edema) of the vitreous body. The basis for this point of view is that some organs in different functional states can significantly change their volume due to changes in blood supply or functional edema. For the vitreous, the situation associated with edema of its substance is unlikely. Hyaluronic substances, which form a vitreous body, have very high hydrophilicity. In normal situations, the hyaluronic substances

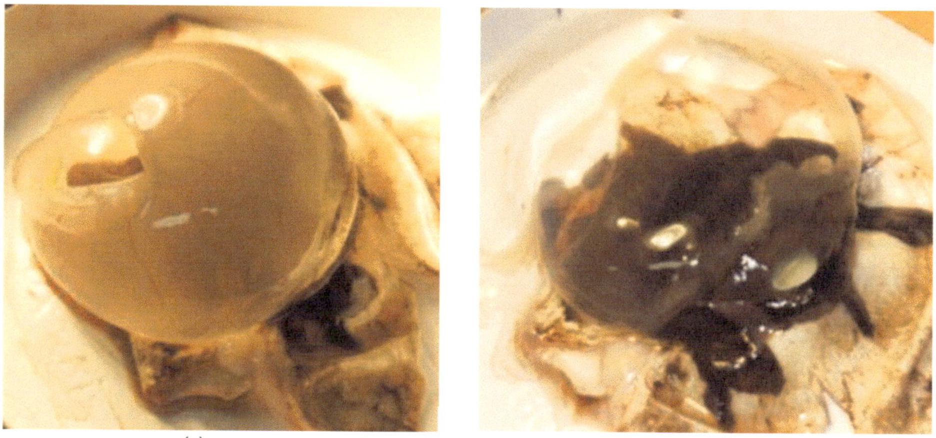

(a) (b)

Figure 4.
(a, b) Cadaver's eye vitreous body specimens. Vitreous body can keep its shape and volume for some time after the specimen preparation due to resilience of vitreous (specimens preparation and photos of the author). (a) Specimen of vitreous body with retina after sclera and choroid elimination. There is the opening in the place of optic nerve entrance. (b) Specimen of vitreous body after retina elimination.

bind interstitial water in the intercellular spaces (according to various sources, in a ratio of up to 1: 4000), while forming very viscous solutions. This is necessary for the stable maintenance of the volume of the vitreous body inside the vitreous cavity throughout life (**Figure 4**).

It is known that the universal response of vitreous to a violation of its chemical composition is a decrease in its volume (vitreosyneresis). The edema of the vitreous body and its increase in volume are highly unlikely. For this reason, a vitreous substance in normal condition is in a state of maximum hydration and cannot additionally increase its volume [9]. (If edema of vitreous can be possible, any situation associated with a functional increase in ocular blood flow could be accompanied by an increase of vitreous volume, and as a result, in anatomically predisposed eyes, this would be accompanied by obligate IOP increase, which does not happen in reality.)

Thus, there is a need to find other reasons for the development of hydrodynamic blocks in addition to increase in thickness of the lens and hypothetical vitreous edema.

One of the diagnostic methods that allow you to accurately say whether anatomically predisposed eyes have a real form of PACG (and active treatment is needed) or while the eyes are still at risk group (and you can limit the tactic by monitoring only), is the Hyams stress test [10].

The Hyams stress test is carried out as follows: IOP is measured with the patient in recumbent position (e.g., with a Schiotz or a Maklakov ophthalmic tonometer [11]. After that, the patient is asked to turn over and lie in the "face down" position for 1 hour. After this time, the patient is again asked to turn over on his back and IOP is measured again. If during this time IOP has increased by 5 mm Hg or more, the test is considered positive, and the diagnosis of PACG is confirmed. If IOP remains unchanged or increases by less than 5 mm Hg, then the test is considered negative.

The Hyams test makes it possible to divide eyes with an anatomical predisposition to PACG into two groups. In a group with negative results, the eyes can be left in the risk group without any treatment, with monitoring only. In a group with positive results, the real form of PACG is confirmed. In such cases, the patients need to receive active treatment (laser iridectomy act).

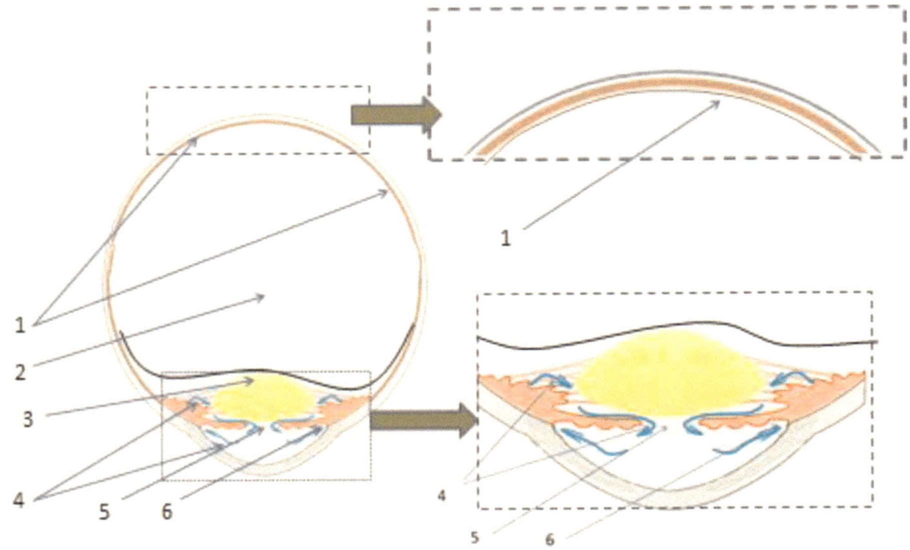

Figure 5.
Cross section of the eye at the beginning of the Hyams test or in the case of negative result (Scheme). 1. Vitreoretinal interface is normal. The posterior hyaloid membrane is in close contact with the retina. 2. Vitreous body (fixed to the retina). 3. Lens. 4. Free intraocular fluid movement. 5. Pupil. 6. Anterior chamber angle. Good vitreoretinal interface gives fixation of vitreous body inside vitreous cavity. There is no pressure of vitreous on the iris-lenticular diaphragm and it is not displaced. Hydrodynamic blocks are absent. Intraocular fluid can freely pass from posterior chamber through the pupil into anterior chamber to drainage zone direction.

In the issue of PACG pathogenesis, there is no clear opinion in which cases the ILD has ability to displace forward and create conditions for hydrodynamic blocks, and in which cases ILD remains stable in its normal position.

From our point of view the mechanism of IOP increases on "angle-closured" type in eyes with an anatomical predisposition to PACG largely depends on the VRI condition. In eyes that have full-fledged VRI, the vitreous body is tightly fixed in its place in the vitreous cavity and does not have a compressive effect on the ILD under the influence of gravitational load in "face down" position (**Figure 5a** and **b**). Due to this, hydrodynamic blocks do not occur, IOP remains normal, and the results of the Hyams test are NEGATIVE.

If VRI condition is unsatisfactory, there are PVD and retrohyaloid space, which gives the opportunity for vitreous body micro-displacement in the vitreous cavity in sagittal direction. In the "face down" position, under the influence of a gravitational load, vitreous begins to press on the ILD. In eyes with an unfavorable anatomical predisposition to PACG, it can be a cause of hydrodynamic blocks described above, and the results of Hyams test are POSITIVE (**Figure 6a** and **b**). When the patient returns to the vertical position, the gravitational load vector changes and this allows ILD to return to its normal position. The hydrodynamic blocks are eliminated and IOP is reduced.

6. Clinical research

To confirm this concept, we conducted a clinical study, the results of which were partly published earlier [12]. For 4 years we supervised a group of patients (135 people —259 eyes, aged 37 up to 88 years, of which 87 women and 48 men) in whose eyes

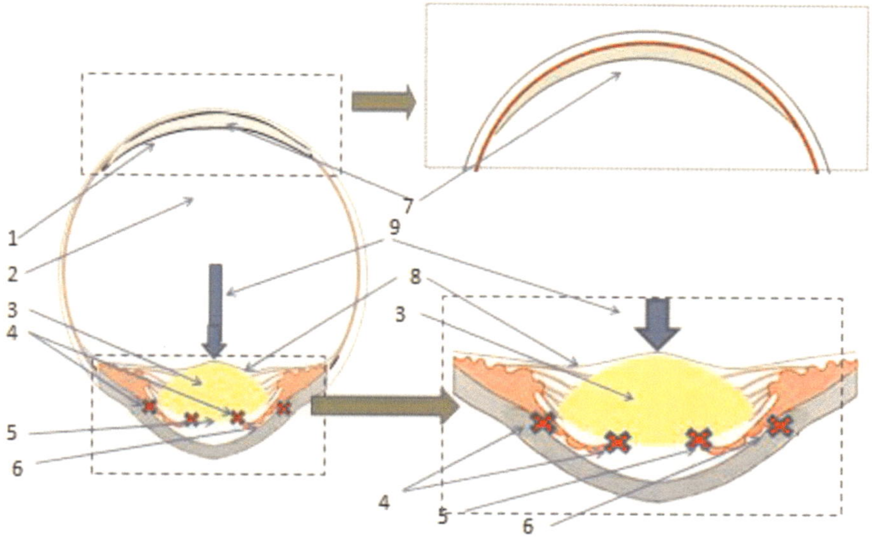

Figure 6.
Cross section of the eye at the Hyams test with a positive result (Scheme). 1. Vitreoretinal interface is violated. Posterior hyaloid membrane is detached. 2. Vitreous body. (Fixation vitreous to retina is disrupted). 3. Lens. 4. Hydrodynamic blocks for the intraocular fluid movement. 5. Pupil is blocked. 6. Narrowing and blocking of anterior chamber angle. 7. Retro-hyaloid space. 8. Anterior hyaloid membrane is pressing on the iris-lenticular diaphragm. 9. Gravity load vector. Due to violation of vitreoretinal interface, posterior vitreous detachment occurred and retrohyaloid space appeared. The vitreous body fixation at the posterior pole of the eye is disturbed, which makes it possible for its micro-displacement in sagittal direction. When the patient is positioned "face down" during the Hyams test, the vitreous body (which has lost its fixation with the retina at the posterior pole of the eye) under the influence of a gravitational load, begins to put pressure on the iris-lenticular diaphragm. As a result, the iris-lenticular diaphragm is displaced forward. This leads to the formation of irido-lenticular, pupillary and angular hydrodynamic blocks. As a result there is IOP increases.

there was an anatomical predisposition to PACG (narrow ACA and an unfavorable ratio between the size of the axial length of the eye, the depth of the anterior chamber of the eye and the thickness of the lens). In all eyes, the Lowe and Chirshikov predictive coefficients were calculated in order to objectively confirm the anatomical predisposition to PACG. In 91.0% of the examined eyes, there was hypermetropic refraction (from +0.5 to +16.0D).

In 36 eyes the diagnosis of PACG had already been confirmed before and treatment was prescribed earlier. The remaining 223 eyes without confirmed PACG where IOP increases had not been detected yet were taken for the research group.

In 88 patients, both paired eyes (176 eyes) were examined. In 47 patients only one eye was examined (because in the fellow eye, the diagnosis of PACG had already been confirmed or it was unsuitable for our research or the eye was absent).

The aim of the research was to study the influence of VRI condition on the development of PACG in anatomically predisposed eyes. Hyams test, OCT, and ultrasound examination were performed on all examined eyes. Depending on the results of the Hyams test, the examined eyes were divided into two groups: with a positive and negative results of the test. It is important to note that in some cases fellow eyes of one patient were attributed to different groups.

PVD and a well-visualized retrohyaloid space were found in all eyes with a positive Hyams test. In the group with negative Hyams test, the plane and very low PVD were detected in four cases. In other eyes from the group with negative results, the PVD was not detected.

In the next stage of the research, we focused attention and took dynamic monitoring of the eyes from the group where despite predisposition to PACG the Hyams test was negative. These eyes were taken for monitoring (4 years). Every 6 months a planned examination was carried out, which included the repeats of the Hyams test, as well as ultrasound examination and OCT for targeted detection of signs of PVD.

During the monitoring process, it was discovered that in 27 eyes from this group the Hyams test transformed from negative to positive over time. We considered such transformation as a non-alternative sign of the eye's transitions from the risk group to the group with real, confirmed PACG. In 23 eyes from this group, where initially PVD could not be detected, PVD appeared during the monitoring process (**Figure 7a** and **b**).

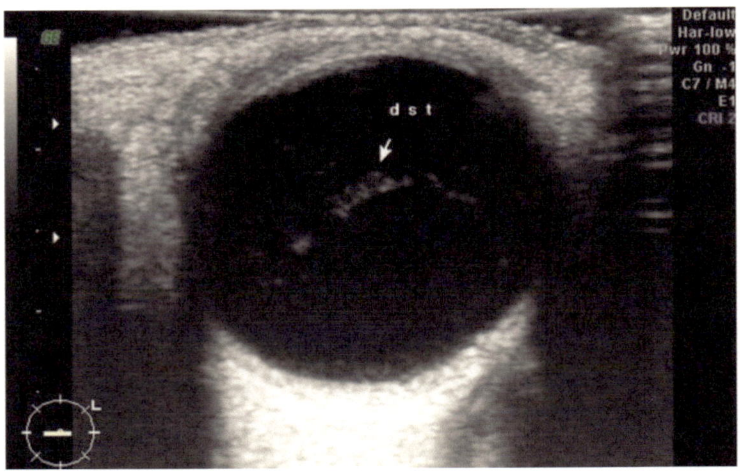

(a)

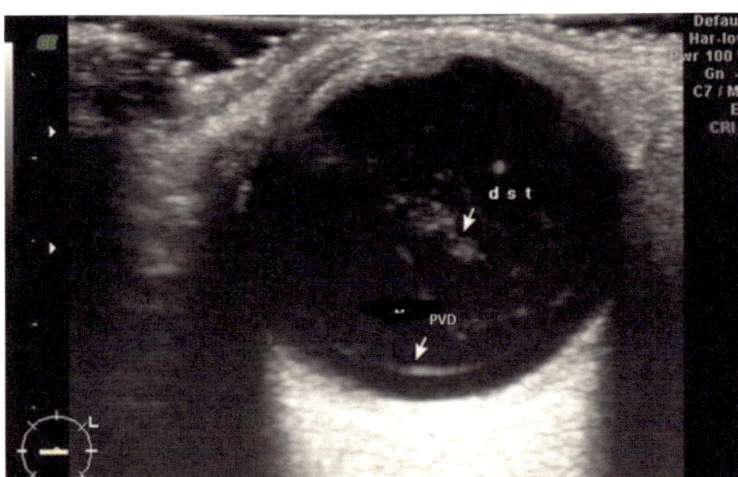

(b)

Figure 7.
(a, b) The eye of patient K. (68 years old) with anatomical predisposition to PACG there was a transition from risk group to the real PACG form. Dynamic monitoring. US B-scan (author'photos). (a) The eye of the patient K. at the first examination. Hyams test is negative, PVD is absent. The risk group. (b) The same eye of the Patient K. after 1.5 years. Transformation of the Hyams test result from negative to positive. The plane PVD was detected. A diagnosis of PACG was confirmed. The patient was sent for laser iridectomy.

In 4 eyes with low-plane PVD (described above), we observed an increase in them to a clinically significant size.

The result of the research has shown that PVD is an obligate feature for the manifested PACG. At the same time, we tried to understand the role of the lens thickness increase factor in the development of PACG. In 9 eyes out of 27 (from the group where the Hyams test was transformed from negative to positive), during monitoring, the lens thickness increased by 0.1–0.15 mm was noted, in the other 18 eyes, the lens thickness remained unchanged. In 16 eyes, in which the Hyams test remained negative, in five cases the thickness of the lens increase by 0.1–0.15 mm was also noted, however, in these eyes, IOP remained within the normal range.

7. Conclusion

VRI condition is important factor in determining the vitreous body fixation inside the vitreous cavity. PVD (and as a result—retrohyaloid space appearance) in the eyes, and anatomically predisposition to PACG are factors that can be a reason for vitreous body and iris-lenticular membrane displacement to the anterior chamber direction in unfavorable situations (e.g., as a result of Hyams probe). Such displacement can provoke the occurrence of iris-lenticular, pupillary, and angular hydrodynamic blocks and IOP increase on "angle-closed" type.

VRI in the eyes with normal or short size (in cases of absence of another problem), for many years, provides good fixation of the vitreous body inside the vitreous cavity. Age-related syneresis processes in the vitreous body are factors determining the VRI violation and as a result the transition of eyes predisposed to PACG from a risk group to a group with a really confirmed form of PACG.

The age-related increase of the lens thickness, of cause, also contributes to the destabilization of ILD location and hydrodynamic processes in the eyes predisposed to PACG, but this should be considered only as one of the factors leading to the development of PACG.

An important and repeating question when we are talking about eyes with narrow ACA and predisposition to PACG is the question—at what moment it is necessary to make a laser iridectomy. Do we have to do it now or we can wait and only monitor the patient?

Based on the foregoing, it is possible to give a recommendation for this issue solution: the detection of PVD is a signal for the transition from passive monitoring to the start of active treatment (laser iridectomy, etc.). And if VRI continues to reliably fix the position of the vitreous body inside the vitreous cavity and the examination does not detect signs of PVD, we can leave the patient under monitoring.

Note

The text is based on data obtained during the work of the author at the Research Institute of Eye Diseases of the Russian Academy of Sciences from 2008 to 2018.

Author details

Alexey Ermolaev
Research Institute of Eye Diseases of Russian Academy of Science, Moscow, Russia

*Address all correspondence to: ermolaev.alexey9@gmail.com

References

[1] Lowe RF. Etiology of anatomical basis for primary angle-closure glaucoma. Biometrical comparisons between normal eyes and eyes with primary angle-closure glaucoma. The British Journal of Ophthalmology. 1970;**54**:161-169

[2] Chirshikov YK. The ratio of certain parameters of the eye in primary glaucoma. Vestnik Ophthalmology. 1979; **1**:13-17

[3] Sebag J. The Vitreous: Structure, Function and Pathobiology. New York: Springer; 1989

[4] Gass JDM. Stereoscopic Atlas of Macular Diseases. St. Louis: Mosby; 1970. p. 201

[5] Worst JGF. The bursa intravitreal premacularis. New Developments in Ophthalmology. 1975;**1975**:275-279

[6] Worst JGF. Cisternal systems of the fully developed vitreous body in the young adult. Transaction on Ophthalmological Society UK. 1977;**97**: 550-554

[7] Krasnov MM. Surgery in glaucoma: Development, current status, and possibilities of pathogenic effect. Vestnik Oftalmologii. 1967;**80**(5):21-28

[8] Chang B, Liebmann J, Ritch R. Angle closure glaucoma in younger patients. Transactions of the American Ophthalmological Society. 2002;**100**: 201-214

[9] Pirie R, Van Heyningem A. Biochemistry of the Eye/Hardcover— Import. Thomas, Biochemistry; 1956. p. 323

[10] Hyams S, Friedman Z, Neumann E. Elevated intraocular pressure in the prone position. A new provocative test for angle-closure glaucoma. American Journal of Ophthalmology. 1968;**66**(4): 661-672

[11] Cordero I. Understanding and caring for a Schiotz tonometer. Community Eye Health Journal. 2014;**27**(87):57

[12] Ermolaev AP. On a connection of early manifestations of angle closure glaucoma and development of posterior vitreous detachment. Vestnik Oftalmologii. 2013;**129**(2):24-28

Chapter 6

Basis, Diagnosis, and Treatment of Uveal Melanoma

Songlin Sun and Liang Xu

Abstract

Uveal melanoma (UM) is the most common primary intraocular malignancy with a strong tendency to metastasize. The prognosis is poor once metastasis occurs. The treatment remains challenging for metastatic UM, even though our understanding of UM has advanced. Risk factors for developing UM include ages, skin colors, and genetic mutations. Many therapies that have applied to cutaneous melanoma have little or no success in UM. Various forms and combinations of radiotherapy, phototherapy, and local resection are utilized for advanced cases. The treatment aims to preserve the eye and useful vision and prevent metastases. This chapter aims to introduce the current study for UM.

Keywords: ophthalmology, uveal melanoma, pathogenesis, diagnosis, pathological features, staging, treatment, prognosis

1. Introduction

Uveal melanoma (UM) is the most common primary malignant intraocular tumor in adults. As a highly aggressive and fatal tumor, it mostly occurs in the choroid (90.0%), followed by the ciliary body (6.0%) and the iris (4.0%). The mean patient age at diagnosis was between the ages of 50 and 60, mostly in Europeans, Americans, and Caucasians, and more men than women. Despite effective treatment of the primary tumor and metastases, 50% of patients develop liver metastases within a median of 2.4 years [1]. Once UM metastasizes throughout the body, there is no effective treatment. Overall, 90% of patients die within 6 months of diagnosis of metastases [2, 3]. However, metastases are detectable in only 1–3% of diagnosed cases. Because the survival rate of patients is closely related to the size of the primary tumor, early diagnosis and early local treatment are crucial. At present, the main treatment methods include enucleation and applicator radiotherapy, but no standard treatment plan has been established for postoperative adjuvant therapy and systemic treatment for advanced patients.

2. Pathogenesis of UM

The occurrence and development of UM involve multi-factors, multi-stages, and multi-gene variation accumulation.

1. **Cytogenetics:** One of the risk factors for UM metastasis is chromosomal variation, including gain of chromosome 1q, 6p, 8q and deletion of chromosome 1p, 3, 6q, 8p, 9p [4]. Chromosome 3 deletion exists in more than 50% of primary UM and is a high-risk prognostic factor for tumor metastasis [5]. Meanwhile, chromosome 3 deletion can also be accompanied with other chromosomal abnormalities. Studies have shown that when chromosome 3 and 1p are deleted, the survival time of UM patients is significantly shortened [6], and if chromosome 3 deletion and chromosome 8q gain are found in tumors, the prognosis is poor [7]. The combination of chromosome 3 deletion and chromosome 6p gain in UM patients has a better prognosis than the presence of chromosome 3 alone [8].

2. **Gene expression profile:** A number of research results have confirmed that gene expression profiles can provide people with more accurate prognostic assessment than cytogenetic, pathological features, and clinical information [9]. Onken et al. [10] detected the expression of 12 differential genes and 3 control genes in UM, and found the gene expression profile of UM. According to these genes, they divided UM into 2 types: type 1 has a lower risk of metastatic spread, while type 2 has a higher risk of metastatic spread. Their founding provided an accurate, practical, and convenient method for predicting the prognosis of UM metastasis. In more than 100 clinical research centers in the United States and Canada, the 15-gene detection chip (trade name: Decision Dx-UM) has been used as a routine examination to screen high-risk groups for early metastasis of UM [11].

3. **Gene mutation:** Currently, the most studied mutated genes in UM are GNAQ, GNA11, and BAP1. Other mutated genes include EIF1AX and SF3B1. While EIF1AX and SF3B1 are associated with good and better prognosis in UM, respectively, BAP1 mutations predict poor prognosis and risk of tumor spread [12–15]. Van Raamsdonk CD et al. found that the mutation frequency of oncogene GNAQ in UM was 40%, and the mutation frequency of GNA11 was 45% [16, 17]. The mutation frequency of GNAQ gene in Chinese UM was as high as 51.9%, and the mutation rate of GNAll gene was 25.9% [18]. Chen et al. [19] found that mutations in GNAQ or GNA11 genes lead to the development of UM through the activation of their downstream signaling pathways PKC and MAPK. Yu et al. [20] and Feng et al. [21] found that GNAQ or GNAll gene mutations lead to excessive activation of YAP protein, resulting in uncontrolled tumor cell proliferation and malignant tumors.

BAP1 (BRCA1-Associated Protein 1) is an important tumor suppressor gene. Wiesner et al. [22] found that the patients suffering from uveal and skin melanoma are related to the abnormal expression of the BAP1 family. BAP1 can regulate the cell cycle, cell differentiation, apoptosis, DNA damage response, and gene expression [23]. Due to the key regulatory role of BAP1 on cells, the decreased gene expression or gene mutation is related to the occurrence and development of various malignant tumors, but its specific mechanism has not yet been elucidated [24]. The loss of BAP1 is associated with the loss of chromosome 3 in UM cells, and the loss of chromosome 3 in UM cells is a risky prognostic factor for the occurrence of metastasis in

UM [25–29]. SF3B1 mutation exists in 19% of UM, which suggests that UM has a better prognosis [30]. Mutations in SF3B1 cause a large amount of mRNA alternative splicing, but how it promotes UM remains unclear. Martin et al. [31] found that 24% of UM had mutations in EIFIAX, which had a good prognosis. The protein encoded by EIF1AX is involved in protein translation, but the specific mechanism between its mutation and the development of UM is still unclear.

4. **Non-coding RNA:** Both miRNA and long non-coding RNA (lncRNA) belong to non-coding RNA, and both play a regulatory role in the occurrence and development of UM.

miRNAs are a group of endogenous RNAs that can directly bind to mRNA and regulate gene expression after transcription. miRNAs are involved in the development process of almost all malignant tumors, including cell proliferation, differentiation, apoptosis, and metastasis mechanisms. In recent years, miRNA has attracted much attention in the field of tumor research. Scientists have analyzed the miRNA expression profile of UM, and a variety of miRNAs have been found to be associated with the prognosis of UM. The genes encoding these miRNAs are considered novel oncogenes and tumor suppressors. For example, both miRNA-130a and miRNA26a exhibit tumor suppressor properties when overexpressed [32, 33].

lncRNAs play a crucial role in the maintenance of cellular homeostasis and participate in many key cellular pathways. In cancer, lncRNAs are associated with apoptosis evasion, proliferation, invasion, and drug resistance. Among them, autophagy-related lncRNA plays an important role in predicting the prognosis of UM patients. The lncRNA RHPN1-AS1 is oncogenic and can suppress UM cell proliferation by silencing its expression [34].

3. Diagnosis

3.1 Symptoms and signs

UM includes melanoma that occurs in the iris, ciliary body, and choroid, and can spread outside the eye, with various clinical symptoms and many complications. Various symptoms and signs appear depending on the site of occurrence. UM can be divided into four stages according to clinical manifestations: intraocular stage, glaucoma stage, extraocular extension stage, and systemic metastasis stage.

The clinical symptoms of choroidal melanoma are diverse, and the ocular symptoms are the most prominent. Symptoms such as vision loss, visual obstruction, metamorphopsia, or discoloration often appear, and the symptoms vary with the location of the tumor. If the tumor is located in the macular area, the early subjective symptoms are metamorphopsia, microopia or macroopia, changes in color vision. Visual field defects may have relative or absolute scotoma, or persistent hypermetropia, or floating in front of the eyes. When the tumor is located in the peripheral part of the fundus, there may be no symptoms. The morphology of choroidal melanoma is divided into three types, namely dome-shaped, mushroom-shaped, and flat diffuse. The melanoma in the choroid often causes exudative retinal detachment, sometimes with vitreous hemorrhage, causing blurred vision.

In iris melanoma, raised lesions in dark brown with clear edges can be seen on the surface of the iris, and dilated "sentinel vessels" can be seen on the surface of the sclera. The OCT examination of the anterior segment showed that there was a circular raised lesion on the surface of the iris, and the anterior surface of the tumor was echogenic; the internal echo of the tumor was attenuated, and imaging could not be performed on the posterior surface.

The location of the ciliary body is hidden and difficult to observe. It is difficult to detect tumors in its location early, because ciliary body melanoma may not have any specific clinical manifestations in the early stage. Ciliary body melanoma can grow forward, backward, and toward the vitreous cavity and sclera, and the clinical manifestations of ciliary body tumors can be different depending on the extent of ciliary body tumor invasion. Ciliary body melanoma can lead to clinical manifestations such as glaucoma, uveitis, lens displacement to varying degrees, diopter changes, vitreous hemorrhage, retinal detachment, and macular edema.

Intraorbital spread of UM: (1) spread along the scleral duct and scleral vortex vein; (2) directly invade the sclera and spread to the outside of the eyeball; (3) directly spread along the cribriform plate; (4) invade the retina, ciliary body, and iris, conjunctiva. The way of extraocular extension of UM is related to the growth location of the tumor. Extraocular extension occurred in the front of the equator, and black nodules can be seen in the conjunctiva, which can be misdiagnosed as scleral staphyloma. The posterior part of the globe spreads, with exophthalmos, eyelid edema, and ocular motility disturbances. Although no tumor was palpable on the orbital rim, the orbital pressure was high and the eyeball could not move back. In severe cases, the eyeball protrudes outside the palpebral fissure, and the surface structure of the eyeball is damaged and uneven. Due to massive necrosis of tumor tissue, panophthalmitis, hypopyon, and orbital cellulitis may occur.

3.2 Eye examination

A comprehensive examination should be performed including vision, intraocular pressure, anterior segment, and fundus. Slit-lamp microscopy and indirect ophthalmoscopy are the main examination methods in ophthalmology, and sometimes gonioscopy or transillumination examination is also required. All patients underwent evaluation of the anterior segment using slit-lamp microscopy and the posterior segment using indirect ophthalmoscopy to determine tumor location, shape, pigmentation, vascularity, tumor margin morphology, distance from the macula, optic disc, and ciliary body and corneal involvement, anterior scleral extension. The evaluation is required to determine whether there are secondary lesions such as malignant transformation of choroidal nevi, such as sentinel vessels on the surface of the sclera, cataracts, subretinal fluid, or orange pigment in the tumor. Gonioscopy can identify involvement of the anterior chamber angle by iris or ciliary body melanoma. Transillumination is performed by transscleral or pupillary illumination to determine the degree of ciliary body involvement.

3.3 Auxiliary inspection

In recent years, with the development of imaging technology, especially the application of ocular ultrasound, CT, MRI, and fundus angiography, the diagnostic accuracy of UM has been greatly improved.

1. Compared with other imaging examinations, B-ultrasound and color Doppler blood flow imaging ultrasonography have unique advantages such as fast, accurate, economical, non-invasive, and repeatable operations. When applying B-ultrasound examination, the main features of UM are as follows: (a) The tumor grows in a fungating or dome-like shape; (b) on the sonogram, the echo is dense and strong at the front edge of the mass, and the echo intensity gradually decreases backward. An echo-free area is formed close to the bulb wall, which is the so-called "hollow out phenomenon;" (c) choroidal indentation sign; and (d) melanin cells in the tumor body carcinogenic sound wave reversal reaction are blocked and the image of the corresponding orbital area is covered. Color Doppler flow imaging (CDFI) can directly display the blood supply of the lesion and clarify the source of the blood supply, which is of great significance for the differential diagnosis of benign and malignant lesions. UM is a solid tumor composed of pigmented cells such as spindle cells and epithelioid cells. The blood supply in the tumor comes from the posterior ciliary vasculature of the branch of the ophthalmic artery. CDFI detection shows that the rich blood flow signals in the UM can be distributed in the whole tumor body in the form of "branches," showing a pure arterial blood flow spectrum, which is the same as the blood flow characteristics of the posterior ciliary artery. The emergence of CDFI technology makes up for the lack of blood flow imaging in ordinary ultrasound diagnosis and provides a new diagnostic method for eye diseases, especially diseases related to blood flow.

2. CT and MRI: UM in the early CT plain scan only shows localized thickening of the eye ring; when the tumor protrudes into the vitreous cavity, it appears as an iso-density or slightly high-density hemispherical or spherical shape with uniform density and clear boundaries. Tumors in enhanced CT scans often show different degrees of enhancement. MRI is radiation-free, multi-parameter, and multi-directional imaging, with high resolution of soft tissue, no bone artifact interference, and dynamic enhancement, which has great advantages in the examination of eye lesions. The main MRI manifestations of UM are as the following: Compared with the cerebral cortex signal, the tumor body mostly shows high signal on T1WI and low signal on T2WI, that is, short T1 signal and short T2 signal. Most of the UM showed mild enhancement after enhanced scanning. The UM-specific signal change is mainly due to the fact that melanin contained in the tumor is a paramagnetic substance that shortens the relaxation time of T1 and T2. Therefore, CT and MRI have important application value in the diagnosis of UM.

3. Fluorescein fundus angiography (FFA) and indocyanine green angiography (ICGA): A large number of melanin granules in UM tumors cause fluorescence shielding. In the early phase of FFA examination, the local manifestations are weak fluorescence, and the fluorescent spots in the tumor body gradually increase in the arterial-venous phase, forming mottled fluorescence with alternating intensity and weak fluorescence in the low fluorescence area. Tumors can be seen tortuous, spiral-shaped tumor blood vessels and retinal blood vessels can be imaged at the same time as a double loop phenomenon, and in the late phase, the imaging shows diffuse fluorescence. ICGA plays an important role in the diagnosis of UM. In the ICGA examination tumors always have no fluorescence, or no fluorescence in the early phase, and weak fluorescence or spot-like fluorescence

or fusion fluorescence in the late phase. In some patients, large blood vessels can be seen during angiography, and in the late phase, fluorescence leakage occurs in tumors. Advanced tumors have emptying phenomenon or three-ring images in some patients. ICGA and FFA are the effective diagnostic and differential means for diagnosing UM. FFA can show the double circulation of the tumor and retinal telangiectasia, and ICGA is used as a supplementary inspection method of FFA. Both of them have important clinical value.

4. Optical coherence tomography (OCT): OCT can show subtle retinal abnormalities, such as subretinal fluid, intraretinal edema, irregular photoreceptor layer, choroidal capillaries compressed by tumors, and orange pigment and cross-sectional architecture of choroidal lesions. Compared with ultrasonography, OCT is more advantageous in measuring small choroidal melanoma (thickness < 3 mm) [35]. OCT of the anterior segment is suitable for the detection of iris melanoma, but the basal margin of the tumor may be blurred by hyperpigmentation. The OCT angiography in Fundus can also be used to monitor macular microangiopathy after radiotherapy providing evidence for clinical treatment [36].

5. Positron emission computed tomography (PET) CT: PET-CT scanning has high sensitivity and predictive value for monitoring systemic metastasis in UM patients. For patients with suspected UM metastasis, PET-CT examination should be performed. It can detect metastasis early and stage the tumor, which is of great value for the treatment and follow-up of patients. In addition, PET-CT can also be used to find the primary tumor of choroidal metastases [37].

4. Pathological features

UM originates from uveal melanocytes, which is limited in the early stage, and further develops into typical fungal changes. Under the electron microscope, UM tumors are composed of round and spindle cells with rich cytoplasm, large nuclei, and frequent mitotic phases. New blood vessels are scattered in the tumor. Most tumors contain melanin, and a few tumors do not. The histopathological classification of UM is currently widely adopted in the world according to the classification standard developed by the WHO in 1980, and it is divided into four categories: (a) spindle cell type: composed of spindle-shaped type A and type B tumor cells in different proportions. Tumor cells are relatively dense, arranged in bundles or swirls. (b) Epithelial cell type: The tumor body is mainly composed of epithelioid tumor cells. Epithelioid cells account for more than 75%, and the rest are spindle-shaped A cells or spindle-shaped B cells. (c) Mixed cell type: composed of spindle-shaped and epithelioid melanoma cells in different proportions. (d) Others: those that do not meet the above classification, such as necrotic type, balloon-like cell type.

Spindle cell melanoma accounts for 40% of all UM, of which more than 90% are spindle cells, and the 15-year mortality rate of patients is 20%; epithelial cell melanoma accounts for 3–5% of all UM, of which more than 90% are epithelial cells, and the 15-year mortality rate of patients is 75%; the remaining 50% are mixed cell melanoma. At present, it is believed that epithelioid cell type UM is the most malignant and has the greatest risk of metastasis, followed by mixed type UM, and spindle cell type UM is the least malignant. The main immunohistochemical markers of UM include S-100, Melan-A, and Vimentin, etc.

5. Differential diagnosis

1. Scleral ciliary nevus: Scleral ciliary nevus is also called benign melanoma. It often occurs in the optic nerve area, followed by the uvea and conjunctiva. In terms of histology, this tumor is similar to benign tumors of the choroid, and its biological behavior is similar to that of pigmented nevus, and very few of them can become malignant. It can be distinguished by FFA, CT, and magnetic resonance examination. Despite this, if the intraoperative conditions permit, the scope of surgery should be determined after local excision of the tumor and frozen examination.

2. Iris implantation cyst: Malignant melanoma of the iris is clinically manifested by rich blood vessels in the tumor, a large amount of pigment loss, hemorrhage in the anterior chamber, pigment granules behind the cornea, inflammatory reaction on the surface of the iris, atrophy, and discoloration of the iris near the tumor. Traumatic implantation of iris cysts is the most common, mostly caused by penetrating eyeball injuries or intraocular surgery.

6. Staging

There are two main staging systems for UM, both based on tumor thickness and maximal basal diameter. The first staging system was formulated by the Collaborative Ocular Melanoma Study Group (COMS) [37], and the second was the TNM staging system proposed by the American Joint Committee on Cancer (AJCC) in 1968 [38]. In COMS staging, tumors are classified according to their thickness and largest basal diameter as small (1.5–2.4 mm thickness with the largest basal diameter 5–16 mm), medium (2.5–10.0 mm thickness with the largest base ≤16 mm in diameter), and large (thickness > 10.0 mm or maximal basal diameter > 16 mm). In TNM staging, tumors are classified into T1, T2, T3, and T4 stages, where "T" indicates the characteristics of the primary tumor, including tumor volume and its infiltrating relationship with surrounding tissues; "N" indicates the degree and scope of regional lymph node involvement; and "M" indicates distant metastasis of the tumor. There is partial overlap between small and medium tumors in the COMS staging and T1 and T2 in the TNM staging, and between large tumors in the COMS staging and T3 and T4 in the TNM staging. In the 8th edition of the TNM staging system launched by AJCC in 2018, more detailed staging was carried out for iris melanoma and the extrascleral extension of the tumor. The primary tumor is divided into T1-T4 stages according to clinical features, T1 stage is tumor limited to iris; T2 stage is tumor invaded ciliary body and (or) choroid; T3 stage is tumor invaded ciliary body and (or) choroid, with scleral infiltration; T4 stage is tumor with extrascleral extension. For ciliary body and choroidal melanoma staging, the eighth edition of the TNM staging system was also updated (**Table 1**).

UM is divided into N0 stage without lymph node involvement and N1 stage with lymph node involvement; M0 stage without metastasis; and M1 stage with metastasis, and is divided into M1a ~ M1c stage according to the size of metastatic lesions.

AJCC assessed the prognosis of patients according to TNM staging, and divided patients into 7 categories according to the assessed prognosis (**Table 2**) [39, 40].

T1 tumors: T1a: The T1-size tumor is not growing into the ciliary body or growing outside the eyeball. T1b: The T1-size tumor is growing into the ciliary body. T1c: The T1-size tumor is not growing into the ciliary body but is growing outside of the eyeball. The part of the tumor that is outside the eyeball is 5 mm (about 1/5 of an inch) or less across. T1d: The T1-size tumor is growing into the ciliary body and also outside of the eyeball. The part of the tumor that is outside the eyeball is 5 mm (about 1/5 of an inch) or less across.
T2 tumors: T2a: The T2-size tumor is not growing into the ciliary body or growing outside the eyeball. T2b: The T2-size tumor is growing into the ciliary body. T2c: The T2-size tumor is not growing into the ciliary body but is growing outside the eyeball. The part of the tumor that is outside the eyeball is 5 mm (about 1/5 of an inch) or less across. T2d: The T2-size tumor is growing into the ciliary body and also outside the eyeball. The part of the tumor that is outside the eyeball is 5 mm (about 1/5 of an inch) or less across.
T3 tumors: T3a: The T3-size tumor is not growing into the ciliary body and is not growing outside the eyeball. T3b: The T3-size tumor is growing into the ciliary body. T3c: The T3-size tumor is not growing into the ciliary body but is growing outside the eyeball. The part of the tumor that is outside the eyeball is 5 mm (about 1/5 of an inch) or less across. T3d: The T3-size tumor is growing into the ciliary body and also outside the eyeball. The part of the tumor that is outside the eyeball is 5 mm (about 1/5 of an inch) or less across.
T4 tumors: T4a: The T4-size tumor is not growing into the ciliary body or growing outside the eyeball. T4b: The T4-size tumor is growing into the ciliary body. T4c: The T4-size tumor is not growing into the ciliary body but is growing outside the eyeball. The part of the tumor that is outside the eyeball is 5 mm (about 1/5 of an inch) or less across. T4d: The T4-size tumor is growing into the ciliary body and also outside the eyeball. The part of the tumor that is outside the eyeball is 5 mm (about 1/5 of an inch) or less across. T4e: The tumor can be any size. It is growing outside the eyeball and the part of the tumor that is outside the eyeball is greater than 5 mm across.

Table 1.
AJCC TNM staging system (T categories for ciliary body and choroidal melanoma [39]).

Stage I	T1a, N0, M0
Stage IIA	T1b to T1d, N0, M0 OR T2a, N0, M0
Stage IIB	T2b or T3a, N0, M0
Stage IIIA	T2c or T2d, N0, M0 OR T3b or T3c, N0, M0 OR T4a, N0, M0
Stage IIIB	T3d, N0, M0 OR T4b or T4c, N0, M0
Stage IIIC	T4d or T4e, N0, M0
Stage IV	Any T, N1, M0 OR Any T, any N, M1

Table 2.
AJCC stage grouping.

7. Treatment

The individualized and comprehensive treatment should be applied to UM patients. The appropriate methods or a combination of multiple methods should be selected according to tumor size, location, shape, growth rate, visual acuity of the affected eye and fellow eye, and general conditions. Given that UM is not sensitive to traditional radiochemotherapy (referred to as radiochemotherapy), enucleation was the only and effective treatment, but this operation has caused great damage to the patient's physiology and psychology, seriously affecting the quality of life. With the advancement of science and technology, new types of radiotherapy such as patch radiotherapy and particle radiotherapy can not only effectively kill tumors and preserve eyeballs, but also preserve part of effective vision. Compared with traditional radiotherapy, the local control rate is higher and complications are fewer. Therefore, eye protection therapy represented by patch radiotherapy and particle radiotherapy has become the first-line treatment for UM. Other treatments include transpupillary thermotherapy (TTT), photodynamic therapy (PDT), local resection of ocular tumors, enucleation, orbital content extraction, and immunotherapy.

7.1 Adhesive radiation therapy

Brachytherapy is a type of radiotherapy in which the radiation source is located next to the treatment target. It is the preferred treatment method for small and medium tumors in UM (the maximal diameter of the tumor base is ≤18 mm and the thickness is ≤10 mm). The goal is to deliver a higher localized radiation dose to the tumor with less damage to surrounding tissue. Currently, the radioactive isotopes commonly used in ophthalmology are 106 ruthenium, 125 iodine, 103 palladium, and 131 cesium [41, 42]. Brachytherapy can continue to give a lower radiation dose, and its radiation dose attenuates with distance (radiation dose = $1/(\text{radiation distance})^2$), so the dose distribution is roughly decreasing from the base of the tumor (adjacent to the applicator) to the apex of the tumor [43]. After radiation exposure, tumor cell DNA breaks, cell membrane permeability increases, cell division cycle arrests, cell proliferation decreases, and necrosis and apoptosis occur [44]. The 5-year and 12-year survival rates of the plaster treatment group for medium-volume (thickness 2.5–10 mm and maximal tumor base diameter < 16 mm) tumors reported by the famous Collaborative Ocular Melanoma Study Group (COMS) were 82% and 57% [45], which were no different from those in the enucleation group; at the same time, the 5-year cumulative local recurrence rate and enucleation rate were only 10.3% and 12.5% [46], and 1/3 of the patients could still retain better vision [47]. The main complications of patch radiotherapy are cataract, retinal detachment, glaucoma, radiation retinopathy, radiation optic neuropathy, etc.

7.2 Particle radiation therapy

Unlike previous photon radiotherapy (including X-rays, alpha, beta, and gamma rays released by isotopes, etc.), particle radiotherapy is a radiation therapy that uses charged particles as radiation sources, including protons, carbon ions, helium ions, etc. Particle radiotherapy has the characteristics of the Bragg peak; that is, after the particle beam obtains energy through the accelerator, it is injected into the human body under precise control and the energy is concentratedly released to the lesion, killing the lesion cells, and at the same time, the energy decays sharply and falls back, forming the Bragg peak [48]. Therefore, particle radiation therapy has little damage to surrounding normal tissues. Due to its good targeting, and uniform dose distribution, it becomes the first choice for UM radiation therapy. It is reported that the eye protection rate of proton radiotherapy is above 85%, the 5-year survival rate is above 80% [49–51], and the 5-year local control rate and disease-related survival rate after heavy ion therapy are 92.8% and 82.2% [52]. It is more suitable for the treatment of difficult tumors near the macula or optic disc [53, 54]. Compared with patch radiotherapy, particle radiotherapy represented by protons and heavy ions has a higher local tumor suppression rate and a lower tumor recurrence rate, which provides an important reference for clinicians to choose treatment in the future. Common complications of particle radiotherapy include cataract, retinal detachment, ocular surface changes, glaucoma, macular degeneration, and radiation-induced fundus lesions.

7.3 Transpupillary thermotherapy (TTT)

TTT is a non-invasive treatment. The 810 nm infrared diode laser is delivered to the inside of the choroidal tumor through the pupil, raising the temperature of the tumor to 45–60°C, resulting in vascular occlusion and tumor necrosis in the tumor. The maximal penetration depth of TTT is 4 mm. It is suitable for small tumors with a thickness of <4 mm that are located outside the optic disc and macula or local recurrence after vitrectomy of the entire tumor. It is more effective for choroidal melanoma with a thickness of <2.5 mm. Tumors with a thickness > 3 mm should be treated with patch radiation therapy combined with TTT, that is, “sandwich” therapy. The advantages of TTT include the precise focus of the laser, which can cause immediate necrosis of the tumor and less damage to the surrounding normal choroid. It is easy to operate. The treatment can be completed in an outpatient clinic, and the treatment can be repeated. The disadvantage of TTT is that it is more likely to recur, and potential complications include occlusion of epiretinal membrane and branch retinal vein, retinal stretch, and secondary rhegmatogenous retinal detachment.

7.4 Photodynamic therapy (PDT)

PDT is a non-thermal laser that activates a photosensitizing dye (verteporfin) to induce vascular closure, tumor necrosis, and cell apoptosis, and can be used to treat small choroidal melanoma [55]. However, tumor pigmentation can affect the effectiveness of PDT, so PDT is mainly used in the treatment of small amelanotic choroidal melanoma, adjuvant treatment of radiotherapy, and supplementary treatment after radiotherapy failure.

7.5 Local tumor resection

Local tumor resection was first used for the residual tumor after radiotherapy, and later it was also reported as the first choice for the treatment of UM [56]. There are two types of surgery to remove the entire tumor through an incision in the sclera (excision) and to remove the entire tumor through the vitreous (endectomy). External resection is suitable for iris, ciliary body, and peripheral choroidal melanoma; internal resection is suitable for choroidal melanoma located retroequatorially. Local tumor resection can provide fresh tissue samples for histopathological diagnosis and genetic testing, and preserve the eyeball and vision. During local excision of the tumor, if there is residual tumor on the scleral surface or the tumor is close to the edge of the surgical resection area, radiotherapy can also be supplemented to prevent tumor recurrence. The effect of local tumor resection is usually ideal, but it is difficult and requires high surgical experience and technical requirements for the surgeon.

At present, the routine surgical indications for clinical UM local resection: (a) The maximal diameter of the tumor base is ≤15 mm; (b) the tumor has no local invasion, or involvement of the sclera and orbit; (c) the tumor has no systemic metastasis. Contraindications to surgery: (a) extraocular invasion or distant metastasis of the tumor; (b) general conditions that cannot tolerate surgery; (c) flat diffuse tumors. The main complications of local tumor resection include retinal detachment, proliferative vitreoretinopathy, and hemorrhage.

7.6 Enucleation

Enucleation is required for large and advanced UM (maximal diameter of tumor base >20 mm or thickness > 12 mm), optic nerve involvement or orbital involvement, and/or secondary glaucoma [57].

7.7 Removal of orbital contents

For UM that invaded the orbit, orbital content extraction was used, and the eyelids were preserved as much as possible during the operation to facilitate rapid healing.

7.8 Immunotherapy

In recent years, with the rapid development of immunotherapy, the tumor microenvironment plays a pivotal role in cancer progression and treatment response. A study of the UM tumor microenvironment based on a public database found that people with high-risk UM risk scores were more sensitive to anti-programmed death receptor 1 immunotherapy [58]. Prostaglandin endoperoxide synthase can be used as an immunotherapy target for UM, and its inhibitor, celecoxib, can effectively inhibit UM cell growth and promote tumor cell apoptosis [59].

8. Prognosis

The 20 to 50% of patients with UM eventually die of tumor metastasis. Tumors metastasize through the blood circulation, with the liver taking the first place (64.86%), followed by the skin, stomach, lung, and bone.

Factors affecting the prognosis of patients with UM include: (1) Patient age. Those over 50 years old have a poor prognosis, which may be related to their reduced immune function. Reduced immune defenses in patients may contribute to tumor metastasis. (2) The largest basal diameter of the tumor. The prognosis of tumor base diameter ≤ 12 mm is better than that of >12 mm. The larger the tumor base, the greater the possibility of destroying blood vessels, the greater the contact area with the sclera, the greater the possibility of spreading outside the eyeball, leading to an increased risk of tumor metastasis. (3) The maximal height of the tumor. The prognosis of tumors whose maximal height exceeds 12 mm is significantly worse than that of those less than 12 mm. (4) The location of the tumor. If the front edge of the tumor is located in front of the equator, the prognosis is worse than that in the back of the equator; if the tumor invades the ciliary body further forward, the prognosis is even worse. (5) With or without ball spread. If the tumor invades the scleral duct and scleral wall tissue, its prognosis is poor. (6) Tumor cell type. Cell type is the most important factor influencing the prognosis of UM. The prognosis of the spindle cell type is better, and the prognosis of mixed cell type and epithelioid cell type is poor. Small tumors are often of spindle cell type, while epithelioid and mixed types are dominant in large tumors.

Author details

Songlin Sun[1] and Liang Xu[2*]

1 Department of Orbit, Yuncheng Eye Hospital, Shanxi Medical University, Yuncheng, Shanxi Province, China

2 Research Center for Translational Medicine, Shanghai East Hospital, Tongji University School of Medicine, Shanghai, China

*Address all correspondence to: xuliang_east@126.com

References

[1] Amirouchene-Angelozzi N, Schoumacher M, Stern MH, Cassoux N, Desjardins L, Piperno-Neumann S, et al. Upcoming translational challenges for uveal melanoma. British Journal of Cancer. 2015;**113**:1746

[2] Pandiani C, Béranger GE, Leclerc J, Ballotti R, Bertolotto C. Focus on cutaneous and uveal melanoma specificities. Genes & Development. 2017;**31**:724-743

[3] Yang J, Manson DK, Marr BP, Carvajal RD. Treatment of uveal melanoma: Where are we now. Therapeutic Advanced Medicine Oncology. 2018;**10**:1758834018757175

[4] Kaur J, Malik MA, Gulati R, Azad SV, Goswami S. Genetic determinants of uveal melanoma. Tumour Biology. 2014;**35**:11711-11717

[5] Shields CL, Ganguly A, Bianciotto CG, Turaka K, Tavallali A, Shields JA. Prognosis of uveal melanoma in 500 cases using genetic testing of fine-needle aspiration biopsy specimens. Ophthalmology. 2011;**118**:396-401

[6] Kilic E, Naus NC, van Gils W, Klaver CC, van Til ME, Verbiest MM, et al. Concurrent loss of chromosome arm 1p and chromosome 3 predicts a decreased disease-free survival in uveal melanoma patients. Investigative Ophthalmology & Visual Science. 2005;**46**:2253-2257

[7] Sisley K, Rennie IG, Parsons MA, Jacques R, Hammond DW, Bell SM, et al. Abnormalities of chromosomes 3 and 8 in posterior uveal melanoma correlate with prognosis. Genes, Chromosomes & Cancer. 1997;**19**:22-28

[8] Parrella P, Sidransky D, Merbs SL. Allelotype of posterior uveal melanoma: Implications for a bifurcated tumor progression pathway. Cancer Research. 1999;**59**:3032-3037

[9] Gill HS, Char DH. Uveal melanoma prognostication: From lesion size and cell type to molecular class. Canadian Journal of Ophthalmology. 2012;**47**:246-253

[10] Onken MD, Worley LA, Ehlers JP, Harbour JW. Gene expression profiling in uveal melanoma reveals two molecular classes and predicts metastatic death. Cancer Research. 2004;**64**:7205-7209

[11] Harbour JW. A prognostic test to predict the risk of metastasis in uveal melanoma based on a 15-gene expression profile. Methods in Molecular Biology. 2014;**1102**:427-440

[12] Ewens KG, Kanetsky PA, Richards-Yutz J, Purrazzella J, Shields CL, Ganguly T, et al. Chromosome 3 status combined with BAP1 and EIF1AX mutation profiles are associated with metastasis in uveal melanoma. Investigative Ophthalmology & Visual Science. 2014;**55**:5160-5167

[13] Koopmans AE, Verdijk RM, Brouwer RW, van den Bosch TP, van den Berg MM, Vaarwater J, et al. Clinical significance of immunohistochemistry for detection of BAP1 mutations in uveal melanoma. Modern Pathology. 2014;**27**:1321-1330

[14] Decatur CL, Ong E, Garg N, Anbunathan H, Bowcock AM, Field MG, et al. Driver mutations in uveal Melanoma: Associations with gene expression profile and patient outcomes. JAMA Ophthalmology. 2016;**134**:728-733

[15] Yavuzyigitoglu S, Drabarek W, Smit KN, van Poppelen N, Koopmans AE, Vaarwater J, et al. Correlation of gene mutation status with copy number profile in uveal Melanoma. Ophthalmology. 2017;**124**:573-575

[16] Van Raamsdonk CD, Griewank KG, Crosby MB, Garrido MC, Vemula S, Wiesner T, et al. Mutations in GNA11 in uveal melanoma. The New England Journal of Medicine. 2010;**363**:2191-2199

[17] Xiaolin X, Bin WW, Bin L, Fei G, Zhibao Z, Jonas JB. Oncogenic GNAQ and GNA11 mutations in uveal melanoma in Chinese. PLoS One. 2014;**9**:e109699

[18] Chen X, Wu Q, Tan L, Porter D, Jager MJ, Emery C, et al. Combined PKC and MEK inhibition in uveal melanoma with GNAQ and GNA11 mutations. Oncogene. 2014;**33**:4724-4734

[19] Yu F, Luo J, Mo J, Liu G, Kim YC, Meng Z, et al. Mutant Gq/11 promote uveal Melanoma tumorigenesis by activating YAP. Cancer Cell. 2014;**25**:822-830

[20] Feng X, Degese MS, Iglesias-Bartolome R, Vaque JP, Molinolo AA, Rodrigues M, et al. Hippo-independent activation of YAP by the GNAQ uveal Melanoma oncogene through a trio-regulated rho GTPase Signaling circuitry. Cancer Cell. 2014;**25**:831-845

[21] Thomas W, Obenauf AC, Rajmohan M, Isabella F, Griewank KG, Peter U, et al. Germline mutations in BAP1 predispose to melanocytic tumors. Nature Genetics. 2011;**43**:1018-1021

[22] Onken MD, Worley LA, Char DH, Augsburger JJ, Correa ZM, Nudleman E, et al. Collaborative ocular oncology group report number 1: Prospective validation of a multi-gene prognostic assay in uveal Melanoma. Ophthalmology. 2012;**119**:1596-1603

[23] Harbour JW, Onken MD, Roberson ED, Duan S, Cao L, Worley LA, et al. Frequent mutation of BAP1 in metastasizing uveal melanomas. Science. 2010;**330**:1410-1413

[24] Neil F, Sophie T, Coupland SE, Coulson JM, Sacco JJ, Yamini K, et al. Patterns of BAP1 protein expression provide insights into prognostic significance and the biology of uveal melanoma. The Journal of Pathology. Clinical Research. 2018;**4**:26-38

[25] William HJ, Roberson EDO, Hima A, Onken MD, Worley LA, Bowcock AM. Recurrent mutations at codon 625 of the splicing factor SF3B1 in uveal melanoma. Nature Genetics. 2013;**45**:133-135

[26] Smit KN, van Poppelen NM, Jolanda V, Robert V, van Marion R, Helen K, et al. Combined mutation and copy-number variation detection by targeted next-generation sequencing in uveal melanoma. Modern Pathology. 2018;**31**:763-771

[27] Coupland SE, Thornton S, Kalirai H. Importance of partial losses of chromosome 3 in uveal Melanoma in the BAP1 gene region. JAMA Ophthalmology. 2020;**138**:188-189

[28] Figueiredo CR, Helen K, Sacco JJ, Azevedo RA, Andrew D, Slupsky JR, et al. Loss of BAP1 expression is associated with an immunosuppressive microenvironment in uveal melanoma, with implications for immunotherapy development. The Journal of Pathology. 2020;**250**:420-439

[29] Hongrun Z, Helen K, Amelia A, Xiaoyun Y, Yalin Z, Coupland SE. Piloting a deep learning model for predicting nuclear BAP1 Immunohistochemical expression of uveal Melanoma from Hematoxylin-and-eosin sections. Science and Technology. 2020;**9**:50

[30] Marcel M, Lars M, Petra T, Sven R, Claudia M, Norbert B, et al. Exome sequencing identifies recurrent somatic mutations in EIF1AX and SF3B1 in uveal melanoma with disomy 3. Nature Genetics. 2013;**45**:933-936

[31] Shuai W, Mei H, Chao Z. Overexpression of microRNA-130a represses uveal melanoma cell migration and invasion through inactivation of the Wnt/β-catenin signaling pathway by downregulating USP6. Cancer Gene Therapy. 2022;**29**:930-939

[32] Lu L, Yu X, Zhang L, Ding X, Pan H, Wen X, et al. The long non-coding RNA RHPN1-AS1 promotes uveal Melanoma progression. International Journal of Molecular Sciences. 2017;**18**:226

[33] Yao L, Mingmei Z, Huayin F, Shaya M. The tumorigenic properties of EZH2 are mediated by MiR-26a in uveal melanoma. Frontiers in Molecular Biosciences. 2021;**8**:713542

[34] Shields CL, Marco P, Ferenczy SR, Shields JA. Enhanced depth imaging optical coherence tomography of intraocular tumors: from placid to seasick to rock and rolling topography--the 2013 Francesco Orzalesi Lecture. Retina. 2014;**34**:1495-1512

[35] Shields CL, Say EAT, Samara WA, Khoo CTL, Arman M, Shields JA. Optical coherence tomography angiography of the macula after plaque radiotherapy of choroidal melanoma: Comparison of irradiated versus nonirradiated eyes in 65 patients. Retina. 2016;**36**:1493-1505

[36] Lucia CM, Vittoria MM, Antonietta BM, Gianluigi P, Grazia SM, Luca I, et al. A prospective analysis of ^{18}F-FDG PET/CT in patients with uveal melanoma: Comparison between metabolic rate of glucose (MRglu) and standardized uptake value (SUV) and correlations with histopathological features. European Journal of Nuclear Medicine and Molecular Imaging. 2013;**40**:1682-1691

[37] Singh AD, Tero K. The collaborative ocular melanoma study. Ophthalmology Clinics of North America. 2005;**18**: 129-142

[38] Amin MB, Edge SB, Greene FL, Byrd DR, Brookland RK, Washington MK, et al., editors. AJCC Cancer Staging Manual. 8th ed. Chicago IL: American Joint Committee on Cancer, Springer; 2017

[39] Kivelä T, Simpson ER, Grossniklaus HE, Jager MJ, Singh AD, Caminal JM, et al., editors. Uveal Melanoma in AJCC Cancer Staging Manual, Chicago IL. 8th ed. Chicago IL: American Joint Committee on Cancer, Springer; 2017. pp. 813-825

[40] Amin MB, Greene FL, Edge SB, Compton CC, Gershenwald JE, Brookland RK, et al. The eighth edition AJCC Cancer staging manual: Continuing to build a bridge from a population-based to a more "personalized" approach to cancer staging. CA: a Cancer Journal for Clinicians. 2017;**67**:93-99

[41] The COMS randomized trial of iodine 125 brachytherapy for choroidal melanoma: V. Twelve-year mortality rates and prognostic factors: COMS report No. 28. Archives of ophthalmology (Chicago, Ill. : 1960). 2006;**124**:1684-1693

[42] Chang MY, McCannel TA. Local treatment failure after globe-conserving therapy for choroidal melanoma. The British Journal of Ophthalmology. 2013;**97**:804-811

[43] Wang Z, Nabhan M, Schild SE, Stafford SL, Petersen IA, Foote RL, et al. Charged particle radiation therapy for

uveal melanoma: A systematic review and Meta-analysis. International Journal of Radiation Oncology, Biology, Physics. 2013;**86**:18-26

[44] Groenewald C, Konstantinidis L, Damato B. Effects of Radiotherapy on Uveal Melanomas and Adjacent Tissues: Eye. London, England; 2013. p. 27

[45] DienerWest M, Earle JD, Fine SL, Hawkins BS, Moy CS, Reynolds SM, et al. The COMS Randomized Trial of Iodine 125 Brachytherapy for Choroidal Melanoma, III: Initial Mortality Findings: COMS Report No. 18. Archives of Ophthalmology. 2001;**119**:969-982

[46] Jampol LM, Moy CS, Murray TG, Reynolds SM, Albert DM, Schachat AP, et al. The COMS randomized trial of iodine 125 brachytherapy for choroidal melanoma. Ophthalmology. 2020;**127**:S148-S157

[47] Melia BM, Abramson DH, Albert DM, Boldt HC, Earle JD, Hanson WF, et al. Collaborative ocular melanoma study (COMS) randomized trial of I-125 brachytherapy for medium choroidal melanoma. Ophthalmology. 2001;**108**:348-366

[48] Laurence D, Livia LR, Christine L, Nathalie C, Remi D, Alexandro M, et al. Treatment of uveal melanoma by accelerated proton beam. Developments in Ophthalmology. 2012;**49**:41-57

[49] Lane AM, Kim IK, Gragoudas ES. Long-term risk of Melanoma-related mortality for patients with uveal Melanoma treated with proton beam therapy. JAMA Ophthalmology. 2015;**133**:792-796

[50] Juliette T, Sophie J, Jean-Pierre C, Celia M, Stéphanie B, Gaelle A, et al. Cataract avoidance with proton therapy in ocular melanomas. Investigative Ophthalmology & Visual Science. 2017;**58**:5378-5386

[51] David B, Pascal R, Laurent K, Thibaud M, Minh NA, Joël H, et al. 20-year assessment of metastatic latency and subsequent time to death after proton therapy for uveal melanomas. Melanoma Research. 2020;**30**:272-278

[52] Toyama S, Tsuji H, Mizoguchi N, Nomiya T, Kamada T, Tokumaru S, et al. Long-term results of carbon ion radiation therapy for locally advanced or Unfavorably located choroidal Melanoma: Usefulness of CT-based 2-port orthogonal therapy for reducing the incidence of Neovascular Glaucoma. International Journal of Radiation Oncology, Biology, Physics. 2013;**86**:270-276

[53] Caroline B, Valerie O, Mary D, Moya C, Giuseppe G, Susan K, et al. Uveal Melanoma in Ireland. Occultation Oncology Pathology. 2019;**5**:195-204

[54] Rumana H, Moritz HF, Heinrich H. OCT changes in peri-tumour normal retina following ruthenium-106 and proton beam radiotherapy for uveal melanoma. The British Journal of Ophthalmology. 2021;**105**:648-652

[55] Turkoglu EB, Renelle P, Arman M, Shields CL. Photodynamic therapy AS primary treatment for small choroidal melanoma. Retina. 2019;**39**:1319-1325

[56] Damato B, Groenewald C, McGalliard J, Wong D. Endoresection of choroidal melanoma. The British Journal of Ophthalmology. 1998;**82**:213-218

[57] Chandrani C, Won KD, Gombos DS, Junna O, Yong Q, Williams MD, et al. Uveal melanoma: From diagnosis to treatment and the science in between. Cancer. 2016;**122**:2299-2312

[58] Qianwen G, Qi W, Anqi L, Yubin Y, Xiangyu D, Lei L, et al. Development and validation of an immune and stromal prognostic signature in uveal melanoma to guide clinical therapy. Aging (Albany NY). 2020;**12**:20254-20267

[59] Zhenxi Z, Jingyu S, Li L, Wenjing D. Identification of precise therapeutic targets and characteristic prognostic genes based on immune gene characteristics in uveal melanoma. Frontiers in Cell Developmental Biology. 2021;**9**:666462

Chapter 7

Retinal Dysfunction Caused by Autoimmune Mechanisms

Toshiaki Hirakata

Abstract

Autoimmune retinal disorders have been identified, including acute zonal occult outer retinopathy (AZOOR), AZOOR complex, autoimmune retinopathy (AIR) comprising paraneoplastic AIR (pAIR), cancer-associated retinopathy (CAR), melanoma-associated retinopathy (MAR), and non-paraneoplastic AIR (npAIR). Patients with autoimmune retinal disorders typically present with sudden or acute onset of photopsia, photophobia, night blindness, rapid visual loss, and visual field abnormalities. The combination of multimodal imaging and electrophysiology is crucial because these diseases are challenging to diagnose. In particular, electroretinograms (ERGs) are essential for diagnosis. However, no treatment has been established to date. Additionally, a case of inner retinal dysfunction, thought to be a type of AIR, was recently reported. The diagnosis is difficult because most cases occur in one eye, and although the patient complains of severe photophobia, retinal imaging is almost normal, vision is preserved and there is almost no progression. The ERG is very characteristic, with cone-rod dysfunction and negative ERG. This chapter describes in detail the characteristics of AZOOR, AIR, and acute inner retinal dysfunction as new phenotypes of AIR.

Keywords: acute zonal occult outer retinopathy, autoimmune retinopathy, cancer-associated retinopathy, melanoma-associated retinopathy, electroretinogram, bipolar cell

1. Introduction

Retinal diseases related to autoimmunity include acute zonal occult outer retinopathy (AZOOR), AZOOR-associated diseases, and autoimmune retinopathy (AIR). These disease conditions are often difficult to diagnose even with the recent retinal imaging tests that have been developed, and it is crucial to combine retinal electrophysiological tests and systemic examinations in treating these diseases. The pathogenesis of these diseases remains unclear and they have no established treatment; however, it has been suggested that often-identified anti-retinal antibodies may play a key role.

Although previous reports have shown that autoimmune-mediated retinopathies often involve the outer retinal layers, current studies have revealed a rare type of retinopathy involving the inner retinal layers. Since it is difficult to diagnose this type of retinopathy using retinal imaging examinations, the use of electroretinograms (ERGs) is important. In this chapter, AZOOR and AIR are reviewed, and this unusual disease type is discussed.

2. AZOOR

AZOOR was first described by J.D. Gass in 1993 [1], and he described it as a disease characterized by the sudden onset of subjective scotomas and photopsia due to loss of areas of the outer retina with a normal fundus aspect [2]. The aggregated data on AZOOR show that it affects young to middle-aged patients, is largely predominant in women, and starts with an acute onset of visual field defects in one or both eyes combined with photopsia, decreased contrast sensitivity, and photophobia [3, 4].

The diagnosis of AZOOR is challenging, and the differential diagnosis includes AIR, syphilitic outer retinopathy, retinal dystrophy, uveitis, and optic nerve disease. Therefore, comprehensive retinal imaging examinations, especially optical coherence tomography (OCT), electroretinograms (ERGs), and systemic examinations, are vital for correct diagnosis.

2.1 Patient demographics

According to studies, the majority of patients with AZOOR are women. Monson et al. reported that 76% of patients with AZOOR were women (n = 99) and 24% were men (n = 31) in 130 published cases [4]. Similarly, Gass et al. demonstrated that women (37 cases, 73%) were more often affected than men (14 cases, 27%) [2]. Saito et al. also reported that among Japanese patients, the population of females (n = 31, 81.6%) with AZOOR was higher than the male (n = 7, 18.4%) [5].

Additionally, most patients with AZOOR are young to middle-aged individuals. The average age at presentation of 103 published AZOOR cases was 36.7 years, with an age range of 13 to 79 years [4]. The median age of 51 patients with AZOOR was 33 years (mean, 36 years; range 13–63 years), and the mean presumed age of AZOOR onset was 33.2 ± 8.7 years (range, 15–47 years), including in Caucasian (39 cases, 91%), Hispanic (3 cases, 7%), and Asian (1 case, 2%) [2]. In 38 Japanese patients with AZOOR, the mean presumed age of AZOOR onset was 33.2 ± 8.7 years (range, 15–47 years) [5].

2.2 Symptoms

Patients presented with acute vision loss affecting one or more zones of the visual field in one or both eyes usually experience photopsia [2, 4, 5]. Moreover, patients occasionally suffer from photophobia and night blindness. Scotomas are often described as dark blind spots or zones involving one or several aspects of the visual field. Interestingly, most patients reported worsening visual function under brightly illuminated conditions, and the temporal relationship between photopsia and visual field defects varied.

2.3 Visual acuity and visual field

Although most patients retained visual acuity of 20/20, the course and severity of AZOOR may vary by race. Saito et al. reported that the final best-corrected visual acuity (BCVA) (logMAR; logarithm of the minimum angle of resolution) was 0.0 or less in 85% of Japanese patients [5]. In contrast, Gass et al. reported that final visual acuity of 39%, 29%, and 10% of the eyes was between 20/10 and 20/20, 20/25 and 20/40, and worse than 4/200, respectively [2].

Moreover, blind spot enlargement and central scotoma can sometimes be observed using visual field tests [2]. Visual field defects remain stable when the disease stabilizes within 4–6 months; however, it can progress in some patients [4].

2.4 Findings in slit lamp test and ophthalmoscopy

A relative afferent pupillary defect was found in 21% of 131 patients with AZOOR [4], and 23.5% of 51 eyes of Japanese patients with AZOOR [5]. Specific abnormalities of the anterior segment are rarely observed in AZOOR, whereas vitreous cells are sometimes observed [2, 4, 5]. Gass et al. suggested that patients without cellular infiltration of the vitreous were more likely to recover vision and less likely to develop clinically apparent retinal pathology [2].

2.5 Multimodal imaging

In most cases, the fundus is normal at initial presentation; however, retinal pigment epithelial (RPE) changes are occasionally observed [2, 4, 5]. Notably, after long-term follow-up, fundus changes, including diffuse retinal, choroidal atrophy resembling retinitis pigmentosa (RP), regional retinal, choroidal atrophy, follicular macular edema, and leukocoria of the retinal vessels are increasingly observed.

OCT is one of the essential ophthalmic examinations for AZOOR diagnosis [6–8], and it shows irregularities of the outer retinal line, including missing or obscured ellipsoid zone (EZ) and the absence of interdigitation zones (IZ). Spaide et al. reported that OCT images showed loss of the EZ, loss of the outer nuclear layer, and thinning of the inner nuclear layer, which could be correlated with the area of visual field loss [9]. Notably, it is crucial to observe the outer retinal layers at the highest possible resolution in OCT.

Adaptive optics scanning laser ophthalmoscopy (AOSLO) revealed focal abnormal cone reflectivity and cone loss regions in patients with AZOOR, corresponding to visual field defects and reduced multifocal electroretinogram (mfERG) responses [10].

Fluorescein angiography (FA) and indocyanine green angiography (ICGA) show abnormalities [5, 11]. FA sometimes shows optic disc and retinal vascular wall staining with leakage in the late phase and hyperfluorescent punctate lesions, while ICGA occasionally indicates diffuse choroidal hyperfluorescence from the posterior pole to the mid-peripheral region during the middle phase. ICGA revealed punctate patchy hypofluorescence at the posterior pole to the mid-peripheral region and hyperfluorescence along the choroidal middle or large vessels.

2.6 ERG change

Electroretinograms (ERGs) are essential for the diagnosis of AZOOR. AZOORs frequently have a strong cone response reduction when comparing rod and cone responses in full-field ERGs; hence, detailed observation of cone and 30-Hz flicker responses is helpful for diagnosis [12]. The severity of the ERG abnormalities varied and generally correlated with the degree of visual field loss. Patients with bilateral AZOOR frequently demonstrated asymmetry in the affected parameters [2].

Moreover, mfERG may be essential for AZOOR diagnosis. Full-field ERG sometimes shows normal results, which may be due to a narrow AZOOR lesion area or mild severity of AZOOR. However, mfERG shows a decrease in the near fixation point or diffuse reduction [13]. Saito et al. showed a normal amplitude in more than half of the patients with single-flash full-field ERG, and there were noticeably reduced mfERG responses corresponding to visual field loss in all eyes examined [5]. Since mfERG reflects retinal function, it is useful for differentiating AZOOR from optic nerve disease near the central visual field.

2.7 Pathophysiology

The etiology of AZOOR is speculative, including the hypothesis of the involvement of an unknown infective viral agent with subsequent autoimmune alteration of photoreceptors. Indeed, some patients reported flu-like symptoms before the onset of AZOOR [5], and the development of AZOOR after hepatitis B vaccination, a Mantoux skin test, and a tick bite has been reported [4].

Patients with AZOOR often have a history of autoimmune disease. Gass et al. reported that 28% of 51 patients with AZOOR with long-term follow-up had a history of experiencing autoimmune diseases, including Hashimoto's disease, multiple sclerosis, transverse myelopathy, Addison's disease, myasthenia gravis, Graves' disease, diabetes, CREST syndrome, and Sjogren syndrome [2].

Based on previous reports, there are two possible hypotheses regarding the mechanism of AZOOR [14]. The first hypothesis is that choroidal circulatory impairment is involved in the pathogenesis of AZOOR [15]. Notably, ICGA has revealed hypofluorescence in areas related or unrelated to AZOOR lesions [5, 11, 15]. Subfoveal choroidal thickness in the AZOOR-affected area decreased significantly as the AZOOR condition improved, suggesting that this anatomic change is correlated with functional recovery [16]. Moreover, in AZOOR-affected eyes, the choroid flow velocity in the affected area significantly increased along with improved visual functions [15]. The choriocapillaris supplies oxygen and nutrition to the outer retinal layers, and OCT images in AZOOR clearly show abnormalities in the outer retinal layers [9]. However, whether the pathogenesis begins with a choroidal circulation disorder remains unclear. The second hypothesis was that anti-retinal antibodies trigger AZOOR onset. Several anti-retinal antibodies are detected in patients with AZOOR [14, 17]. However, the relationship between AZOOR and disease pathology and severity has not yet been clearly proven. The relationship between AZOOR and anti-retinal antibodies is discussed in more detail in the next section.

2.8 AZOOR and anti-retinal antibody

The detection of retinal autoantibodies has been reported in the sera of patients with AZOOR. However, it is unclear how retinal autoantibodies are involved in AZOOR pathogenesis. A previous report showed anti-retinal antibody activity against a 45 kDa antigen in one patient with AZOOR [10]. In 18 Chinese patients with AZOOR, all (100%) were detected with anti-retinal antibodies from serum samples by western blot assay, including recoverin, α-enolase, carbonic anhydrase II, and collapsin response-mediated protein 5 [17]. In contrast, the report detected anti-retinal antibodies in presumed AIR (78.2%), patients with RP (35.0%), bilateral uveitis (63.3%), and healthy donors (33.3%).

Hashimoto et al. assessed the clinical characteristics of patients with AZOOR according to the presence or absence of anti-retinal antibodies [14]. They detected autoantibodies for recoverin, carbonic anhydrase II, and α-enolase in the serum of 33 patients with AZOOR using immunoblot analysis, and at least one serum anti-retinal antibody was detected in 42% of these patients. Interestingly, there were no significant differences in clinical factors between patients with AZOOR who exhibited anti-retinal antibodies and those who did not, including BCVA and mean deviation, a-wave amplitude on single-flash electroretinography, and frequencies of improvement of the macular ellipsoid zone and AZOOR recurrence.

2.9 Treatment

Currently, there is no established treatment for AZOOR. Owing to the presumed involvement of autoimmunity and inflammation in the pathogenesis of AZOOR, systemic corticosteroids are often administered intravenously or orally, especially in severe cases of AZOOR. Some reports have shown successful cases of the treatment of AZOOR using systemic steroids and/or immunosuppressive agents [18, 19]. A study reported the efficacy of intravitreal injection of Ozurdex (corticosteroid) in a patient with AZOOR whose vision did not improve after initial treatment with systemic corticosteroids and calcium channel blockers, which was consistent with the recovered ellipsoid zone disruption [20].

Chiba et al. reported that infliximab was effective in treating retinitis similar to AZOOR in a patient with ulcerative colitis [21]. Takeuchi et al. reported a case of disruption of the external limiting membrane (ELM), EZ, and IZ shown on the spectral domain (SD)-OCT, such as AZOOR in Behcet's disease-associated uveitis reconstituted by continuous infliximab treatment, which led to the improvement of visual acuity [22]. These findings reveal the importance of carefully examining background factors and drug administration.

However, Gass et al. found no difference in final visual function between patients treated and those not treated with corticosteroids [2]. It is unclear whether the recovery was spontaneous or due to the effects of steroids. Further clarification of the pathogenesis of AZOOR and the establishment of treatment for AZOOR are required in the future.

3. Autoimmune retinopathy

AIR is an acquired retinal dysfunction caused by anti-retinal antibodies. It was first described in 1976 by Sawyer et al. when degenerative retinopathies were diagnosed in three elderly females with bronchial carcinoma following the onset of symptoms, including transitory visual obscuration and visual field loss [23]. AIR is usually characterized by bilateral, sudden progressive, painless visual deterioration, scotomas, visual field defects, and retinal (photoreceptor) dysfunction. Despite several years of studies, the underdiagnosis of AIR, a rare inflammatory condition that can lead to blindness, persists. The diagnosis of AIR is challenging and often delayed owing to its rarity and variety of clinical manifestations, including an unrevealing examination in many early stages [24].

AIR can be divided into two main forms: presumed non-paraneoplastic AIR (npAIR) and paraneoplastic AIR. The first category is probably the most prevalent and unrelated to cancer, while the second includes cancer-associated retinopathy (CAR) and melanoma-associated retinopathy (MAR).

3.1 Patient demographic

However, there is a lack of population-based epidemiological studies on AIR. CAR and npAIR occur predominantly in females (63–66%), whereas MAR occurs more frequently in men [24, 25]. Additionally, histories of autoimmune disease are common among patients with npAIR [24, 26]. The combined AIR group (CAR and npAIR with or without cystoid macular edema) had a median age of 51 years (range, 11–85 years) [27]. One large case series of 141 patients with npAIR reported a younger mean age at presentation (55.9 years) than that of another report for patients with paraneoplastic AIR, including CAR and MAR [28].

Essential elements for the diagnosis of npAIR include no evidence of malignancy after a thorough work-up, absence of degenerative eye diseases such as RP, a positive screen for serum anti-retinal antibodies, and an abnormality in ERG findings with or without visual field abnormalities [26]. Additionally, supportive criteria included the presence of symptoms, including photopsia, scotomas, nyctalopia or photo aversion, and dyschromatopsia.

3.2 Symptoms

AIR is usually characterized by bilateral, sudden progressive, painless visual deterioration, scotomas, visual field defects, and retinal (photoreceptor) dysfunction. Patients are typically presented with subacute vision loss, scotomas, photopsia, photophobia, night blindness, and dyschromatopsia [26]. Notably, the disease is usually bilateral but can be asymmetric.

3.3 Visual acuity and visual field

Visual acuity can be quite good in the early stages of the disease [26, 29], and visual field tests reveal constriction and central or paracentral scotomas. However, severe cases can lead to blindness and rapid disease progression. The course of vision condition depends on whether npAIR, CAR or MAR, and the type of retinal autoantibody.

3.4 Multimodal imaging

Fundus ophthalmoscopy shows normal or minimal changes in the early stages of AIR, and the fundus may appear unremarkable or demonstrate retinal vascular attenuation, diffuse retinal atrophy, RPE changes, and waxy disc pallor [26]. OCT can reveal cystoid macular edema, typically in the form of cystic spaces. Moreover, fundus autofluorescence (FAF) shows an abnormal autofluorescence pattern, primarily in the form of a hyperautofluorescent ring in the parafoveal region [30], in which OCT shows loss of ISE and thinning of the outer nuclear layer [31]. FA is performed to exclude other potential causes of vision loss [32]. Because AIR often shows the retinal artery attenuation, retinal ischemic diseases such as retinal artery occlusion should be ruled out by FA.

3.5 Electroretinogram

ERGs are essential ophthalmic examinations used for the diagnosis of AIR, and the full-field ERG, conducted under various conditions, provides information about activity in the rod and cone systems and other neural elements. The mfERG indicates the topographical location of the disease within the retina, while the electro-oculogram (EOG) provides a measurement of the integrity of the RPE layer [31, 33]. In particular, in early cases, more severe ERG changes in the presence of relatively normal retinas or larger visual field sizes contribute to AIR diagnosis [29].

Full-field ERG can show abnormalities in the dark- or light-adapted responses, bipolar cell responses, or a combination of these responses [27], and negative waveforms were often observed [29]. Moreover, different electroretinographic patterns help differentiate between diseases affecting different retinal layers and cell types [31].

3.6 Cancer-associated retinopathy

CAR was first described in three elderly females with bronchial carcinoma in 1976 [23], and it is characterized by sudden and progressive loss of vision associated with photosensitivity, reduced visual acuity, defects in color vision, constriction of visual fields, ring scotoma, and attenuated retinal arterioles [34]. It affects the photoreceptors, cones, and rods. A review of 209 patients with CAR and MAR reported a mean age of 65 years (range, 24–85 years) at diagnosis, with twice as many women affected as men [34]. Major cancer was associated with included breast (16%), lung (16%), melanoma (16%), hematological (15%; such as lymphomas, leukemias, and myelomas), gynecological (9%), prostate (7%), and colon (6%) cancers. Importantly, some patients were diagnosed with cancer during a systemic examination after AIR was presented. A systemic search is crucial when AIR is suspected, notwithstanding the rarity. Although most CAR is bilateral, some are unilateral [35].

3.7 Melanoma-associated retinopathy

MAR is a rare paraneoplastic autoimmune manifestation of malignant melanomas, and the first MAR case was reported in 1988 by Berson and Lessell [36]. MAR is typically defined as the following triad: (i) symptoms of night blindness (nyctalopia), positive visual phenomena, or visual field defects; (ii) ERG findings of a reduction in b-wave amplitude; and (iii) presence of serum autoantibodies that are reactive with retinal bipolar cells [37].

Melanomas express rhodopsin, transducin, recoverin, arrestin, and other phototransduction proteins [38]. Furthermore, when sera and IgG fractions are tested using indirect immunofluorescence, autoantibodies against a melanoma antigen are observed, which cross-react with bipolar cells of the retina [39]. Transient receptor potential cation channel subfamily M member 1 (TRPM1), also known as melastatin, is a member of the melastatin-related transient receptor channel family. Notably, TRPM1 was originally identified as a candidate gene for melanoma metastasis suppression [40].

Previous studies have revealed a relationship between MAR, anti-TRPM1 antibody, and ON bipolar cells. Staining of mouse and primate retinas with MAR sera revealed immunoreactivity in all types of ON bipolar cells, while MAR serum did not stain ON bipolar cells in *Trpm1*$^{-/-}$ mice [41]. Ueno et al. injected serum including anti-TRPM1 antibodies from a patient intravitreally into mice, and then ERGs of the mice were altered acutely, and the shape of the ERGs, including rod response disappearance, negative ERG, and severely affected cone response resembled that of the patient [42].

Immunohistochemical analysis of the eyes injected with serum showed immunoreactivity against bipolar cells only in wild-type animals and not in TRPM1 knockout mice, which was consistent with the serum containing anti-TRPM1 antibodies [42].

Histology also showed that some of the bipolar cells were apoptotic 5 h after the injection in wild-type mice; however, no bipolar cell death was found in TRPM1 knockout mice. At 3 months, the inner nuclear layer was thinner, and the amplitudes of the ERGs remained reduced. These results indicated that the serum of a patient with MAR contained an antibody against TRPM1, which caused acute death of retinal ON bipolar cells in mice.

Patients with MAR suffer from night blindness, photophobia, and bilateral photopsia, and unilateral cases have also been reported though it is rare [43]. Visual acuity and color vision are relatively preserved [44]; however, decreased color discrimination has been reported.

Fundal examination results are usually normal at the onset. Nevertheless, studies have reported some abnormal findings, including white or atrophic retinal spots or diffuse retinal pigment epithelium loss [37, 45, 46]. Moreover, MAR is associated with different patterns of visual field loss, including central and paracentral scotomas, generalized depression or constriction of the peripheral field, and arcuate defects [37, 47].

ERGs are among the most vital ophthalmic examinations that reflect ON bipolar cell dysfunction. The typical ERG pattern is a normal photopic response and markedly reduced scotopic response [48], the rod responses of the ERGs are absent, and the bright-flash ERGs are electronegative. Additionally, ON responses of focal macular ERGs and full-field long-flash ERGs are absent.

3.8 Anti-retinal antibody

The demonstration of anti-retinal antibodies is crucial for the diagnosis of AIR [27]. They can be detected using western blotting, immunohistochemistry, or enzyme-linked immunosorbent assay (ELISA). Possible causes for the generation of autoantibodies that react with retinal antigens include antimicrobial responses (infection) against similar antigens released after infection, antitumor responses (tumor) against upregulated similar proteins, or anti-retinal responses to released sequestered proteins (retinal injury) from dying retinal cells [49].

Notably, autoantibodies may trigger retinal degeneration, exacerbate the degenerative process in response to the release of sequestered antigens, and influence disease progression.

Numerous retinal autoantibodies have been reported to be involved in both npAIR and pAIR. Antibodies against recoverin [50], the inner plexiform layer [51], the inner retinal layer (35-kDa antibody against retinal Müller cell–associated antigen) [52], α-enolase [28, 53], carbonic anhydrase II [54], and rod transducin-α [55, 56] have been described in npAIR. Moreover, antibodies against recoverin [57, 58], enolase [59, 60], tubby-like protein 1 (TULP1) [61], heat shock cognate protein 70 (HSC 70) [62], carbonic anhydrase II [63] have been described in CAR. Autoantibodies against bestrophin [64], Transient receptor potential cation channel, subfamily M, member 1 (TRPM1, also known as melastatin 1 or MLSN1) [41, 65, 66], aldolase A and C [46], and interphotoreceptor retinoid-binding protein [67] have been found in MAR.

Considering the great diversity of anti-retinal antibodies, it is likely that some antibodies have a greater pathogenic potential than others. Anti-recoverin-associated CAR progresses to severe vision loss, often to no light perception [68, 69]. Andoh et al. reported that logMAR BCVA at the final visit was 0.0 or less in 18 eyes (37%), and compared with baseline, the final LogMAR BCVA of 37 eyes (76%) stably maintained vision [53]. They classified α-enolase-positive patients with AIR into three groups as follows: multiple drusen (48%), retinal degeneration (36%), and normal fundus

(16%). Their study showed no significant differences in the initial or final BCVA between the drusen and degeneration groups.

3.9 Treatment

AIR can progress rapidly and cause diffuse retinal degeneration; therefore, its early diagnosis and treatment are critical to lowering the risk of irreversible immunological damage to retinal cells [24]. Many clinicians aim to modulate the immune system and reduce autoimmune attacks on the retina before irreversible damage occurs [70]. Various immunomodulatory approaches have been tried because of the presumed autoimmune nature of AIR; however, the evidence base for therapeutic intervention comprises only a small number of retrospective case series and case reports, and there is no established treatment protocol for CAR, MAR, or presumed npAIR.

Generally, AIR is suggested, to begin with, steroids (local or systemic) and/or with antimetabolites/T-cell inhibitors as the first or second-line treatment, respectively [24, 27, 71]. In a cohort of 24 patients with npAIR who received therapy of various combinations of prednisone, cyclosporine, azathioprine, mycophenolate mofetil, and periocular or intravitreal steroid injections, 15 of the 24 (62.5%) patients showed varying degrees of improvement in visual acuity or visual field, and cystoid macular edema improved in approximately half of them [27].

The best approach for pAIR is to reduce the tumor burden through surgery, chemotherapy, or radiation, as applicable [26]. However, the removal of cancer alone may not be sufficient to affect the course of CAR [72]. Intravenous methylprednisolone has been frequently used as a more effective treatment than oral steroids for the initiation of treatment [73, 74]. Contrastly, Mizobuchi et al. reported the effectiveness of oral prednisolone therapy in patients with CAR who exhibited progressive retinal degeneration [75]. Despite the aggressive immunomodulatory therapy, some patients still progress to experience significant vision loss [68].

Notably, it is important to make an early diagnosis based on ophthalmologic and systemic examinations and early treatment intervention. Further clarification of the pathogenesis of AIR will lead to the development of more effective treatment methods.

4. Acute inner retinal dysfunction

AIR often affects the outer retinal layers; however, recently, a rare type of AIR has been reported, which damages the inner retinal layers is suspected. Moreover, Hirakata et al. reported eight cases of unilateral retinopathy [76], Kido et al. reported four cases [77], and Ueno et al. reported three cases of bilateral retinopathy [78]. All these cases have been reported in Japan. ERGs are essential for AIR diagnosis because vision is preserved, and there are virtually no changes in fundus photographs or OCT. Although the cause of the disease remains known, retinal autoantibodies have been detected in several cases, indicating it is acquired, acute at onset, and autoimmune-related to its pathogenesis. Interestingly, the affected eyes have been observed to be unprogressive over a long observation period.

4.1 Patients' demographic

AIR is characterized by an older age of onset. In unilateral cases, five males and three females, seven Japanese, and one Caucasian were reported by Hirakata et al.

[76], and two males and two females, four Japanese, were reported by Kido et al. [77]. Patients' demographic of unilateral retinopathy is shown in **Table 1**. Additionally, the mean age at the onset of symptoms was 62.2 ± 7.9 years (range 48–76), and three patients had a history of systemic autoimmune diseases, including asthma, palmoplantar pustulosis, and polymyalgia rheumatic [76, 77].

4.2 Symptoms

The majority of the patients experienced sudden and severe photophobia in one eye [76, 77], and some patients required dark glasses to walk under light-adapted conditions. Additionally, some patients developed visual field loss in the affected eye, which was especially severe under light-adapted conditions. Interestingly, photopsia was not observed in any of the patients, and bilateral cases also experienced acute-onset photophobia in both eyes [78].

4.3 Visual acuity and visual field

Although patients suffered from photophobia, visual acuity was relatively well preserved in most patients [76, 77]. Additionally, visual field patterns of Goldmann perimetry (GP) varied in the affected eyes, from almost normal to narrow isopters and scotomas compared with the fellow eye. Humphrey field analyzer (HFA) was also identified in affected patients with atypical abnormalities, possibly due to photophobia.

4.4 Multimodal imaging

Ophthalmoscopy and FAF showed a normal fundus appearance, except for attenuation of the retinal arteries (**Figure 1A** and **B**) [76]. Therefore, performing FA is crucial to rule out ischemic signs, such as the presence of broad non-perfused areas and delayed arm-to-retina time. The OCT images showed three patterns in the affected eye as follows: normal appearance, outer retinal degeneration, and reduced inner nuclear layer (INL) thickness (**Figure 1C** and **D**).

4.5 Electroretinogram

The full-field ERGs of the affected eyes were characterized as having severe cone-rod system dysfunction with negative ERGs in all patients [76–78]. The ERGs of the fellow eyes were either normal or mildly abnormal, and the rod ERGs (DA 0.01), cone, and 30 Hz flicker ERGs were severely reduced or undetectable. The mixed rod-cone ERG (DA 10.0 or 30.0) had slightly to moderately reduced a-waves and severely reduced b-waves, resulting in a negative-type ERG. Additionally, the a-, b-, and d-waves elicited by long-duration stimuli (300.0 cd $m-^{2}$) were also either severely reduced or undetectable in all affected eyes (**Figure 2A**), and mfERG responses were almost absent in the periphery and relatively preserved in the central retinas of the affected eyes (**Figure 2B**).

4.6 Pathophysiology

The patient was elderly at the time of onset and was aware of the sudden photophobia at the time of onset [76–78]. No obvious genetic mutations have been

	Case	Eye	Sex	Onset age	Chief complaints (Onset)	VA (Initial)	VA (Latest)	Past history (Age)
Hirakata et al. [76].	Case 1	R	M	55	None	1.0	1.0	Parkinsonism (65)
		L			Photophobia, night blindness	**0.6**	**0.6**	
	Case 2	R	F	48	Photophobia, VA loss	**h.m.**	**h.m.**	Breast cancer operation (47, 49), Depression
		L			None	0.02	0.04	
	Case 3	R	M	59	None	1.2	1.2	Color blindness, HL
		L			Photophobia	**1.2**	**1.2**	
	Case 4	R	F	52	None	1.2	1.2	Head bone fracture (22), TIA (36)
		L			VF loss, dyschromatopsia	**1.2**	**1.2**	
	Case 5	R	M	60	Photophobia	**1.2**	**1.2**	Asthma, Gout
		L			None	1.2	1.2	
	Case 6	R	M	68	Photophobia	**0.8**	**0.9**	HT, colon bening tumor (65, 70)
		L			None	1.0	1.0	
	Case 7	R	M	62	None	1.2	1.2	Asthma, HT, Coronary stenosis, Palmoplantar pustulosis
		L			Photophobia, dyschromatopsia, VF loss	**0.8**	**1.2**	
	Case 8	R	M	76	Night blindness	1.2	—	Auditory disorder, polymyalgia rheumatica, Colon begnig tumor (80)
		L			None	**1.2**	—	

	Case	Eye	Sex	Onset age	Chief complaints (Onset)	VA (Initial)	VA (Latest)	Past history (Age)
Kido et al. [77].	Case 9	R	M	65	Greying of vision, photophobia	**0.8**	**0.8**	colon cancer (62)
		L			None	0.8	—	
	Case 10	R	F	61	None	1.5	—	HL
		L			Photophobia	**1.5**	—	
	Case 11	R	F	68	None	0.6	1.0	normal tension glaucoma
		L			Decreased vision, photophobia	**1.0**	**0.9**	
	Case 12	R	M	73	None	1.2	—	normal tension glaucoma
		L			Blurred vision, photophobia	**1.0**	—	

A, abnormal; CSC, central serous chorioretinopathy; h.m., hand motion; HL, hyperlipidemia; HT, hypertension; L, left; N, normal; R, right; TIA, transient ischemic attack; VA, visual acuity; and VF, visual field.
Bold type indicates the affected eye.

Table 1.
Patient chracteristics of unilateral acute inner retinal dysfunction.

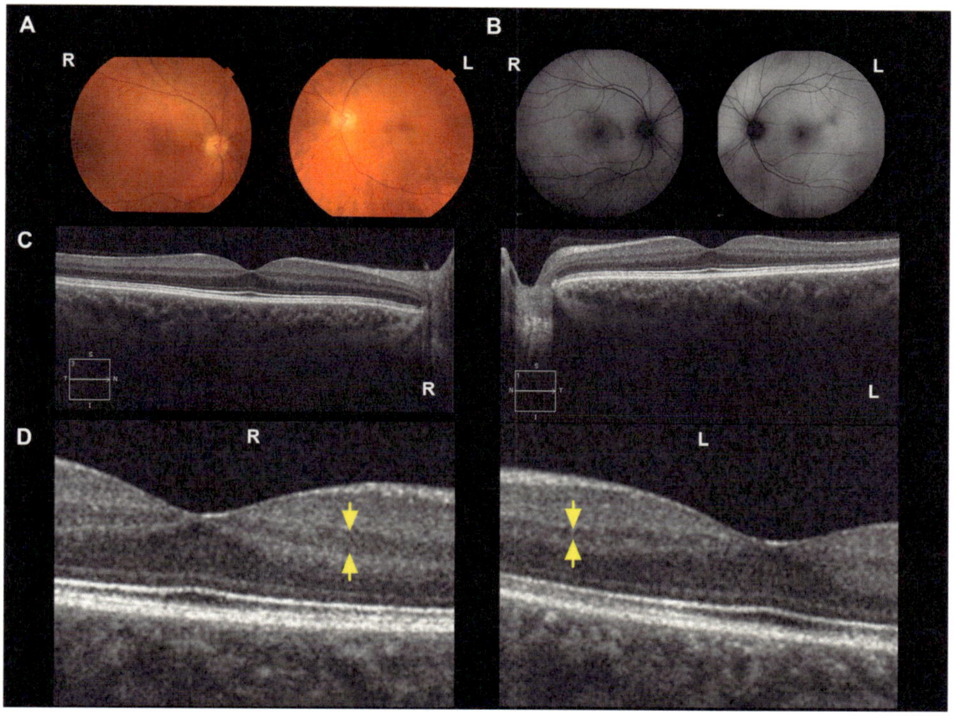

Figure 1.
Multimodal imaging. (A) Fundus photographs and (B) fundus autofluorescence (FAF) images of a 66-year-old caucasian man (Case 1) were shown. (C) OCT images show almost normal in both eyes. (D) Reduced inner nuclear layer (INL) thickness was observed in the affected left eye compared to the fellow right eye. Yellow arrows show INL thickness. R, right; L, left. These data were previously reported by Hirakata et al [76].

revealed as far as we could examine [76]. Anti-retinal antibodies from some patients were detected using western blot analysis in the sera as follows: 63 and 66 kDa anti-retinal specific antibodies, 64 and 47 kDa nonspecific antibodies, 29 kDa anti-retinal specific antibody (anti-CAII antibody), and 46 kDa anti-retinal specific antibody (an anti-α enolase antibody) [76, 77]. Notably, there is a gap between retinal multimodal imaging and ERGs. Despite the almost normal findings of retinal imaging studies, the following ERG changes were significant: severe cone-rod dysfunction with negative ERG configuration and bipolar cell response dysfunction. Moreover, OCT images showed thinning of the INL in the affected eyes of some patients. There were no obvious systemic diseases, such as malignancy, associated with retinal dysfunction. Therefore, these findings suggested AIR and bipolar cell dysfunction. Moreover, retinopathy is not progressive in most patients; thus, there are no reports of treatment yet. Although the syndrome has progressed without progression during follow-up, there has been a report of one case of npAIR with the development of bilateral eyes after more than 10 years [79]; therefore, follow-up should be performed with caution.

4.7 Diagnosis

These patients share some common features as follows: (1) sudden onset of (almost unilateral) photophobia at an older age, (2) preserved visual acuity,

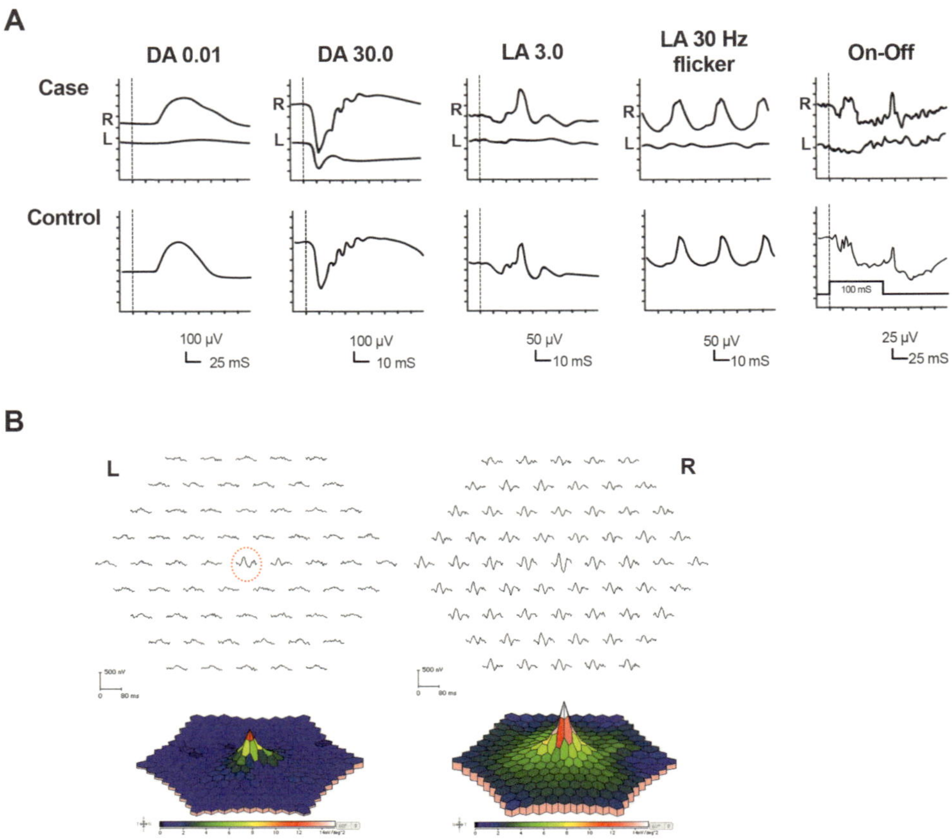

Figure 2.
Electroretinograms of unilateral inner retinal dysfunction. (A) Full-field electroretinograms (ERGs) of a 66-year-old Caucasian man (Case 1) were shown in the upper side. ERGs in the lower side were shown as a normal control. The full-field ERGs of the affected left eye were classified as severe cone-rod system dysfunction with negative ERGs. On the other hand, the ERGs of the fellow eye were normal. (B) Multifocal ERGs (mfERGs) of a 54-year-old Japanese man (Case 3) showed almost absent in the periphery and relatively preserved responses in the central retina of the affected left eye, while mfERG of the right eye was normal. Upper panel shows the mfERG responses and lower panel shows the mfERG 3D map. These data were previously reported by Hirakata et al [76].

(3) negative ERG with well-preserved a-wave, (4) severe cone and rod dysfunction (particularly cone) on ERG, (5) minimal abnormality on multimodal imaging, and (6) no progression after a relatively long-term observation period. Additionally, detection of retinal autoantibodies is helpful for AIR diagnosis, and systemic scrutiny is necessary to rule out pAIR. Since unilateral negative ERG is sometimes caused by retinal ischemia, evidence of the absence of retinal ischemia with FA is also a diagnostic aid.

5. Conclusions

Autoimmune retinal disorders have been described previously, and a combination of multimodal imaging and electrophysiology is crucial because its diagnosis is challenging. Therefore, systemic scrutiny is important. Further clarification of the pathogenesis of this disease is required as there is no established treatment yet in this field.

Acknowledgements

This work was supported by grants from MEXT/JSPS KAKENHI (19K23851 and 20K18395) to T.H.

Conflict of interest

There are no conflicts of interest to declare.

Notes/thanks/other declarations

None.

Author details

Toshiaki Hirakata
Faculty of Medicine, Department of Ophthalmology, Juntendo University, Tokyo, Japan

*Address all correspondence to: t-hirakata@juntendo.ac.jp

References

[1] Gass JD. Acute zonal occult outer retinopathy. Donders Lecture: The Netherlands Ophthalmological Society, Maastricht, Holland, June 19, 1992. Journal of Clinical Neuro-Ophthalmology. 1993;**13**(2):79-97

[2] Gass JD, Agarwal A, Scott IU. Acute zonal occult outer retinopathy: A long-term follow-up study. American Journal of Ophthalmology. 2002;**134**(3):329-339

[3] Herbort CP Jr, Arapi I, Papasavvas I, Mantovani A, Jeannin B. Acute Zonal Occult Outer Retinopathy (AZOOR) results from a clinicopathological mechanism different from choriocapillaritis diseases: A multimodal imaging analysis. Diagnostics (Basel). 2021;**11**(7):1184

[4] Monson DM, Smith JR. Acute zonal occult outer retinopathy. Survey of Ophthalmology. 2011;**56**(1):23-35

[5] Saito S, Saito W, Saito M, Hashimoto Y, Mori S, Noda K, et al. Acute zonal occult outer retinopathy in Japanese patients: Clinical features, visual function, and factors affecting visual function. PLoS One. 2015;**10**(4):e0125133

[6] Tsunoda K, Fujinami K, Miyake Y. Selective abnormality of cone outer segment tip line in acute zonal occult outer retinopathy as observed by spectral-domain optical coherence tomography. Archives of Ophthalmology. 2011;**129**(8):1099-1101

[7] Matsui Y, Matsubara H, Ueno S, Ito Y, Terasaki H, Kondo M. Changes in outer retinal microstructures during six month period in eyes with acute zonal occult outer retinopathy-complex. PLoS One. 2014;**9**(10):e110592

[8] Li D, Kishi S. Loss of photoreceptor outer segment in acute zonal occult outer retinopathy. Archives of Ophthalmology. 2007;**125**(9):1194-1200

[9] Spaide RF, Koizumi H, Freund KB. Photoreceptor outer segment abnormalities as a cause of blind spot enlargement in acute zonal occult outer retinopathy-complex diseases. American Journal of Ophthalmology. 2008;**146**(1):111-120

[10] Mkrtchyan M, Lujan BJ, Merino D, Thirkill CE, Roorda A, Duncan JL. Outer retinal structure in patients with acute zonal occult outer retinopathy. American Journal of Ophthalmology. 2012;**153**(4):757-768

[11] Saito A, Saito W, Furudate N, Ohno S. Indocyanine green angiography in a case of punctate inner choroidopathy associated with acute zonal occult outer retinopathy. Japanese Journal of Ophthalmology. 2007;**51**(4):295-300

[12] Francis PJ, Marinescu A, Fitzke FW, Bird AC, Holder GE. Acute zonal occult outer retinopathy: Towards a set of diagnostic criteria. The British Journal of Ophthalmology. 2005;**89**(1):70-73

[13] Takai Y, Ishiko S, Kagokawa H, Fukui K, Takahashi A, Yoshida A. Morphological study of acute zonal occult outer retinopathy (AZOOR) by multiplanar optical coherence tomography. Acta Ophthalmologica. 2009;**87**(4):408-418

[14] Hashimoto Y, Saito W, Kanaizumi S, Saito M, Noda K, Kanda A, et al. Comparison of clinical characteristics in patients with acute zonal occult outer retinopathy according to anti-retinal antibody status. Graefe's

Archive for Clinical and Experimental Ophthalmology. 2021;**259**(10):2967-2976

[15] Saito M, Saito W, Hashimoto Y, Yoshizawa C, Shinmei Y, Noda K, et al. Correlation between decreased choroidal blood flow velocity and the pathogenesis of acute zonal occult outer retinopathy. Clinical & Experimental Ophthalmology. 2014;**42**(2):139-150

[16] Hashimoto Y, Saito W, Saito M, Hasegawa Y, Takita A, Mori S, et al. Relationship between choroidal thickness and visual field impairment in acute zonal occult outer retinopathy. Journal of Ophthalmology. 2017;**2017**:2371032

[17] Zeng HY, Liu Q, Peng XY, Cao K, Jin SS, Xu K. Detection of serum anti-retinal antibodies in the Chinese patients with presumed autoimmune retinopathy. Graefe's Archive for Clinical and Experimental Ophthalmology. 2019;**257**(8):1759-1764

[18] Neri P, Ricci F, Giovannini A, Arapi I, De Felici C, Cusumano A, et al. Successful treatment of an overlapping choriocapillaritis between multifocal choroiditis and acute zonal occult outer retinopathy (AZOOR) with adalimumab (Humira). International Ophthalmology. 2014;**34**(2):359-364

[19] Kitakawa T, Hayashi T, Takashina H, Mitooka K, Gekka T, Tsuneoka H. Improvement of central visual function following steroid pulse therapy in acute zonal occult outer retinopathy. Documenta Ophthalmologica. 2012;**124**(3):249-254

[20] Kuo YC, Chen N, Tsai RK. Acute Zonal Occult Outer Retinopathy (AZOOR): A case report of vision improvement after intravitreal injection of Ozurdex. BMC Ophthalmology. 2017;**17**(1):236

[21] Chiba-Mayumi M, Hirakata T, Yamaguchi M, Murakami A. Infliximab recovers central cone dysfunction with normal fundus in a patient with ulcerative colitis. American Journal of Ophthalmological Case Report. 2022;**25**:101244

[22] Takeuchi M, Harimoto K, Taguchi M, Sakurai Y. Reconstitution of disrupted photoreceptor layer in uveitis associated with Behcet's disease by infliximab treatment. BMC Ophthalmology. 2015;**15**:177

[23] Sawyer RA, Selhorst JB, Zimmerman LE, Hoyt WF. Blindness caused by photoreceptor degeneration as a remote effect of cancer. American Journal of Ophthalmology. 1976;**81**(5):606-613

[24] Dutta Majumder P, Marchese A, Pichi F, Garg I, Agarwal A. An update on autoimmune retinopathy. Indian Journal of Ophthalmology. 2020;**68**(9):1829-1837

[25] Keltner JL, Thirkill CE, Yip PT. Clinical and immunologic characteristics of melanoma-associated retinopathy syndrome: Eleven new cases and a review of 51 previously published cases. Journal of Neuro-Ophthalmology. 2001;**21**(3):173-187

[26] Grange L, Dalal M, Nussenblatt RB, Sen HN. Autoimmune retinopathy. American Journal of Ophthalmology. 2014;**157**(2):266-272

[27] Ferreyra HA, Jayasundera T, Khan NW, He S, Lu Y, Heckenlively JR. Management of autoimmune retinopathies with immunosuppression. Archives of Ophthalmology. 2009;**127**(4):390-397

[28] Adamus G, Ren G, Weleber RG. Autoantibodies against retinal proteins in paraneoplastic and autoimmune

retinopathy. BMC Ophthalmology. 2004;**4**:5

[29] Heckenlively JR, Ferreyra HA. Autoimmune retinopathy: A review and summary. Seminars in Immunopathology. 2008;**30**(2):127-134

[30] Canamary AM Jr, Takahashi WY, Sallum JMF. Autoimmune retinopathy: A review. International Journal of Retina Vitreous. 2018;**4**:1

[31] Braithwaite T, Vugler A, Tufail A. Autoimmune retinopathy. Ophthalmologica. 2012;**228**(3):131-142

[32] Rahimy E, Sarraf D. Paraneoplastic and non-paraneoplastic retinopathy and optic neuropathy: Evaluation and management. Survey of Ophthalmology. 2013;**58**(5):430-458

[33] Holopigian K, Hood DC. Electrophysiology. Ophthalmology Clinics of North America. 2003;**16**(2):237-251

[34] Adamus G. Autoantibody targets and their cancer relationship in the pathogenicity of paraneoplastic retinopathy. Autoimmunity Reviews. 2009;**8**(5):410-414

[35] Javaid Z, Rehan SM, Al-Bermani A, Payne G. Unilateral cancer-associated retinopathy: A case report. Scottish Medical Journal. 2016;**61**(3):155-159

[36] Berson EL, Lessell S. Paraneoplastic night blindness with malignant melanoma. American Journal of Ophthalmology. 1988;**106**(3):307-311

[37] Elsheikh S, Gurney SP, Burdon MA. Melanoma-associated retinopathy. Clinical and Experimental Dermatology. 2020;**45**(2):147-152

[38] Hartmann TB, Bazhin AV, Schadendorf D, Eichmuller SB. SEREX identification of new tumor antigens linked to melanoma-associated retinopathy. International Journal of Cancer. 2005;**114**(1):88-93

[39] Milam AH, Saari JC, Jacobson SG, Lubinski WP, Feun LG, Alexander KR. Autoantibodies against retinal bipolar cells in cutaneous melanoma-associated retinopathy. Investigative Ophthalmology & Visual Science. 1993;**34**(1):91-100

[40] Duncan LM, Deeds J, Hunter J, Shao J, Holmgren LM, Woolf EA, et al. Down-regulation of the novel gene melastatin correlates with potential for melanoma metastasis. Cancer Research. 1998;**58**(7):1515-1520

[41] Dhingra A, Fina ME, Neinstein A, Ramsey DJ, Xu Y, Fishman GA, et al. Autoantibodies in melanoma-associated retinopathy target TRPM1 cation channels of retinal ON bipolar cells. The Journal of Neuroscience. 2011;**31**(11):3962-3967

[42] Ueno S, Nishiguchi KM, Tanioka H, Enomoto A, Yamanouchi T, Kondo M, et al. Degeneration of retinal on bipolar cells induced by serum including autoantibody against TRPM1 in mouse model of paraneoplastic retinopathy. PLoS One. 2013;**8**(11):e81507

[43] Janaky M, Palffy A, Kolozsvari L, Benedek G. Unilateral manifestation of melanoma-associated retinopathy. Archives of Ophthalmology. 2002;**120**(6):866-867

[44] Chan C, O'Day J. Melanoma-associated retinopathy: Does autoimmunity prolong survival? Clinical & Experimental Ophthalmology. 2001;**29**(4):235-238

[45] Singh AD, Milam AH, Shields CL, De Potter P, Shields JA. Melanoma-associated retinopathy. American Journal of Ophthalmology. 1995;**119**(3):369-370

[46] Lu Y, Jia L, He S, Hurley MC, Leys MJ, Jayasundera T, et al. Melanoma-associated retinopathy: A paraneoplastic autoimmune complication. Archives of Ophthalmology. 2009;**127**(12):1572-1580

[47] Shinohara Y, Mukai R, Ueno S, Akiyama H. Clinical findings of melanoma-associated retinopathy with anti-TRPM1 antibody. Case Report in Ophthalmological Medicine. 2021;**2021**:6607441

[48] Potter MJ, Thirkill CE, Dam OM, Lee AS, Milam AH. Clinical and immunocytochemical findings in a case of melanoma-associated retinopathy. Ophthalmology. 1999;**106**(11):2121-2125

[49] Adamus G. Are anti-retinal autoantibodies a cause or a consequence of retinal degeneration in autoimmune retinopathies? Frontiers in Immunology. 2018;**9**:765

[50] Whitcup SM, Vistica BP, Milam AH, Nussenblatt RB, Gery I. Recoverin-associated retinopathy: A clinically and immunologically distinctive disease. American Journal of Ophthalmology. 1998;**126**(2):230-237

[51] Mizener JB, Kimura AE, Adamus G, Thirkill CE, Goeken JA, Kardon RH. Autoimmune retinopathy in the absence of cancer. American Journal of Ophthalmology. 1997;**123**(5):607-618

[52] Peek R, Verbraak F, Coevoet HM, Kijlstra A. Muller cell-specific autoantibodies in a patient with progressive loss of vision. Investigative Ophthalmology & Visual Science. 1998;**39**(10):1976-1979

[53] Ando R, Saito W, Kanda A, Kase S, Fujinami K, Sugahara M, et al. Clinical features of Japanese patients with anti-alpha-enolase antibody-positive autoimmune retinopathy: Novel Subtype of Multiple Drusen. American Journal of Ophthalmology. 2018;**196**:181-196

[54] Adamus G, Karren L. Autoimmunity against carbonic anhydrase II affects retinal cell functions in autoimmune retinopathy. Journal of Autoimmunity. 2009;**32**(2):133-139

[55] Lerea CL, Somers DE, Hurley JB, Klock IB, Bunt-Milam AH. Identification of specific transducin alpha subunits in retinal rod and cone photoreceptors. Science. 1986;**234**(4772):77-80

[56] Grewal DS, Fishman GA, Jampol LM. Autoimmune retinopathy and antiretinal antibodies: A review. Retina. 2014;**34**(5):827-845

[57] Shiraga S, Adamus G. Mechanism of CAR syndrome: Anti-recoverin antibodies are the inducers of retinal cell apoptotic death via the caspase 9- and caspase 3-dependent pathway. Journal of Neuroimmunology. 2002;**132**(1-2):72-82

[58] Ohguro H, Nakazawa M. Pathological roles of recoverin in cancer-associated retinopathy. Advances in Experimental Medicine and Biology. 2002;**514**:109-124

[59] Dot C, Guigay J, Adamus G. Anti-alpha-enolase antibodies in cancer-associated retinopathy with small cell carcinoma of the lung. American Journal of Ophthalmology. 2005;**139**(4):746-747

[60] Adamus G, Aptsiauri N, Guy J, Heckenlively J, Flannery J, Hargrave PA. The occurrence of serum autoantibodies against enolase in cancer-associated retinopathy. Clinical Immunology and Immunopathology. 1996;**78**(2):120-129

[61] Kikuchi T, Arai J, Shibuki H, Kawashima H, Yoshimura N. Tubby-like protein 1 as an autoantigen in

cancer-associated retinopathy. Journal of Neuroimmunology. 2000;**103**(1):26-33

[62] Ohguro H, Ogawa K, Nakagawa T. Recoverin and Hsc 70 are found as autoantigens in patients with cancer-associated retinopathy. Investigative Ophthalmology & Visual Science. 1999;**40**(1):82-89

[63] Adamus G, Yang S, Weleber RG. Unique epitopes for carbonic anhydrase II autoantibodies related to autoimmune retinopathy and cancer-associated retinopathy. Experimental Eye Research. 2016;**147**:161-168

[64] Eksandh L, Adamus G, Mosgrove L, Andreasson S. Autoantibodies against bestrophin in a patient with vitelliform paraneoplastic retinopathy and a metastatic choroidal malignant melanoma. Archives of Ophthalmology. 2008;**126**(3):432-435

[65] Varin J, Reynolds MM, Bouzidi N, Tick S, Wohlschlegel J, Becquart O, et al. Identification and characterization of novel TRPM1 autoantibodies from serum of patients with melanoma-associated retinopathy. PLoS One. 2020;**15**(4):e0231750

[66] Kondo M, Sanuki R, Ueno S, Nishizawa Y, Hashimoto N, Ohguro H, et al. Identification of autoantibodies against TRPM1 in patients with paraneoplastic retinopathy associated with ON bipolar cell dysfunction. PLoS One. 2011;**6**(5):e19911

[67] Bianciotto C, Shields CL, Thirkill CE, Materin MA, Shields JA. Paraneoplastic retinopathy with multiple detachments of the neurosensory retina and autoantibodies against interphotoreceptor retinoid binding protein (IRBP) in cutaneous melanoma. The British Journal of Ophthalmology. 2010;**94**(12):1684-1685

[68] Shildkrot Y, Sobrin L, Gragoudas ES. Cancer-associated retinopathy: Update on pathogenesis and therapy. Seminars in Ophthalmology. 2011;**26**(4-5):321-328

[69] Adamus G, Guy J, Schmied JL, Arendt A, Hargrave PA. Role of anti-recoverin autoantibodies in cancer-associated retinopathy. Investigative Ophthalmology & Visual Science. 1993;**34**(9):2626-2633

[70] Braithwaite T, Holder GE, Lee RW, Plant GT, Tufail A. Diagnostic features of the autoimmune retinopathies. Autoimmunity Reviews. 2014;**13**(4-5):534-538

[71] Grewal DS, Jaffe GJ, Keenan RT. Sarilumab for recalcitrant cystoid macular edema in non-paraneoplastic autoimmune retinopathy. Retin Cases Brief Rep. 2021;**15**(5):504-508

[72] Chan JW. Paraneoplastic retinopathies and optic neuropathies. Survey of Ophthalmology. 2003;**48**(1):12-38

[73] Katsuta H, Okada M, Nakauchi T, Takahashi Y, Yamao S, Uchida S. Cancer-associated retinopathy associated with invasive thymoma. American Journal of Ophthalmology. 2002;**134**(3):383-389

[74] Jacobzone C, Cochard-Marianowski C, Kupfer I, Bettembourg S, Dordain Y, Misery L, et al. Corticosteroid treatment for melanoma-associated retinopathy: Effect on visual acuity and electrophysiologic findings. Archives of Dermatology. 2004;**140**(10):1258-1261

[75] Mizobuchi K, Katagiri S, Hayashi T, Ninomiya W, Okude S, Asano Y, et al. Unique and progressive retinal degeneration in a patient with cancer associated retinopathy. American Journal of Ophthalmology Case Reports. 2020;**20**:100908

[76] Hirakata T, Fujinami K, Saito W, Kanda A, Hirakata A, Ishida S, et al. Acute unilateral inner retinal dysfunction with photophobia: Importance of electrodiagnosis. Japanese Journal of Ophthalmology. 2021;**65**(1):42-53

[77] Kido A, Ogino K, Miyake Y, Yanagida K, Kikuchi T, Yoshimura N. Unilateral negative electroretinogram presenting as photophobia. Documenta Ophthalmologica. 2016;**133**(1):71-79

[78] Ueno S, Inooka D, Meinert M, Ito Y, Tsunoda K, Fujinami K, et al. Three cases of acute-onset bilateral photophobia. Japanese Journal of Ophthalmology. 2019;**63**(2):172-180

[79] Miura G, Baba T, Iwase T, Ohde H, Kanda A, Saito W, et al. Non-paraneoplastic autoimmune retinopathy that developed in fellow eye 10 years after onset in first eye: A case report. BMC Ophthalmology. 2020;**20**(1):132

Chapter 8

Retinitis Due to Infections

Ruben Rose, Alexey Gorin, Mathias Voß and Helmut Fickenscher

Abstract

Infections are a major cause for retinitis. Whereas Varicella-Zoster and Herpes Simplex viruses are the major reason for acute retinal necrosis, cytomegalovirus retinitis typically occurs in immunocompromised patients. Toxoplasmosis and toxocariasis are the major parasitic pathogens affecting the retina and adjacent tissues. Among the bacterial causes, tuberculosis, syphilis, and bartonellosis are discussed as retinal diseases. The emphasis is laid on the epidemiological and clinical peculiarities, the respective diagnostic procedures, and the therapeutic approaches. Moreover, global disease aspects of infectious retinitis are included.

Keywords: acute retinal necrosis, bartonellosis, chorioretinitis, cytomegalovirus, toxocariasis, toxoplasmosis, tuberculosis, retinis, syphilis, varicella zoster virus

1. Introduction

Retinitis can present in various different forms. Some of them are rather specific for individual pathogens, whereas other phenotypes are rather overlapping (**Table 1**). In this manuscript, the major viral, parasitic, and bacterial pathogens are presented and discussed together with the different clinical manifestations.

Disease form	Main pathogens
Acute retinal necrosis	VZV, HSV
Cytomegalovirus retinitis	CMV
Chorioretinitis	*Toxoplasma gondii, Treponema pallidum*
Chorioiditis with retinitis	Mycobacteria, Toxocara, *T. pallidum*

Table 1.
Classification of retinitis and related disease forms.

2. Virus-induced retinitis

2.1 Acute retinal necrosis

Acute retinal necrosis (ARN) is an infectious inflammation of the retina, the vitreous and the anterior chamber of the eye that can lead to blindness by destruction of the optic nerve and retina in immune competent individuals. The first clinical reports were published by Urayama in 1971 under the designation Kirisawa uveitis. In 1978, the term acute retinal necrosis was introduced by Young and Bird [1, 2].

2.1.1 Pathogen

ARN is primarily caused by the α-herpesviruses Varicella-Zoster virus (VZV) or Herpes-Simplex virus (HSV) 1 and 2, which together account for 97% of cases (95-%-confidence interval (CI) 96–99%). Among ARNs caused by α-herpesviruses, VZV is the leading cause at 69% (95-%-CI 60–76%), followed by HSV-2 and HSV-1. α-herpesviruses carry a large double-stranded DNA genome and establish latency in the nuclei of the sensory and autonomic spinal ganglia of the central nervous system after primary infection. Normally, the virus genome is latently maintained in the sensory ganglia since lytically infected cells are rapidly eliminated by the CD8-positive cytotoxic killer cells of the immune system. The virus genomes persist latently in the nuclei of the sensory neurons in circular extrachromosomal form as episomes. Viral reactivation occurs due to poorly defined stressors such as ultraviolet light, neurosurgical procedures, or steroid or immunspuppressive therapy. Virus reactivation is followed by peripheral viral replication and usually results in herpes zoster, herpes orofacialis, herpes genitalis, or in rare cases also in zoster ophthalmicus or herpes oculi [2, 3].

The roles in ARN development of the β-herpesvirus cytomegalovirus (CMV) and the γ-herpesvirus Epstein–Barr virus (EBV), which establish their latency within myeloid stem cells and quiescent B lymphocytes, respectively, are still controversial. While at least some cases have been reported in which CMV appears to be causal for ARN, EBV has only been detected in some cases in addition to VZV and does not appear to play a causative role in immunocompetent individuals [3, 4].

2.1.2 Epidemiology

ARN is a very rare disease, which affects one individual per 1.5–2.0 million persons per year. In a meta-analysis, men were shown to have a slightly higher risk to be affected by ARN than women [3]. Interestingly, the age of manifestation of ARN depends on the responsible virus species. Patients with ARN due to VZV or HSV-2 have a median age of 48.8 and 47.8 years, respectively, whereas patients with ARN due to HSV-1 have a median age of only 31.1 years [3]. In addition, ARN shows two peaks of manifestation age, the first at age of approximately 20 years and the second at age 50 [4]. In addition, some studies have shown that certain human leukocyte antigen (HLA) types such as HLA-DQw7 as well as HLA phenotype Bw62, DR4, and HLA-DR9 are associated with the occurrence of ARN or its severity, respectively [5, 6].

2.1.3 Clinical peculiarities

Characteristic of ARN is an inflammation of the anterior chamber and vitreous associated with peripheral necrotizing retinitis with focal necrotic lesions that become circular as the disease progresses to the posterior pole. This process is additionally associated with an occlusive vasculitis that leads to arteriolar narrowing. This first phase is followed by a second phase in which retinal atrophy, proliferative vitreoretinopathy, and retinal detachment occur [4]. While some studies have found ARN to be unilateral in nearly 90% of cases, other studies report bilateral involvement in up to one-third of cases [2–4]. In any case, ARN that initially occurs unilaterally may spread to the contralateral eye.

In contrast to ARN, progressive outer retinal necrosis (PORN), now considered a variant of ARN, affects almost exclusively immunocompromised individuals, *e.g.*, human immunodeficiency virus (HIV)-infected individuals in the AIDS stage or organ transplant recipients. It results from reactivation of VZV and spreads extremely rapidly to the deep retinal layers, leading to retinal detachment. However, PORN lacks the vasculitis aspect of classic ARN [2, 4].

2.1.4 Diagnosis

According to the American Uveitis Society, ARN is defined by the following criteria: (1) "focal, well-demarcated areas of retinal necrosis in the peripheral retina (outside the major temporal vascular arcs)"; (2) "rapid, circumferential progression of necrosis (if antiviral therapy has not been administered)"; (3) "evidence of occlusive vasculopathy"; (4) "a marked inflammatory reaction in the vitreous"; and (5) in the "anterior chamber." In addition, symptoms such as optic atrophy, scleritis, and pain are common but not essential [7]. These criteria were established before molecular biological detection methods such as polymerase chain reaction (PCR) were widely available. Therefore, a recent publication proposed a modification of the diagnostic criteria to include serological and PCR-based methods with respect to the responsible viruses. By comparing the antibody concentration against the different herpesviruses in serum with the antibody concentration in vitreous fluid, the Goldmann-Witmer coefficient (GWC) can be determined. A positive GWC is highly specific (100%) at a moderate sensitivity of only 33%. Detection by PCR is both highly sensitive (95%) and only slightly less specific (92%) [8]. Identification of the specific virus is important, as it has therapeutic consequences. The use of PCR-based detection methods has the additional advantage of enabling the identification of viral resistance to the antiviral drugs used by genotyping [9, 10]. Imaging of the eye such as fundus fluorescein angiography or optical coherence tomography is useful to determine the extent and progression of the disease [4].

2.1.5 Therapy

Since the goal of therapy is to inhibit further disease progression driven by viral replication, antiviral therapy should be initiated immediately after clinical diagnosis and not delayed by waiting for laboratory results. However, viral diagnostics are useful because therapy for CMV relies on different antiviral drugs than therapy for VZV, HSV-1, and HSV-2. In addition, as mentioned above, PCR diagnostics allow detection of resistance by genotyping and thus adjustment of therapy. This is particularly important for immunocompromised patients, who are affected, for example, by drug-resistant HSV-1 strains in up to 14% of cases, whereas this is only the case in less than 1% of immunocompetent individuals [11, 12].

The three α-herpesviruses VZV, HSV-1, HSV-2 are treatable with the antiviral drugs aciclovir and its prodrug valaciclovir, penciclovir, and its prodrug famciclovir, as well as by cidofovir and foscarnet. The prodrugs valaciclovir and famciclovir, which must be activated in enterocytes by the first-pass effect, have a good oral bioavailability of 54–60% and 77%, respectively, unlike aciclovir and penciclovir and, thus, can be efficiently administered orally. Aciclovir and penciclovir, as well as their prodrugs, are nucleoside analogs that must be activated by a viral enzyme called thymidine kinase (TK). After activation by viral TK, this group of antiviral drugs causes chain termination during viral replication. Because they act only in virus-infected cells, they are well tolerated, especially in their oral formulation. Nevertheless, there are side effects, which often include headache, rash, and gastrointestinal symptoms in the oral formulations. However, intravenous use of aciclovir may result in neurotoxicity and renal toxicity due to crystalline nephropathy. Therefore, patients with impaired renal function must be treated with lower doses. Because the main cause of viral resistance are mutations within the viral TK, the rate of cross-resistance within this antiviral drug group is high. In case of resistance, cidofovir and foscarnet are alternatives that do not require viral TK activation. The nucleoside analog cidofovir is activated only by cellular kinases and, once activated, acts similarly to the other nucleoside analogs. The drug is excreted exclusively by the kidneys and is nephrotoxic and, therefore, requires renal protection by probenecid administration. Foscarnet, a pyrophosphate analog, directly inhibits the viral polymerase by blocking its pyrophosphate-binding site. The most important side effect of foscarnet is nephrotoxicity. Therefore, the dose must be adjusted in patients with impaired renal function. Both foscarnet and cidofovir must be administered intravenously due to their low oral bioavailability of 20% and 5%, respectively; recommended dosing is 60 mg/kg three times daily and 5 mg/kg over 1 h once weekly for 2 weeks [2, 12].

Traditionally, therapy for ARN consisted of administration of 10 mg/kg aciclovir three times daily or 1500 mg/m^2 per day intravenously for 5–14 days. This should be followed by oral treatment with 800 mg of aciclovir five times daily for 6 weeks, as such treatment has been shown to prevent 90% of contralateral eye infections [2, 4]. However, it has been shown that similar plasma concentrations can be achieved by oral administration of valaciclovir as by intravenous administration of aciclovir, and the visual outcome does not appear to be worse. Therefore, efforts are being made to avoid intravenous therapy completely. Currently, oral therapy regimens with 2000 mg valaciclovir or 500 mg famciclovir three times daily are being used [4, 12]. Regarding the duration of follow-up, some authors recommend extending therapy with 800 mg of aciclovir or 1000 mg of valaciclovir three times daily for 6–12 months, followed by lifelong use of 1000 mg of valaciclovir daily to prevent infestation of the contralateral eye or relapse [12]. During the initial therapy phase, intravitreal use of 2.4 mg/0.1 ml foscarnet or 2.0/0.1 ml ganciclovir two times per week in combination with systemic antiviral therapy appears to have therapeutic benefit [4, 12]. With respect to foscarnet, a recent systematic review based on case–control and cohort studies, as well as case series and case reports, also supports this therapeutic approach [13]. Because vasculitis and inflammation contribute to the progression of ARN, the use of systemic or topical steroids and anticoagulation drugs is under discussion. However, the evidence base for such treatments is low and must be used with caution [12]. In the case of a successful antiviral therapy, no further lesions should be observed from day 2 of therapy, from 4 to 5 days of therapy, the retinal infiltrate should tend to regress, and after 1 month, a complete remission should be observable [2].

Another highly controversial issue is the use of prophylactic procedures such as prophylactic vitrectomy or prophylactic laser retinopexy. It has been shown that the risk of rhegmatogenous retinal detachment after ARN can be significantly reduced by prophylactic vitrectomy [5]. This finding was confirmed by a recent meta-analysis of seven retrospective cohort studies, which included the study by Hillenkamp and colleagues [5, 14]. However, this meta-analysis found that visual outcome was significantly worse in the prophylactic vitrectomy group than in the control group treated with antiviral drugs only. The authors attributed this result to silicone oil tamponade and long-term complications in the vitrectomy group. Although there are also some small studies that see a benefit in terms of visual outcome, there is ultimately no conclusive evidence to support such treatment [12]. Another much debated topic is whether prophylactic laser therapy can reduce the incidence of retinal detachment. Although a meta-analysis of 14 studies found that prophylactic laser retinopexy can significantly prevent retinal detachments after ARN [15], Powell et al. pointed out that prophylactic laser retinopexy is only possible if the vitreous media is clear enough, which means that often only the less severely affected eyes are treated with laser [12]. In addition, the cited meta-analysis by [15] did not examine the question of how the therapy affects visual outcome. Thus, the benefit of prophylactic laser retinopexy remains questionable.

For ARN caused by CMV that lacks TK and instead expresses the kinase UL97, ganciclovir and its orally better bioavailable prodrug valganciclovir, as well as cidofovir and foscarnet, are therapeutic options. Because of its low bioavailability of 5%, ganciclovir must be administered intravenously at a dose of 5 mg/kg. Alternatively, 900 mg of valganciclovir can be administered orally, which has an oral bioavailability of 60%. Because ganciclovir and its prodrug cause neutropenia in approximately 8% of patients, the blood values of patients treated with either of these drugs should be monitored regularly. Cidofovir and foscarnet are alternatives in case of viral resistance to ganciclovir or its prodrug, which is mostly caused by mutations within the UL97 [2].

2.1.6 Prognosis

ARN has often a poor outcome, i.e., two-thirds of affected eyes achieve only a final best-corrected visual acuity of 6/60 or worse. Therefore, early diagnosis and urgent therapy are critical. In PORN, the outcome is even worse. Two-thirds of affected eyes are not even able to perceive light because they often do not respond well to antiviral therapy [4].

2.2 Cytomegalovirus retinitis

In immunocompetent persons, cytomegalovirus (CMV) normally leads only to a rather harmless anterior uveitis. However, in immunocompromised individuals, such as AIDS patients or those who have undergone organ transplantation, CMV can also lead to CMV retinitis, which is distinguishable from ARN but can also cause retinal detachment and blindness [16, 17].

2.2.1 Pathogen

CMV belongs to the beta-herpesviruses and has a large double-stranded DNA genome. It is transmitted perinatally or through any type of close contact via body fluids. The primary infection, which happens usually in young and healthy individuals, is typically mild or asymptomatic. However, primary infection of the pregnant woman may result in severe embryopathy or fetal death. After primary infection, the virus establishes latency within myeloid stem cells. In immunocompetent individuals, reaction is usually asymptomatic. A special but feared transmission of CMV can occur through organ transplantation [3, 4, 17, 18].

2.2.2 Epidemiology

Worldwide, CMV seroprevalence ranges from 60% to 100% and increases with age. In the United States, for example, 36.3% of children aged 6–11 years but 90.8% of adults aged 80 years or older are infected. CMV retinitis affects males more often than females and can occur at any age. However, most cases occur between the ages of 30 and 60. Initially, CMV retinitis was particularly common in AIDS-stage HIV patients, but with the development and widespread use of antiretroviral therapy (ART), its incidence in the AIDS patient group decreased by over 90%, and clinical outcomes in affected individuals improved significantly [4, 17].

2.2.3 Clinical peculiarities

In immunocompetent individuals, CMV reactivation usually results in unilateral, relatively mild, recurrent anterior uveitis with anterior chamber inflammation, elevated intraocular pressure, stromal iris atrophy, and few granulomatous keratic precipitates [16]. However, especially in immunocompromised individuals, CMV can affect the retina and cause unilateral CMV retinitis. In 20% of cases, infection of the contralateral eye occurs over the next 6 months [17]. Retinitis usually consists of two stages. In the first stage, the active retinitis usually shows three types of retinal lesions: First, fulminant and edematous lesions consisting of extensive retinal hemorrhages preceding confluent retinal necrosis; second, indolent and granular lesions consisting of granular satellites with little or no hemorrhage; and third, exudative lesions based on angiitis with extensive vascular sheathing. The second stage is characterized by large necroses and retinal tears. Finally, there is retinal atrophy with fibrosis, calcification, and sclerotic vessels [4].

2.2.4 Diagnosis

The diagnosis of CMV retinitis is made by ophthalmoscopy and should be documented by digital fundus photography. PCR diagnostics can confirm CMV retinitis, which is important with regard to the chosen therapy, and allows monitoring of therapy response and detection of resistant CMV strains by genotyping [4, 12].

2.2.5 Therapy

For retinitis caused by CMV that lacks TK and instead expresses the kinase UL97, ganciclovir and its more orally bioavailable prodrug valganciclovir, as well as cidofovir and foscarnet, are therapeutic options. As mentioned above, ganciclovir and its prodrug cause neutropenia in approximately 8% of patients. Therefore, the blood of patients treated with either of these drugs should be monitored regularly. Cidofovir and foscarnet are alternatives in the event of viral resistance to ganciclovir or its prodrug, which in most cases is caused by mutations within the UL97 [12]. For the therapy of the CMV retinitis, the combination of intravitreal and systemic therapy is recommended [17].

Typical dosage for CMV retinitis therapy: intraveneous ganciclovir, induction by 5 mg/kg 2× daily for 14–21 days, maintenance with 5 mg/kg/day; oral valganciclovir, induction by 900 mg 2× daily, maintenance 900 mg daily; intraveneous foscarnet, 90 mg/kg 2× daily for 14 d, maintenance 120 mg/kg/day; intraveneous cidofovir, 5 mg/kg weekly for 3 weeks, maintenance 5 mg/kg every 2 weeks.

Typical dosage for intravitreal CMV retinitis therapy: ganciclovir, induction by 2 mg 1–4× to stop retinitis, maintenance with 2 mg weekly; foscarnet, induction by 1.2–2.4 mg 1–2× weekly, maintenance with 1.2 mg weekly; cidofovir, induction by 20 μg 1–8×, maintenance with 20 μg every 5–6 weeks.

2.2.6 Prognosis

The consequences of CMV retinitis vary widely and include regression of retinal damage and complications such as retinal detachment or recurrence. In most cases, visual acuity stabilizes or improves, in many cases to complete remission [4].

3. Retinitis forms due to parasites

3.1 Ocular toxoplasmosis

Ocular toxoplasmosis is one of the most frequent causes for infectious uveitis globally, typically presenting as rather unilateral posterior uveitis with chorioretinal lesions and vitritis [19].

3.1.1 Pathogen

The ubiquitously distributed protozoon of the phylum Apicomplexa, *Toxoplasma (T.) gondii* is an obligate intracellular parasite, which invades host cells of a wide range of vertebral species including humans via an apical complex. Specific *T. gondii* genotypes are likely associated with higher prevalence and development of ocular toxoplasmosis [20]. Infection and transmission by *T. gondii* are possible in various stages of the parasitic life cycle. Soil-borne, water-borne, or food-borne uptake of oocysts containing infectious sporozoids and inoculation by tissue cysts containing tachyzoits with undercooked or raw meat, free tachyzoits in milk and eggs are the most common infectious routes besides vertical transmission, organ transplantation, and blood transfusion. *T. gondii* primary infects intestinal epithelial cells, circulates via the blood stream, performs extravasation by forming cysts [21, 22], and develops into different parasitic stages such as free infectious tachyzoits after intracellular replication and cell lysis or rather dormant and inactive encysted bradyzoits. The cell-invading and immune-escaping capacity of *T. gondii* is actively mediated by complex host-parasite interactions via surface ligands. Altered cytokine profiles of targeted macrophages, dendritic, and tissue cells, by intracellular *T. gondii* are the key to immune evasion, organ tropism, and the well balanced pro- and anti-inflammatory signaling of the targeted cells. These mechanisms consequently lead to a constant destructive and protective host tissue and parasite interaction in immunocompetent persons [23].

3.1.2 Epidemiology

Toxoplasmosis is widely spread with an approximately 30% human infection rate and wide geographical variation of seropositive rates up to 80% within certain populations [20, 24, 25]. Recent studies elucidated that endemic *T. gondii* strains play a major role in ocular toxoplasmosis prevalence. Archetypal strains I, II, III are dominant in Europe and North America, and non-archetypal strains are a minority but nevertheless cause the majority of ocular toxoplasmosis cases, approximately 1–2%, in immunocompetent seropositive individuals. In South America and Brazil, non-archetypal strains are dominant, and the ocular toxoplasmosis prevalence is up to 10–20% in the seropositive population [26, 27]. Other important factors related to the endemic seroprevalence of *T. gondii* are climate and socioeconomic factors such as access to clean and not contaminated water, public and institutional surveillance, hygiene and control of parasitic prevalence in life stock and related food products, blood products, and individual host-dependent factors such as food consumption habits, age, and the host's immunocompetence.

Although seroprevalence in populations is rather high, the majority of infected people do not develop symptoms due to immunological parasite-host interactions. Ocular toxoplasmosis can occur month or years after postnatal or congenital infection and might be the first sign of a systemic toxoplasmosis. Therefore, all seropositive individuals are at risk to develop an ocular toxoplasmosis in their lifetime. Age over 40, time of infection, and immunosuppression are risk factors for onset, recurrence, and severity of ophthalmic toxoplasmosis [23].

3.1.3 Clinical peculiarities

In patients with ocular toxoplasmosis, retinochorioditis is the most typical finding. Active intraocular inflammation often presents as focal necrotizing granulomatous retinitis with reactive granulomatous choroiditis and vitritis. The clinical image contains active lesions, often close to a pigmented or atrophic scar, described as whitish foci with obscure borders. Vasculitis can appear close or distant to the lesions and presents mainly as phlebitis and less frequent as arteritis eventually with hemorrhages [28]. In rare cases, Kyrieleis arteritis, a type of arteriolitis with intravascular nodular-like white plaques, can be found [29, 30]. Usually, the active lesions tend to heal within 2–4 month in immunocompetent patients by leaving an atrophic area gradually turning into a hyperpigmented scar due to disruption of retinal pigment epithelium. New active lesions are frequently close to old scars as a sign of recurrence [31]. Especially in immunocompromised patients, the differential diagnosis to other pathogens may be difficult [32].

Nonetheless, there are many atypical and unusual presentations related to the anatomical region of inflammation including anterior uveitis [28] with complication of rise in intraocular pressure, punctate outer retinal toxoplasmosis (PORT) with risk for secondary optic neuropathy and significant visual loss [23], neuroretinitis, and other unspecific features such as scleritis [33], which may delay a timely diagnosis [34] with risk of permanent vitreous opacities, deterioration in visual acuity or even vision loss in case of macular or optic nerve involvement. Recurrences with inflammatory reaction may occur at any time post primary infection resulting from ruptured intraretinal cysts.

Complications are associated with intraocular inflammation and are correlated with older age, retinal lesions larger than one disc size, and extra-macular lesions. Vasculitis-associated complications are proliferative tractional bands, vitreoretinopathy, and retinal vasculitis, which can contribute to tractional retinal detachment and hemorrhages and vascular occlusions. Especially immunocompromised patients with large necrotic areas are at higher risk for retinal cracks and retinal detachment [23].

3.1.4 Diagnostics

Typical ocular toxoplasmosis usually is diagnosed by characteristic clinical findings and serological detection methods. However, imaging technics help to estimate severity of clinical signs, diagnosing atypical ocular toxoplasmosis patterns and surveil the clinical course and treatment efficacy. The diagnostic work-up usually is composed of basic ophthalmological assessments, imaging techniques such as ultrasound, fundus color photography, optical coherence tomography, optical coherence tomography angiography, confocal scanning laser ophthalmoscopy, fundus autofluorescence, fluorescent angiography, indocyanine green angiography, and direct and indirect *T. gondii* detection tests in case of uncertainty after fundus imaging. Therefore, serological methods, immunohistochemical methods, specific PCR methods are commonly used. High sensitivity and specificity of PCR-based assays and detection of specific antibodies from vitreous and aqueous fluid have gained remarkable diagnostic value in diagnosing ocular toxoplasmosis [23]. PCR is the main detection method for determining *T. gondii* infection in ocular inflammation, congenital infections, and immunocompromised patients including HIV-infected patients. Real-time PCR and nested-PCR show consistently good results in detecting parasite DNA in ocular fluids of patients with toxoplasmosis including immunocompromised with high sensitivity and specificity. Detection works best during the first weeks of onset of symptoms.

Serological laboratory tests routinely help to determine whether an infection is recently acquired or chronic according to individual course of IgM, IgG, and IgA titers and IgG avidity patterns. Additionally, serology helps to rule out toxoplasmosis if suspected. Low IgG und absence of IgM antibodies are the regular finding in immunocompetent individuals with typical ocular toxoplasmosis. This highlights that only positive IgG titers are not suitable to confirm the diagnosis. However, solely immune enzyme assays are useful in diagnosing active ocular toxoplasmosis by supporting clinical findings in up to 96% of typical and atypical ocular toxoplasmosis by indicating positivity and significant increase of specific antibodies titers [35]. The approach of combined PCR and antibody detection from aqueous humor has strong predictive power in confirming the clinical diagnosis of ocular toxoplasmosis especially in immunocompromised individuals and atypical cases [36]. Interferon-γ release assays from whole blood for specific *T. gondii* T-cells show reliable results in detecting toxoplasmosis with 96% sensitivity and 91% specificity in seropositive adults with acute or chronic infection and in 94% and 98% for infants with congenital infection by mothers who acquired infection during pregnancy [37, 38].

3.1.5 Therapy

When deciding whether to treat active retinochorioiditis, considerations should include the mostly benign natural course, patients' characteristics (pregnancy, newborns, allergies, etc.) toxicity of potential drugs, the individual clinical course and immune status, presentation of active lesions, visual acuity and vitreous opacity, complications such as vascular occlusion and edema of macular or optic disc. Treatment regimens are combinations of antimicrobial drugs (control of parasite replication) and topical and systemic corticosteroids for 4–6 weeks. The role of treatment in chronic toxoplasmosis remains unclear due to lack of evidence in efficacy against tissue cysts [39]. The main goals of treatment are size reduction of lesions and prevention of adverse complications of active ocular toxoplasmosis. All first-line regimens have no significant effect on recurrences although trimethoprim-sulfamethoxazole might have [40] if substituted for sulfadiazine. Close monitoring of drug-related gastrointestinal, dermatological, and hematological (leukocytopenia, thrombocytopenia) adverse events and allergic side effects is recommended. Weekly blood tests should be performed and depending on the chosen treatment regimen substitution of folic acid is required.

First-line regimens are: (I) pyrimathamine, sulfadiazine, folic acid, and prednisone; (II) pyrimethamine, clindamycin, folic acid, and prednisone; (III) pyrimethamine, sulfadiazine, clindamycin, folic acid, and prednisone "quadruple therapy." Selected alternative regimens are: (IV) trimethoprim-sulfamethoxazole and prednisone; (V) clindamycin, spiramycin, prednisone; (VI) clindamycin, sulfadiazine, prednisone; (VII) pyrimethamine, azithromycin, folic acid, prednisone. Other alternative combinations include atovaquone or tetracycline derivates [41, 42].

The first-line treatments or called classical treatments show better reduction of duration of posterior pole retinitis in comparison to alternative regimens and are more fitting for foveal adjacent and fovea lesions [43]. Systemic corticosteroid therapy usually starts 3 days after and stops 10 days before antimicrobial therapy and is only recommended in immunocompetent individuals [23].

Another therapeutic approach is the intravitreal application of clindamycin and dexamethasone, which show larger lesion size reductions in IgM-positive patients compared with the classic treatment or no treatment. Additional advantages of intravitreal drug application are less systemic side effects what might be beneficial in pregnancy. One of the disadvantages is the risk of fulminant systemic disease in immunocompromised patients. Other supportive measurements include steroid eye drops, mydriatics, and local hypotensive agents to prevent and manage complications of active ocular toxoplasmosis [44]. For immunocompromised or pregnant patients, modified treatment strategies are available, which mostly aim at prevention of severe complications of active ocular toxoplasmosis and toxoplasmosis in general with indications to treat at low thresholds and close treatment supervision by a multidisciplinary team [23].

3.1.6 Prognosis

The prognosis and course are mainly dependent on the timely and appropriate diagnosis and management of active ocular toxoplasmosis, complications, and the frequency of individual recurrences associated with personal and environmental risk factors over time.

3.2 Ocular toxocariasis

Ocular toxocariasis or ocular larva migrans is a worldwide prevalent common zoonotic helminthic infection caused by roundworms, which might cause severe vision impairment or loss.

3.2.1 Pathogen

Toxocara species mainly *T. canis* (dog) and *T. cati/mystax* (cat) are helminths (common ascaris roundworms), which can follow a direct life cycle by infecting definite hosts who shed unembryonated eggs, which become infectious (third-stage larvae, L3) in the environment. Alternatively, they follow indirect life cycles by infecting paratenic hosts where migrating L3 larvae form tissue cysts might finally be inoculated by a definite host. Humans are accidental hosts (L3 larvae cannot complete the life cycle and therefore do not breed eggs) and get infected by accidentally ingesting infectious eggs with contaminated food or water or by consumption of undercooked and raw meat of paratenic hosts containing L3 larvae cysts. After ingestion, L3 larvae penetrate the small intestinal mucosa and circulate via blood to different organs and tissues where the larvae start migrating causing local immunological and inflammatory reactions, which might lead to symptoms. The majority is asymptomatically infected. Symptomatic presentations are either visceral or ocular larva migrans. Severity is a function of parasitic load.

3.2.2 Epidemiology

Toxocariasis is worldwide distributed. The majority of ocular larva migrans infections are related to *T. canis* and less frequent reported by *T. cati/T. mystax*. Seroprevalence rates for Toxocara antibodies vary from approximately 3 to over 70% [45] with lower rates in industrialized countries and higher rates in low- and middle-income countries related to lower standards in water, sanitation and hygiene and public surveillance, prevention, and control. Exceptions are reported, which mostly are related to habitual food consumption than low hygiene standards [45, 46].

Ocular larva migrans affects children and adults with mean age at onset ranging from 6.4 [47] to 51.7 [48, 49] years and is a significant cause for visual impairment during childhood. The age at presentation with symptoms may vary from 1 to 77 years [48–51].

3.2.3 Clinical peculiarities

Ocular larva migrans is mainly unilateral eye involvement but may appear bilateral [52]. One exclusive feature in ocular larva migrans might be present as migrating granuloma, either continuous or discontinuous. The clinical presentations can be categorized as.

i. the most common one as posterior pole granuloma. Imposing as posterior pole located whitish, focal intraretinal, or subretinal mass accompanied by inflammation and mostly less than one disc diameter. Pigmentation can be observed as well as vitreous haze and macular lesions [53].

ii. Peripheral granuloma in the retinal periphery imposing as whitish focal nodule accompanied by diffuse inflammation and sometimes proliferation of fibrocellular bands leading to the optic nerve forming retinal folds, which can cause retinal traction and consecutive retinal detachment.

iii. Nematode endophthalmitis present as panuveitis, sometimes with hypopyon and more often with vitreous haze and diffuse intraocular inflammation and severe pain [60]. When the inflammation and vitreous haze and vitreous opacity subside, retinal granuloma should be actively searched for.

iv. Atypical presentations might show motile retinal larvae, diffuse chorioretinitis, optic neuritis [54–56]. Additionally unspecific findings such as iridocyclitis, keratitis, concunctivitis, or cataract can be found [54].

Vision loss might occur as result to severe intraocular inflammation and consecutive vitritis, aggravation of underlying comorbidities and caused by the location of the granuloma itself.

3.2.4 Diagnostics

Diagnosis can be determined by evaluation of clinical characteristics assessed by basic ophthalmologic methods and supported by imaging via ultrasound and the detection of the typical granuloma in the course. And additionally performed serological tests to detect Toxocara larvae specific serum antibodies via indirect enzyme-linked immunosorbent assay [50, 54, 55]. Titers higher than 1:32 in ELISA indicate toxocariasis with sensitivity of 78% [57]. In contrast, titers lower than 1:8 cannot completely rule out toxocariasis infection in the presence of typical clinical signs. Total IgE serum levels might support diagnosis and can be beneficial in monitoring treatment efficacy when decreasing under therapy [48, 49]. Eosinophilia as seen in visceral larva migrans is usually not present in ocular larva migrans.

3.2.5 Therapy

Standard treatment of active intraocular inflammation is the application of systemic and topic corticosteroids to reduce inflammation, limiting membrane formation and vitreous opacity, and improving vision [48, 49, 53, 58–60]. Antihelminthic treatment with albendazole or diethylcarbamazine in ocular larva migrans is controversially discussed due to lack of knowledge about intraocular efficacy. The combination with albendazole and corticosteroids shows effects with regard to reduction of recurrence [48, 49, 59] compared with corticosteroid-only treatments. Vitreoretinal surgical interventions might improve vision, if structural problems such as vitreous opacity, retinal detachment, or epiretinal membranes persist after medical therapy [48, 49, 61].

4. Bacterial forms of retinitis

4.1 Tuberculosis

4.1.1 Epidemiology

The WHO reports that more than 2 billion people are affected worldwide by tuberculosis [62]. Extrapulmonary tuberculosis occurs in 20%, and ocular tuberculosis develops from 3.5 to 5.1% of infected people. Patients with HIV often develop a generalization of the specific inflammation process, caused by *Mycobacterium tuberculosis* [63–65].

4.1.2 Clinical features

Ocular tuberculosis has no direct relation to the clinical manifestations of pulmonary tuberculosis; moreover, up to 60% of patients with extrapulmonary variants of tuberculosis do not have affected lungs [66]. According to the results of Collaborative Ocular Tuberculosis Study (COTS) [62, 67], the manifestations of tuberculosis with retinal involvement can be divided into a few different forms:

1. Tubercular posterior uveitis (TPU), the inflammation affects retina and/or the choroid. 2. Tubercular panuveitis (TBP), the inflammation affects anterior chamber, vitreous body and retina/choroid. 3. Tubercular retinal vasculitis (TRV), phlebitis, or arteritis with or without vessel occlusion.

Choroidal tubercles can be characterized as the most common intraocular manifestation of TPU. Choroidal tubercles are disseminated ill-defined, oval, grayish-white or yellowish deep lesions, mostly localized in the posterior pole, they show early hypofluorescence and late staining on fluorescein angiography [68]. Choroidal tubercles may develop itself to choroidal tuberculomas, which present a solitary mass with overlying retinal folds or retinal detachment. These may be located anywhere in the choroid and can be misdiagnosed as intraocular tumors or subretinal abscesses [62].

TRV can be described as perivenular cuffing with thick exudates, with or without retinal hemorrhages, focal choroiditis lesions, and moderate vitritis. Because of occlusive nature, TRV leads to peripheral capillary nonperfusion and retinal or optic disc neovascularization. These processes can be complicated by vitreous hemorrhage, traction retinal detachment, iris neovascularization, and neovascular glaucoma [68, 69]. These clinical sings are not very specific for a tuberculous etiology; other ocular pathologies, such as sarcoidosis or ocular infection with Toxoplasma, can also produce similar clinical forms.

4.1.3 Diagnostics

The interferon-γ release assay (IGRA) indicates a latent or active tuberculosis and quantifies interferon-γ released by sensitized T cells when they were exposed to *M. tuberculosis* peptide antigens. IGRA has some advantages in the diagnostics of the ocular tuberculosis, because it allows to overcome the limitations of tuberculin skin test. The early secretory antigen target 6 (ESAT-6) and culture filtrate protein 10 (CFP-10) are not present in the Bacille Calmette-Guérin vaccination strains and non-tuberculous mycobacterium species and provide increased specificity of IGRA versus skin tests [70]. There are two available IGRA test systems: the QuantiFERON-TB Gold Plus (QFT-Plus, Qiagen, Hilden, Germany) and the T-SPOT.TB (Oxford Immunotec, Abingdon, UK) [70, 71].

Some clinical particularities need to be considered, before the antitubercular therapy (ATT) is initiated. The usually applied cutoff values (0.35 IU/ml) for QFT were shown to be too low in the setting of uveitis and may lead to overtreatment [72]. A cutoff value of 2.00 IU/ml was proposed instead, based on receiver operating characteristic (ROC) curve analysis, which showed that a threshold of 2.00 IU/ml had 84% sensitivity and 87% specificity for successful ATT in patients with ocular tuberculosis. Moreover, the best option for optimizing the routine screening, based on QFT, is to adjust the cutoff value on local endemicity and epidemiological data [73]. An analysis conducted by Agrawal and colleagues suggests that QFT levels alone cannot adequately separate tuberculosis-positive and -negative patients among patients with clinical signs suggestive of ocular tuberculosis [74]. Thus, if QFT is used as a routine diagnostic tool, its results cannot be taken and interpreted without context. Even negative IGRA test results should be interpreted with caution because they do not exclude the diagnosis.

The nucleic acid amplification enables diagnostics of ocular tuberculosis without the need to detect acid-fast bacilli, which are rarely presented in ocular samples. The quantitative real-time PCR uses fluorescent probes for fast detection and quantification of *M. tuberculosis* load in the sample. The advantage of this procedure is a decreased rate of contamination [75]. Multi-targeted PCR simultaneously amplifies multiple gene targets to achieve a higher diagnostic sensitivity. The sensitivity and specificity of PCR methods were estimated and documented by [71], and sensitivity was ranging from 37.7 to 85.2% and specificity was at a level of 90–100%. The MTBDRplus assay, which was performed on vitreous fluid samples, could detect rifampicin and isoniazid resistance, confirmed by rpoB and katG gene sequencing [76]. Larger studies must be planned and performed to validate the accuracy and reliability of modern PCR methods [67]. PCR is considered a reliable method, and clinicians should evaluate negative results in correlation with clinical findings, an expected clinical response to ATT supports the PCR results [77].

4.1.4 Therapy

The role of ATT by ocular tuberculosis remains controversial, and there is no international agreement on therapeutic protocols and duration of the ATT [78–82]. Evidence shows efficacy of ATT in reducing the rate of disease recurrences [83].

Results derived from a meta-analysis of 28 studies, which evaluated the effect of ATT on the ocular outcome of 1917 [80] patients, demonstrate that 84% of patients treated with ATT did not experience relapse of inflammation during the follow-up. The role of oral corticosteroids and immunosuppression agents is also still controversial, and there is no agreement on their efficacy in patients with tubercular uveitis treated with ATT [80]. Recent studies show a success of local therapy in the management of tubercular uveitis as an optional adjunctive anti-inflammatory therapy [82, 84, 85].

4.1.5 Prognosis

There is no evidence-based data about long-time prognosis. A low treatment failure rate was shown to occur in patients with tuberculous uveitis treated with ATT. Patients with TBP complicated by vitreous and choroidal involvement had a higher risk of treatment failure [74].

4.2 Ocular syphilis

Syphilis caused by the spirochete bacterium *Treponema pallidum* has an ability to mimic different diseases due to its variety of clinical manifestations.

4.2.1 Epidemiology

The CDC in the United States reported 7.5 cases of primary and secondary syphilis per 100,000 population in 2015; 54% of patients were males, who have practiced sex with other males [86]. The syphilis co-infection of HIV patients ranges from 20% to 70% [87]. Statistical analysis estimates that HIV-positive individuals have an 86 times higher risk of syphilis [63]. Male gender was found to be the only statistically significant risk factor for the development of ocular syphilis; ocular syphilis was seen in 9.5% of men as compared with 1.5% of women [87].

4.2.2 Clinical features

Retinal manifestations of ocular syphilis include following constellations [87]: 1. Chorioretinitis; 2. Necrotizing retinitis; 3. Retinal vasculitis; 4. Retinal vasculitis; 5. Vitritis; 6. Exudative retinal detachment.

Chorioretinitis with vitritis is the most usual finding in syphilitic posterior uveitis and involves the posterior pole and mid-periphery. The inflammatory lesions are initially small, between one-half to one in disc-diameter, but they can become large and confluent [88–90]. The affection of the retina or choroid is usually seen in secondary syphilis, and approximately half of the patients with ocular syphilis experience bilateral involvement [91].

Acute syphilitic posterior placoid chorioretinitis (ASPPC) is a rare manifestation of ocular syphilis [92]. ASPPC is characterized by yellowish, placoid, outer retinal lesions, usually located at or near the macula, with a faded center and stipulation of the retinal pigment epithelium. Such lesions can be seen as the result of active specific inflammation of the chorioretinal complex (choriocapillaris-pigment epithelial-retinal photoreceptor complex). The inflammation can be triggered by dissemination and direct invasion of *T. pallidum*, which causes occlusion of the choriocapillaris or sedimentation of soluble immune complexes, which cause an inflammation of the vessel wall or both of these pathogenetic inflammation ways [92]. Two cases of acute zonal occult outer retinopathy (AZOOR) were reported in which syphilis was identified as the underlying disease [93]. AZOOR presents with a sudden onset of photopsia and scotoma, which are related to loss of outer retinal sectors function. Fundoscopy can be normal in the early phase of the disease.

Necrotizing retinitis is a seldom complication of ocular syphilis and can mimic acute retinal necrosis [94–96]. Usual clinical features of retinitis associated with ocular syphilis are presented by retinal lesions, which tend to heal with minimal disruption of the retinal pigment epithelium [97]. Vasculitis involves retinal arteries, arterioles, capillaries, and veins [98]. The fundus fluorescein angiography can be complex and demonstrates perivascular exudation and fibrosis, occlusive vasculitis [93, 99], isolated or focal retinal vasculitis, which can simulate branch retinal vein occlusion [100, 101].

4.2.3 Diagnostics

The screening tests used for syphilis diagnostics are enzyme immunoassays (EIA) and chemiluminescent immunoassays (CIA), which detect antibodies to treponemal antigens. If positive, a non-treponemal test, rapid plasma reagin (RPR) or Venereal Diseases Research Laboratory (VDRL) test for cardiolipin antibodies should be performed [87]. The *T. pallidum* hemagglutination assay (TPHA) or *T. pallidum* particle agglutination test (TPPA) detects specific treponemal antibodies. Some of HIV-positive patients can show non-reactive serological results. This phenomenon can be avoided by testing diluted serum [87].

Direct detection can be carried out with dark-field microscopy, PCR, and immune histochemistry. Dark-field microscopy directly visualizes *T. pallidum* by investigation of clinical samples (exudates from chancres, condylomata lata, lymph node aspirates, etc.) [102]. The sensitivity and specificity of dark-field microscopy are approximately 90% and 100%, respectively [103]. PCR of vitreous aspirates can be used, for example, to diagnose atypical manifestations of ocular syphilis [104] and can also be used to identify drug resistance of *T. pallidum* [105, 106].

4.2.4 Therapy

The current CDC guidelines recommend penicillin G as the drug of choice. Primary and secondary syphilis: benzathine penicillin G, 2.4 million units intramuscularly (i.m.) in a single dose. Early latent syphilis: benzathine penicillin G 2.4 million units i.m. in a single dose. Late latent syphilis: benzathine penicillin G 7.2 million units, as three doses of 2.4 million units i.m./week. Tertiary syphilis with normal CSF results: benzathine penicillin G 7.2 million units, as three doses of 2.4 million units i.m./week. Neurosyphilis and ocular syphilis: aqueous crystalline penicillin G 18–24 million units/day, as 3–4 million units i.v. every 4 h or continuous infusion for 10–14 days; or alternatively procaine penicillin G 2.4 million units i.m./days plus probenecid 500 mg orally 4× daily, both for 10–14 days. Systemic steroids have not been proven to have clinical benefits in the treatment of syphilis [107]. All patients with ocular or neurosyphilis should be screened for HIV. Highly effective treatment protocols to prevent neurosyphilis in patients with HIV and syphilis are still not available [108]. However, the antiretroviral therapy can improve clinical outcomes in patients with HIV and syphilis [87].

4.2.5 Prognosis

After serological diagnosis, syphilis treatment is associated with good prognosis [109].

4.3 Ocular manifestations of bartonellosis

There are over 30 different Bartonella subspecies. *Bartonella henselae, Bartonella quintana,* and *Bartonella bacilliformis* are responsible for most infections in humans. This organism is a Gram-negative hematotropic pathogen, it affects erythrocytes and/or endothelial cells. The clinical form can manifest as disseminated vascular proliferations throughout the body [110].

4.3.1 Epidemiology

Cats are the main reservoir, and over 90% of patients with Bartonella species infection have had a contact with a cat [111]. The clinical infection with Bartonella species has the term Cat-scratch disease (CSD) as a synonym. A multicenter retrospective study of CSD patients with ocular manifestations was performed between 1996 and 2015 [112]. Seasonal patterns were observed with ocular CSD [112]. Ocular bartonellosis has a broad age distribution [113]. In one clinical study, 141 of 3222 patients (4.4%) have had concomitant ocular manifestation of CSD [114].

4.3.2 Clinical features

The posterior segment manifestations of CSD include intermediate uveitis, optic neuritis, neuroretinitis, focal or multifocal retinitis and/or choroiditis, vascular occlusions, retinal vasculitis, granulomas, exudative retinal detachments, macular exudates, macular hole, white dot syndromes, angiomatous lesions, and acute endophthalmitis [115–117]. Patients may experience a varying severity of unilateral or bilateral visual loss and central scotoma. Neuroretinitis presents as optic disc swelling with serous retinal detachment, and macular exudation, which can be seen 2–4 weeks after the initial observation of optic disc swelling. The macular exudates can take a long time to resolve, up to 12 months [112].

4.3.3 Diagnostics

The diagnosis of CDS is based on the presence of the following clinical criteria [114]: 1. Contact with cats; 2. Positive skin test in response to CSD antigen; 3. Characteristic lymph nodes and lymphadenopathy not caused by other bacteria.

The best screening test for diagnostics of CSD is a serologic testing by either indirect fluorescence assay (IFA) or ELISA [118]. The IFA test has a sensitivity and specificity of 90% in immunocompetent patients and is the more commonly used diagnostic test [115, 119]. PCR is also a useful diagnostic test in particular by negative serology. PCR demonstrates a high specificity, but the sensitivity is lower than serology testing [119].

4.3.4 Therapy

Antibacterial therapy can be performed with the following antimicrobial drugs: doxycycline, macrolide antibiotics (clarithromycin, erythromycin, azithromycin), rifampicin, ciprofloxacin, ceftriaxone, and cotrimoxazole [111]. The usual therapy includes doxycycline 100 mg 2× per day for 4–6 weeks for immunocompetent patients and up to 4 months for immunocompromised patients. Younger patients can be treated with a macrolide antibiotic because of less long-term side effects [119].

Corticosteroids may be used as additional therapy component to antibiotic treatment with the aim to stop and control the inflammatory response. A multivariate logistic regression analysis has shown a significant improvement of visual acuity by a combination therapy (systemic corticosteroids and antibiotics) [112].

4.3.5 Prognosis

Most patients reached a good final visual acuity [112].

5. Conclusions

Several viral, parasitic, and bacterial pathogens form the major causes for infectious retinitis. Since the phenotype is not absolutely specific for the individual infection, specific diagnostic procedures focusing on the major pathogens and, in most cases, on nucleic acid amplification need to be used. Due to the individual pathogen, specific therapy is possible in many cases and increases the quality of the therapeutic outcome. Nevertheless, the current therapeutic results demand further development and improvement of the therapy of infectious retinitis.

Author details

Ruben Rose, Alexey Gorin, Mathias Voß and Helmut Fickenscher*
Institute for Infection Medicine, University Medical Center Schleswig-Holstein, Christian-Albrecht University of Kiel, Kiel, Germany

*Address all correspondence to: fickenscher@infmed.uni-kiel.de

References

[1] Young NJ, Bird AC. Bilateral acute retinal necrosis. The British Journal of Ophthalmology. 1978;**62**:581-590. DOI: 10.1136/bjo.62.9.581

[2] Rautenberg P, Hillenkamp J, Grančičova L, Nölle B, Roider J, Fickenscher H. Virus diagnostics and antiviral therapy in acute retinal necrosis (ARN). In: Arbuthnot P, editor. Antiviral Drugs—Aspects of Clinical Use and Recent Advances. Rijeka: Intech; 2012. pp. 17-34

[3] Rautenberg P, Grančičova L, Hillenkamp J, Nölle B, Roider JB, Fickenscher H. Acute retinal necrosis from the virologist's perspective. Der Ophthalmologe. 2009;**106**:1065-1073. DOI: 10.1007/s00347-009-2048-4

[4] Lee JH, Agarwal A, Mahendradas P, Lee CS, Gupta V, Pavesio CE, et al. Viral posterior uveitis. Survey of Ophthalmology. 2017;**62**:404-445. DOI: 10.1016/j.survophthal.2016.12.008

[5] Hillenkamp J, Nölle B, Bruns C, Rautenberg P, Fickenscher H, Roider J. Acute retinal necrosis: Clinical features, early vitrectomy, and outcomes. Ophthalmology. 2009;**116**:1971-1975. DOI: 10.1016/j.ophtha.2009.03.029

[6] Hillenkamp J, Nölle B, Rautenberg P, Fickenscher H, Roider J. Acute retinal necrosis. Der Ophthalmologe. 2009;**106**:1058-1064. DOI: 10.1007/s00347-009-2047-5

[7] Holland GN. Standard diagnostic criteria for the acute retinal necrosis syndrome. American Journal of Ophthalmology. 1994;**117**:663-667. DOI: 10.1016/s0002-9394(14)70075-3

[8] Takase H, Okada AA, Goto H, Mizuki N, Namba K, Ohguro N, et al. Development and validation of new diagnostic criteria for acute retinal necrosis. Japanese Journal of Ophthalmology. 2015;**59**:14-20. DOI: 10.1007/s10384-014-0362-0

[9] Brunnemann AK, Bohn-Wippert K, Zell R, Henke A, Walther M, Braum O, et al. Drug resistance of clinical varicella-zoster virus strains confirmed by recombinant thymidine kinase expression and by targeted resistance mutagenesis of a cloned wild-type isolate. Antimicrobial Agents and Chemotherapy. 2015;**59**:2726-2734. DOI: 10.1128/AAC.05115-14

[10] Sauerbrei A, Bohn-Wippert K, Kaspar M, Krumbholz A, Karrasch M, Zell R. Database on natural polymorphisms and resistance-related non-synonymous mutations in thymidine kinase and DNA polymerase genes of herpes simplex virus types 1 and 2. The Journal of Antimicrobial Chemotherapy. 2016;**71**:6-16. DOI: 10.1093/jac/dkv285

[11] Gilbert C, Bestman-Smith J, Boivin G. Resistance of herpesviruses to antiviral drugs: Clinical impacts and molecular mechanisms. Drug Resistance Updates. 2002;**5**:88-114. DOI: 10.1016/s1368-7646(02)00021-3

[12] Powell B, Wang D, Llop S, Rosen RB. Management strategies of acute retinal necrosis: Current perspectives. Clinical Ophthalmology. 2020;**14**:1931-1943. DOI: 10.2147/OPTH.S258488

[13] Schoenberger SD, Kim SJ, Thorne JE, Mruthyunjaya P, Yeh S, Bakri SJ, et al. Diagnosis and treatment of acute retinal necrosis. A report by the American Academy of ophthalmology. Ophthalmology. 2017;**124**:382-392. DOI: 10.1016/j.ophtha.2016.11.007

[14] Fan S, Lin D, Wang Y. Role of prophylactic vitrectomy in acute retinal necrosis in preventing rhegmatogenous retinal detachment: Systematic review and meta-analysis. Ocular Immunology and Inflammation. 2022;**30**:515-519. DOI: 10.1080/09273948.2020.1800051

[15] Chen M, Zhang M, Chen H. Efficiency of laser photocoagulation on the prevention of retinal detachment in acute retinal necrosis: A systematic review and meta-analysis. Retina. 2022;**42**:1702-1708. DOI: 10.1097/IAE.0000000000003527

[16] Chan NSW, Chee SP, Caspers L, Bodaghi B. Clinical features of CMV-associated anterior uveitis. Ocular Immunology and Inflammation. 2018;**26**:107-115. DOI: 10.1080/09273948.2017.1394471

[17] Port AD, Orlin A, Kiss S, Patel S, D'Amico DJ, Gupta MP. Cytomegalovirus retinitis: A review. Journal of Ocular Pharmacology and Therapeutics. 2017;**33**:224-234. DOI: 10.1089/jop.2016.0140

[18] Pesch MH, Schleiss MR. Emerging concepts in congenital cytomegalovirus. Pediatrics. 2022;**50**:e2021055896. DOI: 10.1542/peds.2021-055896

[19] Atmaca LS, Simsek T, Batioglu F. Clinical features and prognosis in ocular toxoplasmosis. Japanese Journal of Ophthalmology. 2004;**48**:386-391. DOI: 10.1007/s10384-003-0069-0

[20] Grigg ME, Dubey JP, Nussenblatt RB. Ocular toxoplasmosis: Lessons from Brazil. American Journal of Ophthalmology. 2015;**159**:999-1001. DOI: 10.1016/j.ajo.2015.04.005

[21] Feustel SM, Meissner M, Liesenfeld O. Toxoplasma gondii and the blood-brain barrier. Virulence. 2012;**3**:182-192. DOI: 10.4161/viru.19004

[22] Lachenmaier SM, Deli MA, Meissner M, Liesenfeld O. Intracellular transport of toxoplasma gondii through the blood-brain barrier. Journal of Neuroimmunology. 2011;**232**:119-130. DOI: 10.1016/j.jneuroim.2010.10.029

[23] Kalogeropoulos D, Sakkas H, Mohammed B, Vartholomatos G, Malamos K, Sreekantam S, et al. Ocular toxoplasmosis: A review of the current diagnostic and therapeutic approaches. International Ophthalmology. 2022;**42**:295-321. DOI: 10.1007/s10792-021-01994-9

[24] Montoya JG, Liesenfeld O. Toxoplasmosis, The Lancet. 2004;**363**(9425):1965-1976. DOI: 10.1016/S0140-6736(04)16412-X

[25] Holland GN. Ocular toxoplasmosis: A global reassessment. Part I, epidemiology and course of disease. American Journal of Ophthalmology. 2003;**136**:973-988. DOI: 10.1016/j.ajo.2003.09.040

[26] Soheilian M, Heidari K, Yazdani S, Shahsavari M, Ahmadieh H, Dehghan M. Patterns of uveitis in a tertiary eye care center in Iran. Ocular Immunology and Inflammation. 2004;**12**:297-310. DOI: 10.1080/092739490500174

[27] Balasundaram MB, Andavar R, Palaniswamy M, Venkatapathy N. Outbreak of acquired ocular toxoplasmosis involving 248 patients. Archives of Ophthalmology. 2010;**128**:28-32. DOI: 10.1001/archophthalmol.2009.354

[28] Delair E, Latkany P, Noble AG, Rabiah P, McLeod R, Brézin A. Clinical manifestations of ocular toxoplasmosis. Ocular Immunology and Inflammation. 2011;**19**:91-102. DOI: 10.3109/09273948.2011.564068

[29] Smith JR, Cunningham ET Jr. Atypical presentations of ocular toxoplasmosis.

Current Opinion in Ophthalmology. 2002;**13**:387-392. DOI: 10.1097/00055735-200212000-00008

[30] Pichi F, Veronese C, Lembo A, Invernizzi A, Mantovani A, Herbort CP, et al. New appraisals of Kyrieleis plaques: A multimodal imaging study. The British Journal of Ophthalmology. 2017;**101**:316-321. DOI: 10.1136/bjophthalmol-2015-308246

[31] Bowie WR, King AS, Werker DH, Isaac-Renton JL, Bell A, Eng SB, et al. Outbreak of toxoplasmosis associated with municipal drinking water. The BC toxoplasma investigation team. The Lancet. 1997;**350**(9072):173-177. DOI: 10.1016/s0140-6736(96)11105-3

[32] Hasselbach HC, Fickenscher H, Nölle B, Roider J. Atypical ocular toxoplasmosis with concomitant ocular reactivation of varicella-zoster virus and cytomegalovirus in an immunocompromised host. Klinische Monatsblätter für Augenheilkunde. 2008;**225**:236-239. DOI: 10.1055/s-2008-1027146

[33] Schuman JS, Weinberg RS, Ferry AP, Guerry RK. Toxoplasmic scleritis. Ophthalmology. 1988;**95**:1399-1403. DOI: 10.1016/s0161-6420(88)32998-2

[34] Bosch-Driessen LEH, Berendschot TTJM, Ongkosuwito JV, Rothova A. Ocular toxoplasmosis: Clinical features and prognosis of 154 patients. Ophthalmology. 2002;**109**:869-878. DOI: 10.1016/s0161-6420(02)00990-9

[35] Papadia M, Aldigeri F, Herbort CP. The role of serology in active ocular toxoplasmosis. International Ophthalmology. 2011;**31**:461-465. DOI: 10.1007/s10792-011-9507-z

[36] Previato M, Frederico FB, Murata FH, Siqueira RC, Barbosa AP, Silveira-Carvalho AP, et al. A Brazilian report using serological and molecular diagnosis to monitoring acute ocular toxoplasmosis. BMC Research Notes. 2015;**8**:746. DOI: 10.1186/s13104-015-1650-6

[37] Chapey E, Wallon M, Debize G, Rabilloud M, Peyron F. Diagnosis of congenital toxoplasmosis by using a whole-blood gamma interferon release assay. Journal of Clinical Microbiology. 2010;**48**:41-45. DOI: 10.1128/JCM.01903-09

[38] de Araújo TE, Dos Santos LI, Gomes AO, Carneiro ACAV, Machado AS, Coelho-Dos-Reis JG, et al. UFMG congenital toxoplasmosis Brazilian group UFMG-CTBG, beside the authors. Putative biomarkers for early diagnosis and prognosis of congenital ocular toxoplasmosis. Scientific Reports. 2020;**10**:16757. DOI: 10.1038/s41598-020-73265-z

[39] Stanford MR, Gilbert RE. Treating ocular toxoplasmosis: Current evidence. Memórias do Instituto Oswaldo Cruz. 2009;**104**:312-315. DOI: 10.1590/s0074-02762009000200027

[40] Silveira C, Belfort R Jr, Muccioli C, Holland GN, Victora CG, Horta BL, et al. The effect of long-term intermittent trimethoprim/sulfamethoxazole treatment on recurrences of toxoplasmic retinochoroiditis. American Journal of Ophthalmology. 2002;**134**:41-46. DOI: 10.1016/s0002-9394(02)01527-1

[41] Orefice F, Bonfioli AA. Toxoplasmosis. In: Orefice F, editor. Uveıtis—Clinica e Cirurgica. 1st ed. Rio de Janeiro: Cultura Medica; 2000. pp. 680-784

[42] Bonfioli AA, Orefice F. Toxoplasmosis. Seminars in Ophthalmology. 2005;**20**:129-141. DOI: 10.1080/08820530500231961

[43] Rothova A, Meenken C, Buitenhuis HJ, Brinkman CJ, Baarsma GS, Boen-Tan TN, et al. Therapy for ocular toxoplasmosis. American Journal of Ophthalmology. 1993;**115**:517-523. DOI: 10.1016/S0002-9394(14)74456-3

[44] Holland GN, Lewis KG. An update on current practices in the management of ocular toxoplasmosis. American Journal of Ophthalmology. 2002;**134**:102-114. DOI: 10.1016/s0002-9394(02)01526-x

[45] Stensvold CR, Skov J, Møller LN, Jensen PM, Kapel CM, Petersen E, et al. Seroprevalence of human toxocariasis in Denmark. Clinical and Vaccine Immunology. 2009;**16**:1372-1373. DOI: 10.1128/CVI.00234-09

[46] Fan CK, Hung CC, Du WY, Liao CW, Su KE. Seroepidemiology of Toxocara canis infection among mountain aboriginal schoolchildren living in contaminated districts in eastern Taiwan. Tropical Medicine & International Health. 2004;**9**:1312-1318. DOI: 10.1111/j.1365-3156.2004.01332.x

[47] Biglan AW, Glickman LT, Lobes LA Jr. Serum and vitreous Toxocara antibody in nematode endophthalmitis. American Journal of Ophthalmology. 1979;**88**: 898-901. DOI: 10.1016/0002-9394(79)90568-3

[48] Ahn SJ, Ryoo NK, Woo SJ. Ocular toxocariasis: Clinical features, diagnosis, treatment, and prevention. Asia Pacific Allergy. 2014;**4**:134-141. DOI: 10.5415/apallergy.2014.4.3.134

[49] Ahn SJ, Woo SJ, Jin Y, Chang YS, Kim TW, Ahn J, et al. Clinical features and course of ocular toxocariasis in adults. PLoS Neglected Tropical Diseases. 2014;**8**:e2938. DOI: 10.1371/journal.pntd.0002938

[50] Woodhall D, Starr MC, Montgomery SP, Jones JL, Lum F, Read RW, et al. Ocular toxocariasis: Epidemiologic, anatomic and therapeutic variations based on a survey of ophthalmic subspecialists. Ophthalmology. 2012;**119**:1211-1217. DOI: 10.1016/j.ophtha.2011.12.013

[51] Alabiad CR, Albini TA, Santos CI, Davis JL. Ocular toxocariasis in a seronegative adult. Ophthalmic Surgery, Lasers & Imaging. 2010;**41**:1-3. DOI: 10.3928/15428877-20100325-06

[52] Park SP, Park I, Park HY, Lee SU, Huh S, Magnaval JF. Five cases of ocular toxocariasis confirmed by serology. The Korean Journal of Parasitology. 2000;**38**:267-273. DOI: 10.3347/kjp.2000.38.4.267

[53] Wilkinson CP, Welch RB. Intraocular toxocara. American Journal of Ophthalmology. 1971;**71**:921-930. DOI: 10.1016/0002-9394(71)90267-4

[54] Rubinsky-Elefant G, Hirata CE, Yamamoto JH, Ferreira MU. Human toxocariasis: Diagnosis, worldwide seroprevalences and clinical expression of the systemic and ocular forms. Annals of Tropical Medicine and Parasitology. 2010;**104**:3-23. DOI: 10.1179/136485910X12607012373957

[55] Smith H, Holland C, Taylor M, Magnaval JF, Schantz P, Maizels R. How common is human toxocariasis? Towards standardizing our knowledge. Trends in Parasitology. 2009;**25**:182-188. DOI: 10.1016/j.pt.2009.01.006

[56] Stewart JM, Cubillan LD, Cunningham ET Jr. Prevalence, clinical features, and causes of vision loss among patients with ocular toxocariasis. Retina. 2005;**25**:1005-1013. DOI: 10.1097/00006982-200512000-00009

[57] Schantz PM. Toxocara larva migrans now. The American Journal of Tropical Medicine and Hygiene. 1989;**41**:21-34. DOI: 10.4269/ajtmh.1989.41.21

[58] Shields JA. Ocular toxocariasis. A review. Survey of Ophthalmology. 1984;**28**:361-381. DOI: 10.1016/0039-6257(84)90242-x

[59] Barisani-Asenbauer T, Maca SM, Hauff W, Kaminski SL, Domanovits H, Theyer I, et al. Treatment of ocular toxocariasis with albendazole. Journal of Ocular Pharmacology and Therapeutics. 2001;**17**:287-294. DOI: 10.1089/108076801750295317

[60] Bird AC, Smith JL, Curtin VT. Nematode optic neuritis. American Journal of Ophthalmology. 1970;**69**:72-77. DOI: 10.1016/0002-9394(70)91858-1

[61] Giuliari GP, Ramirez G, Cortez RT. Surgical treatment of ocular toxocariasis: Anatomic and functional results in 45 patients. European Journal of Ophthalmology. 2011;**21**:490-494. DOI: 10.5301/EJO.2010.6118

[62] Abdisamadov A, Tursunov O. Ocular tuberculosis epidemiology, clinic features and diagnosis: A brief review. Tuberculosis (Edinburgh, Scotland). 2020;**124**:101963. DOI: 10.1016/j.tube.2020.101963

[63] Lee JY. Diagnosis and treatment of extrapulmonary tuberculosis. Tuberculosis and Respiratory Diseases (Seoul). 2015;**78**:47-55. DOI: 10.4046/trd.2015.78.2.47

[64] Ramírez-Lapausa M, Menendez-Saldana A, Noguerado-Asensio A. Extrapulmonary tuberculosis: An overview. Revista Española de Sanidad Penitenciaria. 2015;**17**:3-11. DOI: 10.4321/S1575-06202015000100002

[65] Mehta S, Mansoor H, Khan S, Saranchuk P. Isaakidis P (2013) ocular inflammatory disease and ocular tuberculosis in a cohort of patients co-infected with HIV and multidrug-resistant tuberculosis in Mumbai, India: A cross-sectional study. BMC Infectious Diseases. 2013;**13**:225. DOI: 10.1186/1471-2334-13-225

[66] Alvarez S, McCabe WR. Extrapulmonary tuberculosis revisited: A review of experience at Boston City and other hospitals. Medicine (Baltim). 1984;**63**:25-55

[67] Agarwal A, Agrawal R, Gunasekaran DV, Raje D, Gupta B, Aggarwal K, et al. The collaborative ocular tuberculosis study (COTS)-1 report 3: Polymerase chain reaction in the diagnosis and management of tubercular uveitis: Global trends. Ocular Immunology and Inflammation. 2019;**27**:465-473. DOI: 10.1080/09273948.2017.1406529

[68] Gupta V, Shoughy SS, Mahajan S, Khairallah M, Rosenbaum JT, Curi A, et al. Clinics of ocular tuberculosis. Ocular Immunology and Inflammation. 2015;**23**:14-24. DOI: 10.3109/09273948.2014.986582

[69] Gupta V, Gupta A, Arora S, Bambery P, Dogra MR, Agarwal A. Presumed tubercular serpiginouslike choroiditis: Clinical presentations and management. Ophthalmology. 2003;**110**:1744-1749. DOI: 10.1016/S0161-6420(03)00619-5

[70] Diel R, Goletti D, Ferrara G, Bothamley G, Cirillo D, Kampmann B, et al. Interferon-gamma release assays for the diagnosis of latent mycobacterium tuberculosis infection: A systematic review and meta-analysis. The European Respiratory Journal. 2011;**37**:88-99. DOI: 10.1183/09031936.00115110

[71] Ang M, Vasconcelos-Santos DV, Sharma K, Accorinti M, Sharma A,

Gupta A, et al. Diagnosis of ocular tuberculosis. Ocular Immunology and Inflammation. 2018;**26**:208-216. DOI: 10.1080/09273948.2016.1178304

[72] Gineys R, Bodaghi B, Carcelain G, Cassoux N, Boutin LTH, Amoura Z, et al. QuantiFERON-TB gold cut-off value: Implications for the management of tuberculosis-related ocular inflammation. American Journal of Ophthalmology. 2011;**152**:433-440. DOI: 10.1016/j.ajo.2011.02.006

[73] Slater ML, Welland G, Pai M, Parsonnet J, Banaei N. Challenges with QuantiFERON-TB gold assay for large-scale, routine screening of U.S. healthcare workers. American Journal of Respiratory and Critical Care Medicine. 2013;**188**:1005-1010. DOI: 10.1164/rccm.201305-0831OC

[74] Agrawal R, Grant R, Gupta B, Gunasekeran DV, Gonzalez-Lopez JJ, Addison PKF, et al. What does IGRA testing add to the diagnosis of ocular tuberculosis? A Bayesian latent class analysis. BMC Ophthalmology. 2017;**17**:245. DOI: 10.1186/s12886-017-0597-x

[75] Sharma K, Gupta V, Bansal R, Sharma A, Sharma M, Gupta A. Novel multi-targeted polymerase chain reaction for diagnosis of presumed tubercular uveitis. Journal of Ophthalmic Inflammation and Infection. 2013;**3**:25. DOI: 10.1186/1869-5760-3-25

[76] Sharma K, Gupta A, Sharma M, Sharma A, Singh R, Aggarwal K, et al. MTBDRplus for the rapid diagnosis of ocular tuberculosis and screening of drug resistance. Eye (London, England). 2018;**32**:451-456. DOI: 10.1038/eye.2017.214

[77] Sudheer B, Lalitha P, Kumar AL, Rathinam S. Polymerase chain reaction and its correlation with clinical features and treatment response in tubercular uveitis. Ocular Immunology and Inflammation. 2018;**26**:845-852. DOI: 10.1080/09273948.2017.1287925

[78] Lee C, Agrawal R, Pavesio C. Ocular tuberculosis—A clinical conundrum. Ocular Immunology and Inflammation. 2016;**24**:237-242. DOI: 10.3109/09273948.2014.985387

[79] Ang M, Chee SP. Controversies in ocular tuberculosis. The British Journal of Ophthalmology. 2017;**101**:6-20. DOI: 10.1136/bjophthalmol-2016-309531

[80] Kee AR, Gonzalez-Lopez JJ, Al-Hity A, Gupta B, Lee CS, Gunasekeran DV, et al. Anti-tubercular therapy for intraocular tuberculosis: A systematic review and meta-analysis. Survey of Ophthalmology. 2016;**61**:628-653. DOI: 10.1016/j.survophthal.2016.03.001

[81] Agrawal R, Gupta B, Gonzalez-Lopez JJ, Rahman F, Phatak S, Triantafyllopoulou I, et al. The role of anti- tubercular therapy in patients with presumed ocular tuberculosis. Ocular Immunology and Inflammation. 2015;**23**:40-46. DOI: 10.3109/09273948.2014.986584

[82] Agrawal R, Gunasekeran DV, Raje D, Agarwal A, Nguyen QD, Kon OM, et al. Global variations and challenges with tubercular uveitis in the collaborative ocular tuberculosis study. Investigative Ophthalmology & Visual Science. 2018;**59**:4162-4171. DOI: 10.1167/iovs.18-24102

[83] Testi I, Agrawal R, Mehta S, Basu S, Nguyen Q, Pavesio C, et al. Ocular tuberculosis: Where are we today? Indian Journal of Ophthalmology. 2020;**68**:1808-1817. DOI: 10.4103/ijo.IJO_1451_20

[84] Jain L, Panda KG, Basu S. Clinical outcomes of adjunctive sustained-release intravitreal dexamethasone

implants in tuberculosis-associated multifocal serpigenoid choroiditis. Ocular Immunology and Inflammation. 2018;**26**:877-883. DOI: 10.1080/09273948.2017.1383446

[85] Hasanreisoglu M, Gulpinar Ikiz G, Aktas Z, Ozdek S. Intravitreal dexamethasone implant as an option for anti-inflammatory therapy of tuberculosis uveitis. International Ophthalmology. 2019;**39**:485-490. DOI: 10.1007/s10792-018-0831-4

[86] Tsuboi M, Nishijima T, Yashiro S, Teruya K, Kikuchi Y, Katai N, et al. Prognosis of ocular syphilis in patients infected with HIV in the antiretroviral therapy era. Sexually Transmitted Infections. 2016;**92**:605-610. DOI: 10.1136/sextrans-2016-052568

[87] Dutta Majumder P, Chen EJ, Shah J, Ching Wen Ho D, Biswas J, See Yin L, et al. Ocular syphilis: An update. Ocular Immunology and Inflammation. 2019;**27**:117-125. DOI: 10.1080/09273948.2017.1371765

[88] Aldave AJ, King JA, Cunningham ET Jr. Ocular syphilis. Current Opinion in Ophthalmology. 2001;**12**:433-441. DOI: 10.1097/00055735-200112000-00008

[89] Margo CE, Hamed LM. Ocular syphilis. Survey of Ophthalmology. 1992;**37**:203-220. DOI: 10.1016/0039-6257(92)90138-j

[90] Tamesis RR, Foster CS. Ocular syphilis. Ophthalmology. 1990;**97**:1281-1287. DOI: 10.1016/s0161-6420(90)32419-3

[91] Morgan CM, Webb RM, O'Connor GR. Atypical syphilitic chorioretinitis and vasculitis. Retina. 1984;**4**:225-231. DOI: 10.1097/00006982-198400440-00003

[92] Gass JD, Braunstein RA, Chenoweth RG. Acute syphilitic posterior placoid chorioretinitis. Ophthalmology. 1990;**97**:1288-1297. DOI: 10.1016/s0161-6420(90)32418-1

[93] Lima BR, Mandelcorn ED, Bakshi N, Nussenblatt RB, Sen HN. Syphilitic outer retinopathy. Ocular Immunology and Inflammation. 2014;**22**:4-8. DOI: 10.3109/09273948.2013.841960

[94] Kuo A, Ziaee SM, Hosseini H, Voleti V, Schwartz SD, Kim NU, et al. The great imitator: Ocular syphilis presenting as posterior uveitis. American Journal of Case Reports. 2015;**16**:434-437. DOI: 10.12659/AJCR.893907

[95] Mendelsohn AD, Jampol LM. Syphilitic retinitis. A cause of necrotizing retinitis. Retina. 1984;**4**:221-224

[96] Rahman HT, Yeh S. Diffuse infiltrative syphilitic retinitis in an HIV-positive patient. The Journal of Ophthalmic Inflammation and Infection. 2011;**1**:123-123. DOI: 10.1007/s12348-011-0026-x

[97] Fu EX, Geraets RL, Dodds EM, Echandi LV, Colombero D, McDonald HR, et al. Superficial retinal precipitates in patients with syphilitic retinitis. Retina. 2010;**30**:1135-1143. DOI: 10.1097/IAE.0b013e3181cdf3ae

[98] Crouch ER, Goldberg MF. Retinal periarteritis secondary to syphilis. Archives of Ophthalmology. 1975;**93**:384-387. DOI: 10.1001/archopht.1975.01010020396017

[99] Yokoi M, Kase M. Retinal vasculitis due to secondary syphilis. Japanese Journal of Ophthalmology. 2004;**48**:65-67. DOI: 10.1007/s10384-003-0011-5

[100] Lobes LA, Folk JC. Syphilitic phlebitis simulating branch vein occlusion. Annals of Ophthalmology. 1981;**13**:825-827

[101] Savir H, Kurz O. Fluorescein angiography in syphilitic retinal vasculitis. Annals of Ophthalmology. 1976;**8**:713-716

[102] Majumder PD, Sudharshan S, Biswas J. Laboratory support in the diagnosis of uveitis. Indian Journal of Ophthalmology. 2013;**61**:269-276. DOI: 10.4103/0301-4738.114095

[103] Tsang RS, Morshed M, Chernesky MA, Jayaraman GC, Kadkhoda K. Canadian public health laboratory network laboratory guidelines for the use of direct tests to detect syphilis in Canada. Canadian Journal of Infectious Diseases and Medical Microbiology. 2015;**26**:13A-17A. DOI: 10.1155/2015/685603

[104] Troutbeck R, Chhabra R, Jones NP. Polymerase chain reaction testing of vitreous in atypical ocular syphilis. Ocular Immunology and Inflammation. 2013;**21**:227-230. DOI: 10.3109/09273948.2013.770887

[105] Lukehart SA, Godornes C, Molini BJ, Sonnett P, Hopkins S, Mulcahy F, et al. Macrolide resistance in treponema pallidum in the United States and Ireland. The New England Journal of Medicine. 2004;**351**:154-158. DOI: 10.1056/NEJMoa040216

[106] Martin IE, Tsang RS, Sutherland K, Tilley P, Read R, Anderson B, et al. Molecular characterization of syphilis in patients in Canada: Azithromycin resistance and detection of treponema pallidum DNA in whole-blood samples versus ulcerative swabs. Journal of Clinical Microbiology. 2009;**47**:1668-1673. DOI: 10.1128/JCM.02392-08

[107] Workowski KA, Bolan GA. Sexually transmitted diseases treatment guidelines. Morbidity and Mortality Weekly Report. 2015;**64**:1-137

[108] Rolfs RT, Joesoef MR, Hendershot EF, Rompalo AM, Augenbraun MH, Chiu M, et al. A randomized trial of enhanced therapy for early syphilis in patients with and without human immunodeficiency virus infection. The syphilis and HIV study group. The New England Journal of Medicine. 1997;**337**:307-314. DOI: 10.1056/NEJM199707313370504

[109] Cunningham ET Jr, Eandi CM, Pichi F. Syphilitic uveitis. Ocular Immunology and Inflammation. 2014;**22**:2-3. DOI: 10.3109/09273948.2014.883236

[110] Angelakis E, Raoult D. Pathogenicity and treatment of Bartonella infections. International Journal of Antimicrobial Agents. 2014;**44**:16-25. DOI: 10.1016/j.ijantimicag.2014.04.006

[111] Zangwill KM, Hamilton DH, Perkins BA, Regnery RL, Plikaytis BD, Hadler JL, et al. Cat scratch disease in Connecticut. Epidemiology, risk factors, and evaluation of a new diagnostic test. The New England Journal of Medicine. 1993;**329**:8-13. DOI: 10.1056/NEJM199307013290102

[112] Habot-Wilner Z, Trivizki O, Goldstein M, Kesler A, Shulman S, Horowitz J, et al. Cat-scratch disease: Ocular manifestations and treatment outcome. Acta Ophthalmologica. 2018:e524-e532. DOI: 10.1111/aos.13684

[113] Tan CL, Fhun LC, Tai EL, Abdul Gani NH, Muhammed J, Tuan Jaafar TN, et al. Clinical profile and visual outcome of ocular bartonellosis in Malaysia. Journal of Tropical Medicine. 2017;**2017**:7946123. DOI: 10.1155/2017/7946123

[114] Mabra D, Yeh S, Shantha JG. Ocular manifestations of bartonellosis. Current Opinion in Ophthalmology. 2018;**29**:582-587. DOI: 10.1097/ICU.0000000000000522

[115] Roe RH, Michael Jumper J, Fu AD, Johnson RN, Richard McDonald H,

Cunningham ET. Ocular bartonella infections. International Ophthalmology Clinics. 2008;**48**:93-105. DOI: 10.1097/IIO.0b013e31817d7697

[116] Amer R, Tugal-Tutkun I. Ophthalmic manifestations of bartonella infection. Current Opinion in Ophthalmology. 2017;**28**:607-612. DOI: 10.1097/ICU.0000000000000419

[117] Curi AL, Machado D, Heringer G, Campos WR, Lamas C, Rozental T, et al. Cat-scratch disease: Ocular manifestations and visual outcome. International Ophthalmology. 2010;**30**:553-558. DOI: 10.1007/s10792-010-9389-5

[118] Bergmans AM, Peeters MF, Schellekens JF, Vos MC, Sabbe LJ, Ossewaarde JM, et al. Pitfalls and fallacies of cat scratch disease serology: Evaluation of Bartonella henselae-based indirect fluorescence assay and enzyme-linked immunoassay. Journal of Clinical Microbiology. 1997;**35**:1931-1937. DOI: 10.1128/jcm.35.8.1931-1937.1997

[119] Biancardi AL, Curi AL. Cat-scratch disease. Ocular Immunology and Inflammation. 2014;**22**:148-154. DOI: 10.3109/09273948.2013.833631

Chapter 9

Approaches to Retinal Detachment Prophylaxis among Patients with Stickler Syndrome

Ameay V. Naravane and Polly A. Quiram

Abstract

Stickler syndrome is the most common cause of pediatric rhegmatogenous retinal detachments. Given the dramatic long term visual impact and difficult surgical management of these detachments, there is increasing interest in determining whether prophylactic treatment can be used to prevent retinal detachments in this population. However, severity of ocular findings in Stickler syndrome can vary by subtype. Three commonly used modalities to provide prophylactic treatment against retinal detachments in patients with Stickler syndrome include scleral buckle, laser retinopexy, and cryotherapy. While laser retinopexy is the most common approach to prophylactic treatment, treatment settings can vary by specialist. In addition, the decision to treat and manage Stickler syndrome is nuanced and requires careful consideration of the individual patient. After reviewing the literature on prophylactic treatment approaches, this chapter will also over guidelines in management of this complex patient population.

Keywords: Stickler syndrome, pediatric retinal detachment, prophylactic treatment, laser retinopexy, scleral buckle, cryotherapy

1. Introduction

Originally described in 1965, Stickler syndrome is a multiorgan system connective tissue disorder with an estimated incidence between 1:7500–1:9000 births [1, 2].

To date, Stickler syndrome has been reported to be caused by mutations in seven genes including COL2A1, COL11A1, COL11A2, COL9A1, COL9A2, COL9A3, and LOXL3 [3]. Mutations in the first three genes are inherited in an autosomal dominant pattern, while mutations in the latter four genes are inherited in an autosomal recessive pattern. These genes are associated with formation of collagen type II, IX, and XI [4].

Ocular manifestations of Stickler syndrome can be seen in 95% of patients [3]. The hallmark ocular finding of Stickler syndrome is vitreous abnormalities, seen in 40% of patients [4, 5]. Patients also present with high myopia (90%) and congenital cataracts (30%) [4, 5]. 40–80% of Stickler syndrome patients can develop retinal detachments, which makes it the most common cause of inherited pediatric retinal detachments [4–9].

Given its multisystem manifestations, as ophthalmologists, it is important to be aware of both the ocular and systemic clinical manifestations of this disease. Additional common clinical findings often include craniofacial abnormalities (84%), hearing loss (70%), and arthropathy (90%) [3]. Finally, early arthritis is common among all patients with Stickler syndrome. Other spinal abnormalities have also been reported including scoliosis and kyphosis with resulting chronic back pain affects the majority of adults [3].

Stickler syndrome Type 1 (STL1) is primarily due to autosomal dominant mutations in *COL2A1* and accounts for 80–90% of cases [3, 10]. While the majority of individuals with *COL2A1* mutations exhibit systemic signs, individuals with other variants of the COL2A1 mutation may present with only ocular symptoms. Craniofacial abnormalities are common and are typically due to underdevelopment of the maxilla and result in midface hypoplasia, micrognathia, and Pierre Robin Sequence. Sensorineural hearing loss is the most common type of hearing loss seen in Stickler syndrome, however STL1 typically has a milder presentation of hearing loss. On the other hand, STL1 is associated with the highest rate of RD (60–74%) of all the subtypes [7]. A summary of the prevalence of each type of Stickler syndrome and the associated retinal detachment rate can be found in **Table 1**.

Stickler syndrome Type 2 (STL2) is less common than STL1 but is due to autosomal dominant mutations in *COL11A1*. Craniofacial abnormalities such as midfacial and nasal bridge flattening are typically less pronounced. Approximately 1/3 of patients have variable manifestations of midline clefting (for example bivid uvula, high arched palate, or cleft palate). On the other hand, more severe early onset hearing loss is much more common in type 2 than type 1. 45% of patients with STL2 have been estimated to have hearing loss, 80% of whom had high frequency sensorineural hearing loss [8]. STL2 has a reported incidence of RD of 42–50%, 19% of which are bilateral, making it the subtype with the second highest RD rate [8].

Mutations in COL11A2, which cause Stickler Syndrome Type 3 is the only gene not associated with ocular manifestations [4]. It primarily affects joints and can cause mild to moderate hearing loss [9].

Gene	Stickler syndrome subtype	Percent of Stickler syndrome attributed to this gene	Retinal detachment rate
COL2A1	STL1	80–90%	60–74%
COL11A1	STL2	10–20%	42–50%
COL11A2	STL3	Rare	Non ocular form
COL9A1	STL4	Rare	Reported, incidence unknown*
COL9A2	STL5	Rare	Reported, incidence unknown*
COL9A3	STL6	Rare	Reported, incidence unknown*

**Retinal detachments have been reported in patients with this mutation. However, these reports have only been from case reports of families with these disorders.*

Table 1.
Incidence of retinal detachment by Stickler syndrome subtype.

Finally, mutations in *COL9A1, COL9A2, COL9A3* result in the autosomal recessive variants of Stickler syndrome (Stickler syndrome type 4-6). There is more limited data on these rarer forms of Stickler syndrome. Unlike the autosomal dominant forms of Stickler syndrome, cleft palates are commonly not seen in Stickler Syndrome Type 4-6 [4]. Among the recessive types of Stickler syndrome (STL4-6), mild to moderate hearing loss has been reported in STL5, while STL4 and 6 tend to have more severe hearing loss [3].

STL4 has been associated with moderate sensorineural hearing loss most pronounced at higher frequencies, femoral head epiphyseal dysplasia, and spinal abnormalities similar to those seen in STL1-3. Retinal detachments have been reported in the literature in a case series of patients with STL4 but because of how rare STL4 is, incidence is unknown. STL4 has also been associated with exudative retinal detachments exudative retinal detachment [4, 11, 12].

In STL5, hearing loss, midface hypoplasia, and a small chin have been reported in small case series. Retinal detachments have also been reported in patients with this subtype [13].

Finally, STL6 has been associated with moderate to profound progressive sensorineural hearing loss and moderate to high myopia. This rarer type of Stickler syndrome has only been reported in seven total families with the biallelic recessive COL9A3 mutation. Cataracts and retinal detachment have also been reported. In contrast to other subtypes, skeletal involvement appears more variable in STL6 [14].

2. Rationale for prophylactic treatment

Unfortunately, surgical repair of RRDs in patients with Stickler syndrome is technically challenging because of the vitreous abnormalities and early presentation of these patients [7]. Stickler syndrome patients are likely to develop giant retinal tears and have a propensity for developing proliferative vitreoretinopathy [15]. Pediatric retinal surgeons are highly aware of the extensive and often multiple surgeries that these patients may require. Anatomic success rate after one surgery can vary from 19 to 78%, while 97% achieve successful reattachment with an average of 2.3 surgeries [15].

Visual outcomes after these extensive surgeries are moderate at best. One case series reported that best corrected visual acuity at last follow up (>1 year) was 20/103 [15]. Further discussion regarding the best surgical approach to managing these complex retinal detachments is out of the scope of this chapter. Given the long-term impact these extensive pediatric retinal detachments can have on Stickler syndrome patients, many pediatric retinal surgeons have explored approaches to prevent these complex retinal detachments from occurring. In particular, the use of prophylactic treatment to prevent or reduce the morbidity of retinal detachments has become increasingly employed.

Although definitive evidence supporting prophylactic treatment is lacking, several systemic review articles have suggested a decreased incidence of RD with prophylactic treatment [7, 16, 17]. However, there have been no prospective randomized control trials performed looking at prophylactic treatment of patients with Stickler syndrome. In addition, retrospective case series have not found a clear benefit from prophylactic laser retinopexy in reducing the rate of RDs in their patient cohort [18].

One challenge in developing a consensus regarding prophylactic treatment is that wide variability in treatment modality, technique, and timing varies from study to study. In addition, many studies often rely on a clinical diagnosis of Stickler syndrome that has not been verified with genetic testing given lack of access. This makes head-to-head comparison of these different studies challenging from both a treatment and patient selection perspective [19]. The three common approaches for prophylactic treatment include scleral buckle, laser retinopexy, and cryotherapy retinopexy. Some have even reported combined use of these approaches, for example, use of both cryotherapy and scleral buckle [20]. Others, in particular those who report use of laser retinopexy, employ a variety of laser treatment protocols that make it difficult to compare efficacy of one treatment approach to another. Much of the early literature regarding prophylactic treatment stem from robust trials using the Cambridge prophylactic cryotherapy protocol, however, cryotherapy is not widely used, especially the U.S. [11].

Given the wide variation in prophylactic treatment approaches, the purpose of this chapter is to provide an overview of the three primary types of prophylactic treatment (laser retinopexy, cryotherapy, and scleral buckle) and review the literature supporting these approaches.

3. Cryotherapy

Much of the robust data regarding prophylactic treatment of patients with Stickler syndrome comes from two studies that first popularized the Cambridge prophylactic cryotherapy treatment protocol. The prophylaxis approach consisted of 360-degree cryotherapy, transconjunctivally in a contiguous fashion to the post-oral retina while the patient was under general anesthesia. The cryotherapy lesions were applied "shoulder to shoulder" to ensure continuity of treatment without gaps.

The first retrospective review was published in 2008 and examined a cohort of 204 patients with type 1 Stickler syndrome (confirmed with genetic testing). The cohort was divided into three groups: group 1 consisted of patients who received no prophylaxis, group 2 consisted of patients with bilateral 360 prophylactic cryotherapy, and group 3 included patients who had unilateral surgical repair for a retinal detachment and subsequently underwent prophylaxis in the fellow eye [21]. The study found 73% of patients without treatment developed a retinal detachment, 48% of which were bilateral. In patients with bilateral prophylactic treatment, only 8% developed retinal detachments. Finally in patients who underwent unilateral prophylaxis, only 10% developed an RD.

The results of this trial demonstrated a clear benefit from prophylactic cryotherapy treatment. The study was followed up 6 years later with a larger retrospective comparative case series looking at 487 patients with type 1 Stickler syndrome. The study examined patients who received bilateral prophylactic treatment compared to those who received no prophylactic treatment. 53.6% of patients in the bilateral control group (i.e., no treatment) developed retinal detachment, 10.3% of which were unilateral and 43.3% of which were bilateral. In patients with bilateral prophylaxis, 8.3% developed a retinal detachment, of which 7.9% were unilateral and 0.4% were bilateral [11].

Despite their retrospective nature, together these two studies laid a robust foundation indicating the benefits of prophylactic treatment for retinal detachment in patients with Type 1 Stickler syndrome. Unfortunately, the use of cryotherapy as prophylaxis is limited worldwide.

4. Laser retinopexy

One of the first retrospective case series that looked at the use of laser retinopexy as prophylaxis for Stickler syndrome was reported in 1996. The series looked at a small family cohort of patients with Stickler syndrome and compared the incidence of retinal detachments in 10 laser treated eyes to 34 non-treated eyes. The study found a 10% detachment rate in the argon laser retinopexy treated cohort [22].

Since then, several studies have looked at use of laser retinopexy. In 2016, a retrospective case series of 70 eyes from 62 patients found a 36.3% rate of retinal detachment among eyes that received prophylactic retinopexy in Saudi Arabia. However, the study lacked a control group and excluded all Stickler syndrome patients who did not develop RDs [18]. In 2018, a case series of 30 eyes from 15 patients with genetically confirmed Type 1 Stickler syndrome demonstrated a 5% detachment rate in patients with laser prophylaxis compared to 50% of patients who did not receive laser treatment [23]. Neither of these case series reported on their laser retinopexy approach, making it difficult to replicate a similar laser protocol.

In 2021, a small case series of 5 eyes from 4 family members with confirmed Type 2 Stickler Syndrome using a two-step laser retinopexy approach, "ora secunda cerclage" (OSC). OSC involves first a laser burn of moderately high intensity placed in a tight grid pattern (one spot width separation) 2 mm onto the pars plana to the ora serrata and 4 mm posteriorly halfway to the vortex vein ampullae. This is followed by an optional step 2 where the laser grid is posteriorly extended to and between the vortex vein ampullae [24]. Although the case series was limited in size, with 8.7 years of follow up, none of the eyes developed a retinal tear or RRD.

In 2022, two additional studies evaluating laser retinopexy were published. The first retrospective case series examined a cohort of 95 eyes from 48 patients and found that the retinal detachment rate was 26.7% among eyes without previous prophylactic laser retinopexy and only 4.6% among eyes with previous prophylactic laser retinopexy [25]. Laser burns of approximately 500 microns applied with a power titrated to a gray-white color in a nearly confluent pattern of 7–10 rows from the ora serrata for 360 degrees was performed in one session (**Figure 1**). The other retrospective case series evaluated patients receiving either extended vitreous base laser (EVBL), non-protocol laser (NPL) or no laser prophylaxis in a group of 230

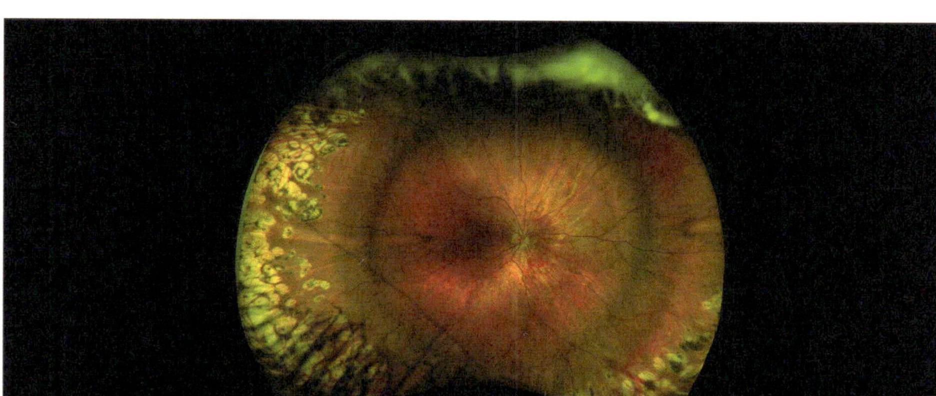

Figure 1.
Example of prophylactic laser Retinopexy used in patient with Stickler syndrome.

eyes. There was a 3% retinal detachment rate in the EVBL treatment group compared to a 73% detachment rate in patients who had received no laser retinopexy [26]. EVBL protocol was to treat from the ora serrata to the equator 360 degrees with laser burn spacing between one half to 1 spot size.

Over the past several years there has been a large increase in the number of series reporting positive outcomes using laser retinopexy as prophylaxis for retinal detachments in patients with Stickler syndrome. Laser retinopexy is often preferred to cryotherapy because of its ease of use and more widely spread familiarity. While the evidence supporting laser retinopexy continues to mount, as with the cryotherapy studies, this data is retrospective in nature. In addition, unlike the studies from the cryotherapy group, many of the large studies presented here are based on a clinical diagnosis of Stickler syndrome making it difficult to determine which patients were inherently at a higher risk because of their Stickler syndrome mutation. Additionally, as previously alluded to, each of the studies presented here have a unique approach to the laser retinopexy performed, making even head-to-head comparisons in the laser group alone difficult.

5. Scleral buckle

The last commonly used prophylactic approach is use of a scleral buckle. Use of scleral buckle to prevent detachments in patients with stickler syndrome has been reported in the literature as far back as 30 years ago. Retrospective case series in 1994 of 22 patients with "Wagner-Stickler" syndrome looked at rates of detachment in patients with various prophylactic treatment approaches. Eight patients were treated with an encircling scleral buckle but none of these patients developed a retinal detachment [27].

Unlike cryotherapy and laser retinopexy which target retinal adhesions, scleral buckle targets the issue of vitreous traction. However, by addressing the risk of vitreous traction, patients undergoing scleral buckle must also consider the increased risks of a more invasive procedure.

A recent retrospective case series published in 2022 assessed the impact of prophylactic scleral buckle in patients with genetically confirmed type 1 Stickler syndrome whose fellow eyes had a retinal detachment. All scleral buckles were performed by the same surgeon and used a 6 mm wide encircling band [20]. Thirty-nine patients underwent a scleral buckle with cryotherapy while 13 patients underwent a scleral buckle alone. In total, with an average of 15 years of follow up, only five patients developed a retinal detachment, all of whom had only received a scleral buckle alone. 0% of patients receiving both a scleral buckle and cryotherapy had a retinal detachment. Although the results of one retrospective case series must be interpreted with caution, these results suggest that the combination of scleral buckle and cryotherapy may significantly reduce the risk of retinal detachment in patients with Stickler syndrome.

6. Management approach

The first step is often determining when to offer prophylactic treatment for RRD prevention in Stickler syndrome patients. Among an International group of pediatric retinal surgeons, the most important factors influencing the decision to offer prophylactic treatment were a history of retinal detachment in the fellow eye, a family history of retinal detachment, and whether the patient had a high-risk genotype (i.e., COL2A). At the same time, almost half of respondents (41%) offered prophylactic treatment to all patients with Stickler syndrome [28].

Once the decision to provide prophylactic treatment is decided, the type of treatment must then be determined. In this international cohort of pediatric retinal surgeons, 76% reporting using laser retinopexy, 12% used scleral buckle, and 12% used cryotherapy [28].

Similar to what has been reported in the literature, the surveyed group of pediatric retinal surgeons reported using a wide variety in laser technique used. For example, 71% applied laser 360 degrees, 23% applied to visible lattice only, and 6% applied to both visible lattice and 360-degree laser to the vitreous base. The number of rows of laser also varied. 58% applied 3–5 rows of laser, 19% applied 5–7 rows of laser, and 32% applied 7–10 rows of laser. Respondents on average used a spot size of 350 microns (range 200–1500 microns, mode: 200 microns) [28].

Use of scleral buckle was less common in the surveyed cohort. Respondents reported use of scleral buckle ranged from in combination with laser retinopexy in all patients with Stickler syndrome to only those with high-risk genotypes. Other respondents reported use of a scleral buckle only if there was a family history of RD or a history of RD in the fellow eye. Finally, some respondents indicated use of SB for patients with high-risk genotypes, if there was a family history of RD or if there was a history of RD in the fellow eye. Of the respondents using both laser retinopexy and scleral buckle, 50% performed laser retinopexy at the same time as buckle placement while the other 50% performed the two procedures in a staged manner [28].

Cryotherapy was also similarly less common. Similar to the results presented above in Section 4.0, 100% of respondents applied cryotherapy confluently for 360 degrees but 50% reported application of 1 row of cryotherapy while the other half reported two rows. This suggests that while cryotherapy is a viable treatment modality that has robust evidence supporting its efficacy in preventing retinal detachments in patients with Stickler syndrome, its use is limited [28].

Another important step in management is determining what age to offer treatment. Patients with Stickler syndrome often start to develop retinal detachments in young adulthood. One study reported an average age of presentation with retinal detachment at 11 years (3–45 years), however others have reported detachments as early as 18 months [18, 21]. This can pose challenges as patients that young are nonverbal and often may present with detachments much later. In the study group that was surveyed, the recommended age of prophylactic treatment was 4.6 years but ranged from 3 months to 12 years old.

After the decision of when and who to treat have been determined, the follow up interval must also be decided. The majority of pediatric retinal surgeons reevaluated patients between 1 to 6 months after prophylactic treatment was performed. However, the decision as to when patients were to follow up was often heavily dependent on individual patient factors. The same factors that influenced pediatric retinal surgeons' decision to offer prophylactic treatment in the first place (i.e., high risk genotype, family history of RD, and history of RD in fellow eye). In addition, the respondents also mentioned the patients age, monocular status, rural location, activities the child was involved in all also impacted their follow up interval.

If prophylactic treatment was not offered, pediatric retinal surgeons, on average, followed patients every 6 months but this ranged from 3 months to 12 months.

7. Conclusions

The overview provided in this chapter offers a starting point into the discussion on prophylactic treatment for retinal detachments in patients with Stickler syndrome. While the evidence for prophylactic treatment of patients with Stickler syndrome is mounting, there is no prospective randomized controlled trial clearly demonstrating this benefit. There are significant challenges to a prospective trial as previously discussed in this chapter including how rare Stickler syndrome is, the varying prevalence of RD depending on subtype, and variations in treatment approach even with the treatment modality. In the interim, this overview can guide ophthalmologists in the treatment of initial management of Stickler syndrome patients.

Acknowledgements

No additional acknowledgements.

Conflict of interest

The authors declare no conflict of interest.

Notes/thanks/other declarations

None.

Author details

Ameay V. Naravane* and Polly A. Quiram

1 Department of Ophthalmology and Visual Neurosciences, University of Minnesota, Minneapolis, United States

2 Retina Consultants of Minnesota, Minneapolis, United States

*Address all correspondence to: ameay.naravane@gmail.com

References

[1] Stickler GB, Belau PG, Farrell FJ, et al. Hereditary progressive arthro-ophthalmopathy. Mayo Clinic Proceedings. 1965;**40**:433-455

[2] Robin NH, Moran RT, Ala-Kokko L. Stickler Syndrome. In: Pagon RA, Adam MP, Ardinger HH, et al., editors. GeneReviews. Seattle, WA: University of; 2000 [updated November 26, 2014] http://www.ncbi.nlm.nih.gov/books/NBK1302/

[3] Boothe M, Morris R, Robin N. Stickler syndrome: A review of clinical manifestations and the genetic evaluation. Journal of. Personalized Medicine. 2020;**105**:1-8

[4] Huang L, Chen C, Wang Z, et al. Mutation Spectrum and De novo mutation analysis in Stickler syndrome patients with high myopia or retinal detachment. Genes. 2020;**11**:1-11

[5] Snead MP, McNinch AM, Poulson AV, et al. Stickler syndrome, ocular-only variants and a key diagnostic role for the ophthalmologist. Eye. 2011;**25**:1389-1400

[6] Stickler GB, Hughes W, Houchin P. Clinical features of hereditary progressive arthro-ophthalmopathy: A survey. Genetics in Medicine. 2001;**3**:192-196

[7] Coussa RG, Sears J, Traboulsi EI. Stickler syndrome: Exploring prophylaxis for retinal detachment. Current Opinion in Ophthalmology. 2019;**30**:06-313

[8] Poulson AV, Hooymans JM, Richards AJ, et al. Clinical features of type 2 Stickler syndrome. Journal of Medical Genetics. 2004;**41**:1-7

[9] EV B, Leijendeckers JM, Huygen PLM, et al. Audiometric characteristics of two Dutch families with non-ocular Stickler syndrome (COL11A2). Hearing Research. 2012;**291**:15-23

[10] Snead MP, Yates JR. Clinical and molecular genetics of Stickler syndrome. Journal of Medical Genetics. 1999;**36**:353-359

[11] Fincham et al. Prevention of retinal detachment in Stickler syndrome. Ophthalmology. 2014;**121**:1589-1597

[12] Nikopoulos K, Schrauwen I, Simon M, et al. Autosomal recessive Stickler syndrome in two families is caused by mutations in the COL9A1 gene. Investigative Ophthalmology and Visual Science. 2011;**52**:4774-4779

[13] Baker S, Booth C, Fillman C, et al. A loss of function mutation in the *COL9A2* gene causes autosomal recessive Stickler syndrome. The American Journal of Medical Genetics - Part A. 2011;**155**:1668-1672

[14] Nash BM, Watson CG, Hughes E, et al. Heterozygous *COL9A3* variants cause severe peripheral vitreoretinal degeneration and retinal detachment. European Journal of Human Genetics. 2021;**29**:881-886

[15] Lee AC, Greaves GH, Rosenblatt BJ, Deramo VA, Shakin EP, Fastenberg DM, et al. Long-term follow-up of retinal detachment repair in patients with Stickler syndrome. Ophthalmic Surgery, Lasers & Imaging Retina. 2020;**51**(11):612-616

[16] Boysen KB, La Cour M, Kessel L. Ocular complications and prophylactic strategies in Stickler syndrome: A systematic literature review. Ophthalmic Genetics. 2020;**41**:223-234

[17] Carroll C, Papaioannou D, Rees A, Kaltenthaler E. The clinical effectiveness and safety of prophylactic retinal interventions to reduce the risk of retinal detachment and subsequent vision loss in adults and children with Stickler syndrome: A systematic review. Health Technology Assessment. 2011;**15**:1-62

[18] Alshahrani ST, Ghazi NG, Al-Rashaed S. Rhegmatogenous retinal detachments associated to Stickler syndrome in a tertiary eye care center in Saudi Arabia. Clinical Ophthalmology. 2016;**10**:1-6

[19] Traboulsi EI. Preventing retinal detachment in patients with Stickler syndrome: The effects of Preemptive laser photocoagulation. Ophthalmology Retina. 2022;**6**:4

[20] Ripandelli G, Rossi T, Cacciamani A, et al. The prophylaxis of fellow-eye retinal detachment in stickler syndrome: A retrospective series. Retina. 2022;**42**:250-255

[21] Ang A et al. Retinal detachment and prophylaxis in type 1 stickler syndrome. Ophthalmology. 2008;**115**:164-168

[22] Leiba H, Oliver M, Pollack A. Prophylactic laser photocoagulation in Stickler syndrome. Eye. 1996;**10**:701-708

[23] Wubben TJ, Branham KH, Besirli, et al. Retinal detachment and infantile-onset glaucoma in Stickler syndrome associated with known and novel COL2A1 mutations. Ophthalmic Genetics. 2018;**39**:615-618

[24] Morris RE, Parma ES, Robin NH, et al. Stickler syndrome (SS): Laser prophylaxis for retinal detachment (modified Ora Secunda cerclage, OSC/SS). Clinical Ophthalmology. 2021;**15**:19-29

[25] Naravane AV, Belin PJ, Pierce B, et al. Risk and prevention of retinal detachments in patients with stickler syndrome. Ophthalmic Surgery, Lasers and Imaging. 2022;**53**:7-11

[26] Khanna S, Rodriguez SH, Blair MA, et al. Laser prophylaxis in patients with Stickler syndrome. Ophthalmology Retina. 2022;**6**(4):263-267

[27] Monin C, Van Effenterre G, Andre-Sereys P, et al. Prevention of retinal detachmet in Wagner-Stickler disease. Comparative study of different methods. Apropos of 22 cases. Journal Français d'Ophtalmologie. 1994;**17**:167-174

[28] Naravane AV, Belin PJ, Quiram PA. Rhegmatogenous retinal detach (RRD) prophylaxis for patients with Stickler syndrome: An international survey of pediatric retinal specialist treatment preferences. 2022. Submitted [unpublished]

Chapter 10

Recent Advances in Optogenetic Retinal Prostheses

Himanshu Bansal and Sukhdev Roy

Abstract

Optogenetics has emerged as a revolutionary technology that enables circuit-specific restoration of neuronal function with millisecond temporal resolution. Restoring vision is one of the most promising and forefront applications of optogenetics. This chapter discusses essential components, mechanisms, present challenges, and future prospects of optogenetic retinal prostheses. The theoretical framework and analysis of optogenetic excitation of retinal ganglion neurons are also presented, which are useful in developing a better understanding and guidance for future experiments. It shows that the newly discovered ChRmine opsin provides control at light powers that are two orders of magnitude smaller than that required with experimentally studied opsins that include ChR2, ReaChR, and ChrimsonR, while maintaining single-spike temporal resolution, in retinal ganglion neurons.

Keywords: optogenetics, computational optogenetics, retinal prostheses, channelrhodopsin, vision restoration

1. Introduction

Loss of vision due to retinal degenerative diseases, including retinitis pigmentosa (RP) and macular degeneration affects millions of people worldwide [1–3]. The degeneration of light-sensitive rod and cone photoreceptors in the retina breaks the process of converting the light signal into an electrical signal. It thus results in partial vision loss or complete blindness. Earlier studies have confirmed that the remaining retinal tissue retains functionality and connections to the brain without these photoreceptors [4, 5]. Direct electrical stimulation of the remaining retinal neurons enables light sensation and visual perception, which confirms that the remaining retinal neural circuits can transmit information to the brain even in the late stage of retinal degenerative diseases [6–8]. However, applications of electrical prosthetic devices are limited due to their poor spatial resolution and highly invasive nature [4, 9, 10]. Although there are alternative methods for treating blindness, that includes pharmaceuticals, gene therapy, and stem cells, they are limited in certain conditions [11–14].

The emergence of optogenetics has revolutionized neuroscience by providing unprecedented spatiotemporal resolution in bidirectionally controlling neural activity with relatively lower invasiveness [15, 16]. In optogenetics, the gene of a light-sensitive protein is introduced into light-insensitive cells. In response to light, the expressed protein generates either inward or outward current and thus depolarizes or hyperpolarizes the cell [17]. It has contributed to our knowledge of how neural circuits operate and holds tremendous prospects in neural prostheses, particularly in vision restoration [18–23]. As one of the most promising technologies, optogenetics has applications in and beyond neuroscience, including cardiac optogenetics, sensory restoration, all-optical manipulation, and imaging of neural circuits in living animals [24]. More recently, a pioneering human clinical study on optogenetic retinal prostheses has reported successful partial vision recovery in a blind patient [25].

2. Optogenetic strategies for retinal prostheses

The method of optogenetic retinal prostheses is fundamentally different from electrical prostheses [26]. In optogenetics, injection of genetically encoded opsin viral vector into the surviving retinal neurons imparts light sensitivity to the light-insensitive retinal neurons. Thus, vision can be restored with the help of an optoelectronic device that converts visual scene pixels into appropriate light pulses and delivers them to the targeted cells. The implantation of optoelectronic headsets does not require the same level of invasiveness as their electronic counterpart [18, 26].

As the retina is a layered structure, the signal from photoreceptor cells in the foremost layer undergoes various processing before reaching the inner most layer *i.e.,* retinal ganglion neurons (RGNs). After that, the processed signal is transmitted to higher visual areas in the brain. As optogenetics allows cell-specific opsin expression, in principle, it would be best to transfect as early as possible in the visual pathway taking advantage of internal signal processing in the retinal circuits [26]. Once transfected, the retinal neurons require spatiotemporal patterns of high-intensity light depending on the dynamic range and spatial configuration of the targeted neurons and the kinetics and photosensitivity of light-sensitive proteins [27–29]. The selection of targeted cell type and opsin construct decides the quality of restored vision. Furthermore, the safety of retinal tissue after the expression of opsin into the desired neural population must be ensured [30].

In patients with RP, cone cells are not necessarily completely destroyed. These cells lose their outer segment and survive until very late stages of the condition [31]. Typically, the cone photoreceptor cells hyperpolarize in the presence of light and get depolarized in the dark. Thus, it would be better to use light-driven chloride pumps to perfectly mimic the signal in response to light [32–34]. Optogenetic excitation of the surviving cone cells through genetic expression of these cells with halorhodopsin has restored visual responses in the mouse with RP [35]. However, a major drawback of targeting cone cells is their very few surviving populations. Furthermore, there might be no chance of survival of these cells in late stages of other retinal dystrophies. Thus, the restored vision will be restricted to tunnel vision similar to mid-stage RP [8, 26]. The next best layer to target is the bipolar cells. There are two types of these bipolar cells, *i.e.,* ON and OFF cells, which depolarize and hyperpolarize in response to light. Thus, these cells need to be expressed with excitatory and inhibitory opsins to avoid conflicting responses to visual stimuli, respectively [28, 34].

Alternatively, direct optogenetic excitation of RGNs is possible. RGNs also come in ON and OFF varieties. A key issue with the direct excitation of inner retinal neurons is the absence of normal retinal processing. A possible solution to overcome the issue is to process the visual scene by the computational circuit of retinal encoding before delivering it to inner retinal neurons [36]. In the case of direct excitation of RGNs, optoelectronic goggles have been used to mimic retinal processing and to modify visual scene intensity and color compatible with the light-sensitive protein expressed in RGNs [26].

To accurately restore vision by direct photostimulation of inner retinal neurons, these neurons are to be driven at their natural frequencies, evoked in response to dynamic visual stimuli [18]. There are at least 16 different types of RGNs having different temporal properties [37]. Recently, monitoring 342 RGNs in the human retina revealed that the maximum neural population fires at ~50 Hz, in response to full-field contrast steps, but it could reach up to 180 Hz in a few cells [37]. Although opsins with fast turn-off kinetics would allow precise spiking in those neurons, they invariably require high irradiances, as light sensitivity and kinetics are inversely correlated. Furthermore, the intensity threshold to evoke spikes in opsin-expressing retinal neurons should be below a safety threshold to reduce the possibility of photochemical damage in the retina [38]. Also, the opsins should respond to large intensity variations [26].

3. The first human clinical trial of retinal prosthesis

The first human clinical study has recently shown partial recovery of visual function in a blind patient with RP using optogenetics [25]. In the study, a serotype AAV encoding ChrimsonR fused to the red fluorescent protein tdTomoto was administered in one eye of the patient to target mainly foveal RGNs. After injecting the opsin into the ganglion cells, the retina was stimulated by an optoelectronic goggle after 7 months, as the expression takes two to six months to get stabilized in the cells [25, 39].

Recovery of visual function was tested under three conditions with three psychophysical tests. The conditions were as follows:

I. Both eyes were open in the absence of the goggles (Natural binoculars).

II. Untreated eye covered and treated eye opened in the absence of the goggles (Natural monocular).

III. Untreated eye covered and treated eye opened in the presence of the goggles (Stimulated monocular).

The conducted psychophysical tests were as follows:

I. Perceiving, locating, and touching a single object on a white table (Test-I)

II. Perceiving, locating, and counting more than one object (two or three tumblers) (Test-II)

III. Combined the assessment of vision with extracranial multichannel electroencephalography (Test-III)

The average response of the patient under the above conditions and psychological tests are summarized in **Table 1**.

The study has shown that wearing the goggle, which transforms the changes in intensity, pixel by pixel, into a monochromatic image and projects them in real time onto the retina, the patient could perceive, locate, count, and touch different objects (**Table 1**) [25].

Tests/Conditions	Success rate		
	Natural binocular	Natural monocular	Stimulated monocular
Test-I	No detection	No detection	92%
Test-II	No detection	No detection	63%
Test-III	5.8%	6%	41%

Table 1.
The success rate of visual perception under different conditions and psychological tests [25].

4. Challenges and limitations in optogenetic retinal prostheses

Channelrhodopsin-2 (ChR2) from *Chlamydomonas reinhardtii* was the first light-sensitive opsin used to restore light responses in blind mice [40]. ChR2 was injected in thalamic projecting RGNs via adeno-associated virus (AAV) serotype 2 [40]. However, the required light intensity to evoke spiking with ChR2, having its maximum absorption at 460 nm, exceeds the standard safety threshold and might cause photochemical damage in the human retina and retinal pigment epithelium [41–43].

To overcome the limitation, new opsins with increased light sensitivity were developed through mutations and discovery that increased the dynamic range of neural activity and, thus, image contrast within regulatory limits. Since the safety limits of light intensity have a strong wavelength dependence, opsins with red-shifted wavelength activation peaks safely allow the use of higher irradiance than their blue-shifted counterparts. Shifting the wavelength from blue o red allows for safely increasing the photon flux by three orders of magnitude. Deeper penetration of longer wavelengths is an additional advantage with the red-shifted opsins [41].

To reduce irradiance requirement, opsin with Ca^{2+} selectivity named CatCh was expressed into RGNs [22, 44, 45]. Although the activation threshold of CatCh-expressing RGNs is below the damage threshold and allows normal displays to evoke responses, CatCh suffers from inherent toxicity associated with Ca^{2+} influx [9]. Engineered mutants of CoChR, developed by optimizing the off-rate through site-directed mutagenesis, have also been used to restore functional vision under normal light conditions. Although the mutants functions at safe irradiances, they do not provide sufficient temporal resolution [46].

At present, red-shifted opsins are being intensively investigated as red-shifted photons can reach deeper areas in the tissue, which is important for noninvasive light delivery in *in vivo* experiments [47–49]. Three orders of magnitude higher irradiance can be used at 590 nm in contrast to light at 470 nm for safe illumination of the retina [41]. The safety threshold shifts on changing wavelengths of light as 7.52×10^{13} photons mm^{-2} s^{-1} at 470 nm to 5.94×10^{15} photons mm^{-2} s^{-1} at 590 nm [41, 50]. Recently, a red-activable variant of ChR2, named ReaChR, has restored light sensitivity in blind rd1 mice, primate retina, and post-mortem human retinae when targeted to RGNs [41, 47]. However, ReaChR could not drive RGNs beyond 30 Hz [41]. Although ReaChR requires similar irradiance as ChR2, it is safe at the red-shifted wavelength [4, 41]. To get high-frequency along with red-shifted activation wavelength, ChrimsonR was used for optogenetic vision restoration [25, 39, 51–53]. Even though ChrimsonR uses a safe wavelength of light, it still requires extremely bright light [4]. ChrimsonR has been used for the first clinical study to restore vision in a human patient [25]. **Table 2** summarizes different opsins, their characteristic features, and their response in retinal neurons [9, 25, 39–41, 47, 54–59].

Opsin	λ_{max} (nm)	τ_{off} (ms)	EPD50 (mW/mm^2)	Peak current (pA)	Target cell type	Animal Model	Operating photon flux in retinal neurons (Photons mm^{-2} s^{-1})	Ref.
ChR2	460	11.6 ± 0.4	1.3 ± 0.2	~200	RGNs	Wide-type, *rd1* mice, RCS rats	>1e+17	[40, 54, 55]
					ON Biopolar Cells	*rd1, rd10, rd16* mice	>1e+16	[56, 57]
ChR2 (H134R)	460	20.9 ± 2.2	0.43 ± 0.04	~1200	ON Bipolar Cells	*rd1* mice	>1e+16	[58]
ReaChR	590	137.2 ± 7	0.8	349 ± 192	RGNs	Mice, macaque and human retina	>1.25e+15	[41]
CoChR(H94E/L112C/K246T)	480	750	0.05	~ 1500	RGNs	Transgenic mice	>1e+14	[46]
CatCh	460	16 ± 3	0.4 ± 0.1	~ 300	RGNs	*rd1* mice, macaque eyes	>1e+15	[9]
*Ps*CatCh2.0	450	—	—	~ 400	RGNs	*rd1* mice	>4e+16	[59]
ChrimsonR	590	16 ± 2.1	~ 1	~ 400	RGNs	Macaque, Human	>7e+14	[25, 39]

Table 2.
Microbial rhodopsins in optogenetic retinal prostheses.

Although recently discovered opsins could allow control at improved light levels, they have not yet been studied for that purpose. To drive opsin-expressing neurons at their firing frequencies, optogenetic approaches are combined with an extraocular device or optoelectronic goggles [26]. These devices consist of a camera and an image processing unit. These devices are crucial for optogenetic retinal prostheses for the following reasons [18]:

i. The light-sensitive opsins used in optogenetics are sensitive to only 3–4 log units of irradiance, which is a very shorter range than at which human vision operates (10 log units).

ii. Microbial opsins have maximal responses at a single wavelength and thus need a monochromatic light source to maximize their response.

iii. The light-sensitive proteins are not sufficiently sensitive to respond to normal daylight.

iv. The optoelectronic goggle converts natural scenes having different wavelengths into monochromatic light pulses.

v. In the case of direct excitation of inner retinal neurons, there is a need for a system that can compensate for the visual processing pathways.

Optogenetic-based retinal prostheses involve the genetic expression of opsin-construct into the retinal neurons. Neurotoxicity and immunogenicity are the key concerns for clinical trials. Attempting functional-level response in the system by enhancing opsin expression is problematic due to the increased risk of cell toxicity and immune response [27, 60]. Although AAVs have a favorable safety profile in gene therapy, their safety is dose-dependent [61]. This limits the expression of microbial opsin with a safe viral dose [9]. Another critical task in clinical trials is to achieve stable opsin expression in the retina. Earlier studies have shown that the virus-mediated expression of ChR2 remained stable beyond 3 months in nonhuman primates [62]. Similar safety and stability checks must be conducted while selecting new opsins for retinal prostheses. Therefore, long-term stability and neurotoxicity with new microbial rhodopsins will need to be carefully evaluated before they can be considered for clinical applications [18].

5. New opsins in optogenetics

In recent years, intense research efforts have been directed to design more efficient opsins with tailored properties, including unitary spectral conductance, retinal binding affinity, faster temporal kinetics, light actuation sensitivity, spectral tuning, and protein stability. Being a primary goal of optogenetics, new opsins are first investigated in neurons in the brain (**Table 3**) [29, 32, 63–68].

CsChrimson is a CsChR-Chrimson chimera, produced by replacing the Chrimson N terminus with the CsChR N terminus. It exhibits more sensitivity than Chrimson, while the spectral and kinetic properties are the same [51]. bReaChES was generated by introducing a Glu123Ser mutation and replacing the first 51 amino-terminal residues with the first 11 amino-terminal residues in the ReaChR construct [63]. It

Opsin	λ_{max} (nm)	τ_{off} (ms)	EPD50 (mW/ mm^2)	Peak photocurrent (pA)	Spiking Frequency in Neurons (Hz)	Ref.
CsChrimson	585	30	0.7	~700	20	[49, 51]
bReaChES	585	39 ± 3.6	0.2	~2000	10	[49, 63]
ChRmine	585	60 ± 20	0.03 ± 0.01	~4000	40	[49]
rsChRmine	530	175	0.22	1.5 ± 0.3 nA	40	[64]
hsChRmine	530	35 ± 15	—	2.5 ± 0.4 nA	40	[64]
Chronos	470	3.5	0.3	1100	60	[51]
ChroME	510	5.5 ± 0.2	0.075	1.5 ± 0.1 nA	40	[65, 66]
ChroME2s	510	13 ± 1	0.06	2.5 ± 0.2 nA	40	[66]
ChroME2f	510	9.6 ± 0.6	0.085	2.3 ± 0.2 nA	40	[66]

Table 3.
Newly discovered or engineered microbial rhodopsins in optogenetics.

has allowed simultaneous stimulation and recording using Ca^{2+} indicators [63]. Most recently, screening of residues forming the cation-conducting ChR pore guided by crystal structure-derived knowledge has resulted in ~1000 suitable new opsin sequences. A sequence of a marine opsin gene optimized for mammalian expression, named ChRmine from *Tiarina fusus*, exhibits a very large inward photocurrent ~4 nA with red-shifted excitable wavelength along with an order of magnitude faster recovery than for other red-shifted opsins [49, 68].

More recent efforts to understand the mechanism of ion transport by ChRmine has been enabled by its cryo-electron microscopy structure at 2.0 A° resolution. The structural knowledge has been used to design new variants with faster speed (hsChRmine) and greater red shift (rsChRmine), while retaining high current and light sensitivity [64]. Along with the development of red-shifted opsins, new efficient blue-activated opsins have also been discovered and engineered. *de novo* sequencing of opsins from over 100 algal species has resulted in Chronos, a blue light-sensitive opsin exhibiting high light sensitivity and unprecedented kinetics, with a turn-off of 3.6 ± 0.2 ms. It is the fastest blue-shifted opsin reported to date [51]. Recent efforts to engineer Chronos have resulted in a mutant, ST-Chronos-M140E, or ChroME. It exhibits rapid decay kinetics while exhibiting photocurrents more than 3-5 times larger than Chronos [65]. More recently, two new mutants have been engineered, namely ChroME2f and ChroME2s, with enhanced properties that can support large-scale, temporally precise multiphoton excitation [66].

Although the newly discovered opsins can significantly improve optogenetic retinal prostheses, developing strategies for safe and sufficient expression of new opsins in retinal neurons and experimentation of each opsin pair with different targeted retinal neurons is a lengthy process and needs repetitive investigation and safety checks before clinical studies.

6. Computational modeling of optogenetic excitation of retinal neurons

Computational modeling of optogenetic systems has made significant contributions in developing a better understanding of the reaction dynamics behind photocurrent generation in the opsin molecules and change in membrane potential in opsin-expressing neurons in response to light. It helps in correctly interpreting experiments and optimizing photostimulation conditions within a complex cell/tissue environment, which is often questionable and challenging [69–74]. Due to the naturally occurring structural and functional diversity in the cell types in living animals, a large data set is required for optogenetics to be used in different environments, which is a challenging task. The problem persists while selecting light-sensitive proteins to get desired control over cellular activity. Computational models can help quick (virtual) testing of newly developed light-sensitive proteins in different cell types and within realistic tissue and organ-level settings.

Initial efforts in the field of computational optogenetics include modeling of the photoresponse of ChR2 considering three, four and six-state models of its photocycle, light-mediated spiking in neurons under continuous and pulsed illumination, the effect of illumination of sub-cellular compartments, analysis of activation threshold of opsin-expressing cell within tissue while considering scattering and absorption [69–74]. Although there were many new opsins with improved kinetics, photocurrent, and light sensitivity, theoretical models of these opsins were not formulated until recently.

In the last few years, theoretical models of optogenetic systems consisting of new light-sensitive proteins have been formulated. Accurate theoretical models of optogenetic excitation of neurons with Chronos, CheRiff, ReaChR, Chrimson, ChrimsonR, CsChrimson, f-Chrimson, vf-Chrimson, bReaChES and ChRmine and inhibition with NpHR, eNpHR3.0, Jaws, and GtACR2 have been reported recently. Using these computational models, a detailed theoretical analysis of the effect of photostimulation and physiological parameters was also conducted, which has provided a better understanding of the mechanism, limitations, and advantages of different types of neurons [75, 76]. Further, accurate theoretical models of bidirectional optogenetic control with spectrally separated excitatory-inhibitory opsin pairs, namely ChR2(H134R)-eNpHR3.0, Chrimson-GtACR2, Chronos-eNpHR3.0, Chronos-Jaws, CheRiff-Jaws, and Vf-Chrimson-GtACR2 were also reported. A comprehensive theoretical study on high-frequency low-power bidirectional optogenetic control of neurons with single spike resolution with already tested opsin pairs and with new

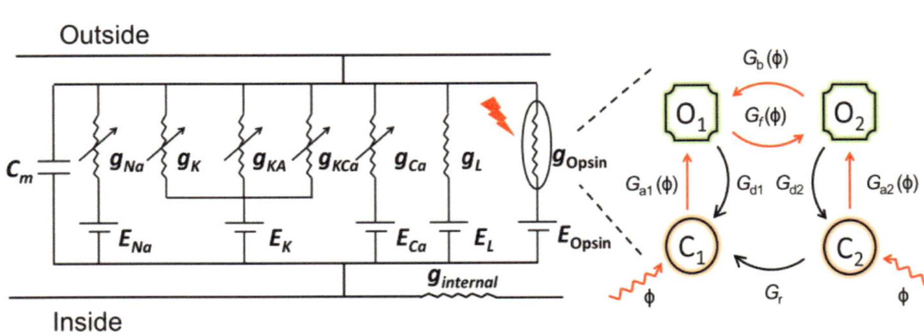

Figure 1.
Equivalent circuit diagram of biophysics model of opsin-expressing retinal ganglion neurons. C_m is the membrane capacitance. g_{Na}, g_K, g_{KA}, g_{KCa}, g_{Ca} and g_L are maximal conductances of naturally occurring sodium, potassium, potassium (A-type), Ca^{2+} activated potassium, calcium, and leak channels. E_{Na}, E_K, E_{Ca}, and E_L are the reversal potential for sodium-, potassium-, calcium-conducting, and leaky channels. g_{Opsin} is the light-dependent conductance through opsin channels having reversal potential E_{Opsin}. C_1 and C_2 are the closed states, and O_1 and O_2 are the open states. G_{a1}, G_{a2}, G_b, and G_f are the light-dependent rate functions, while G_{d1}, G_{d2}, and G_r are the light-independent rate constants. ϕ is the photon flux. (For details, see Ref. [38]).

opsin pairs not experimented till that time for better control was conducted using theoretical models [38]. Recently, computational simulations have proposed a novel method of co-expressing step-function opsins with fast channelrhodopsins to avoid spike failure from desensitization of photocurrent [77]. Integration of theoretical models of photoresponse of ChRmine into biophysical circuit models of cardiac cells has shown that ChRmine could be used for ultra-low power deep sustained optogenetic excitation/suppression of electrical activity in cardiomyocytes [78].

Theoretical simulations of optogenetic visual cortical prosthetic systems have provided a better understanding of the mechanism behind signal encoding by the visual cortex [79, 80]. Theoretical modeling of optogenetic excitation of retinal neurons would be a primary step to design ideal optogenetic prosthetic devices and circuits. Also, the newly discovered light-sensitive proteins have the potential to overcome current challenges. However, designing methods for the efficient and safe delivery of new opsins in the retina is a lengthy process. No mathematical model was reported until recently to study optogenetically evoked spiking in RGNs.

The theoretical framework of the biophysical mechanism of optogenetic excitation of already tested opsins, namely, ChR2, ReaChR, and ChrimsonR, and newly discovered potential opsins, *i.e.,* CsChrimson, bReaChES, and ChRmine has contributed significantly to our knowledge and provided insights into the design of optimized optogenetic retinal prosthetic circuits [38] (**Figure 1**). In the first step, the photocurrent characteristics of different opsins were compared over a wide range of irradiances (**Figure 2**). The variation of photocurrent with time is shown in **Figure 2A**. Peak and plateau photocurrent of these opsins were compared over a wide range of irradiance **Figure 2B** and **C**. Theoretical simulations have helped in determining the minimum pulse width to achieve maximum photocurrent at each irradiance, also called saturating pulse width (SPW), which is important to minimize delivered light power while getting maximum output (**Figure 2D**). SPW decreases on increasing irradiance and saturates at higher irradiances for each opsin [38].

Further, the variation of photocurrent with time on illuminating with repetitive light pulses at different light stimulation frequencies was compared (**Figure 2E**). At higher frequencies, the photocurrent in all the opsins does not reach the baseline before the arrival of the subsequent light pulse, which results in a non-zero photocurrent plateau indicated by an arrow in **Figure 2F**. The percentage of return to baseline (RTB %) plays a crucial role in temporal resolution at high frequencies. In all the opsins, RTB % decreases with stimulation frequency. The potential interactions between pulse width, irradiance, and stimulation frequency can have a profound impact on temporal fidelity due to the inverse relationship between kinetics and photosensitivity of opsins. The study also reported that RTB % does not change with irradiance, while it is lower at longer pulse [38].

To determine the irradiance range at which each opsin-expressing RGN exhibit spiking, the variation of membrane potential with time were simulated on illuminating with long (500 ms) and short (10 ms) light pulses at different irradiances (**Figure 3**). The variation of membrane potential with time on illuminating 500 ms light pulses at increasing irradiances has been shown in **Figure 3A**. From the variation of the number of spikes with pulse irradiance, the study has revealed that ChRmine is most sensitive among the studied opsins and the maximum firing frequency within the safety limit of irradiance is two-three orders of magnitude higher than the opsins tested for retinal prostheses (**Figure 3A**). Further, the response of these RGNs was simulated under randomized photon fluxes of increasing contrast (**Figure 4B**). Interestingly, ChRmine can respond to irradiances changes from one order to four orders (**Figure 3B**).

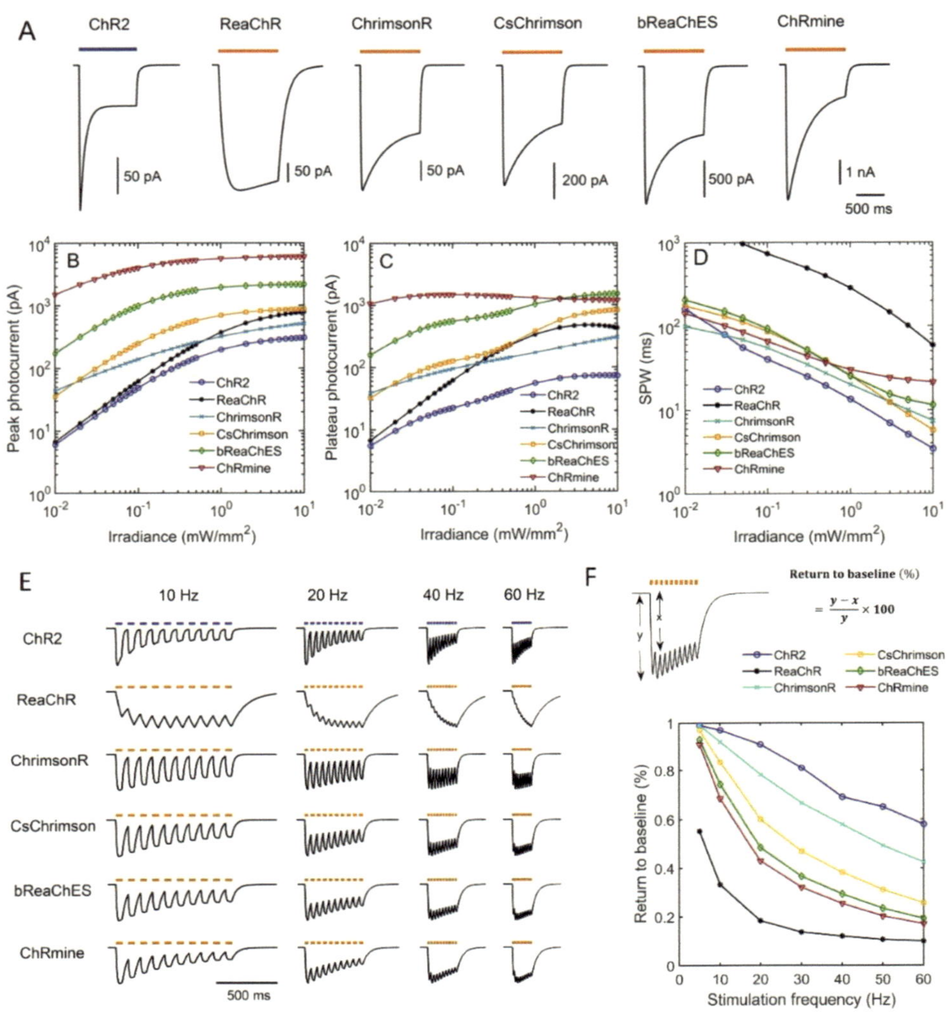

Figure 2.

Photocurrent characteristics of ChR2, ReaChR, ChrimsonR, CsChrimson, bReaChES and ChRmine on illuminating with their peak absorption wavelength i.e., 460 nm for ChR2 and 590 nm for other opsins. (A) Variation of photocurrent with time on illuminating with single light pulse (1 s, 1 mW/mm²), and (B–D) corresponding variation of (B) peak, (C) plateau photocurrent and (D) saturating pulse width (SPW) with irradiance. (E) Variation of photocurrent with time on illuminating with multiple light pulses at indicated frequencies and different pulse widths (50 ms for 10 Hz, 25 ms for 20 Hz, 12.5 ms for 40 Hz, and 8.5 ms for 60 Hz) at 1 mW/mm², and (F) corresponding variation of return to baseline (%) with stimulation frequency, calculated using the formula shown above the box. © IOP Publishing. Reproduced with permission. All rights reserved [38].

In moving picture frames, time-dependent change in irradiances of each pixel is the key photostimulation parameter to encode changes in visual scenes. In optogenetics, irradiances below certain threshold results in spike failure, while pulses longer than a certain limit result in spurious spiking patterns. Thus, it would be necessary to determine how larger fluctuations in irradiance and pulse-width can be tolerated by retinal neural circuits. The theoretical study determined a region in the irradiance-pulse-width plot in which each point is a combination of allowed irradiance and pulse-width, while maintaining single-spike resolution (**Figure 4**).

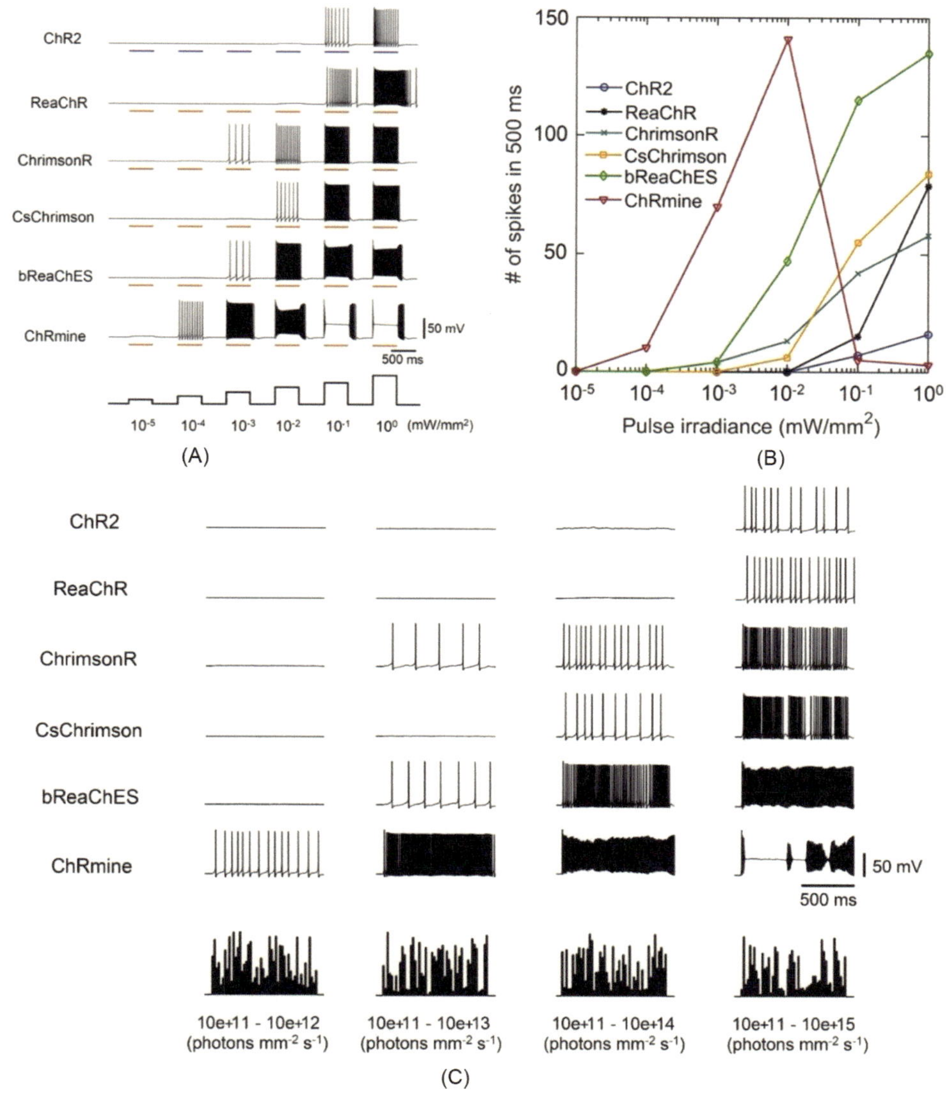

Figure 3.
Frequency response of opsin expressing retinal ganglion neurons in response to long- and short-duration light pulses at different irradiances. (A) Variation of membrane potential with time in response to light pulses (500 ms) at increasing irradiances, and (B) corresponding variation of the number of spikes during illumination at different irradiances. (C) Light-evoked spiking in different opsins-expressing RGNs on illuminating with multiple light pulses each of 10 ms at 50 Hz for 1 s and at randomized photon fluxes of increasing contrast from 10^{11} to 10^{12} photons mm^{-2} s^{-1} to 10^{11} to 10^{15} photons mm^{-2} s^{-1}. © IOP Publishing. Reproduced with permission. All rights reserved [38].

In visual systems, internal delays in signal processing may lead to mislocalization while capturing things changing with time [81]. Thus, the latency of a system is a critical feature for information processing which is determined by the turn-on rate of the opsin photocurrent [48, 81]. Furthermore, due to desensitization of photocurrent in opsins, sustained excitation of opsin-expressing neurons results in spike failure [27]. In the study, they have shown the variation of first spike latency with irradiance

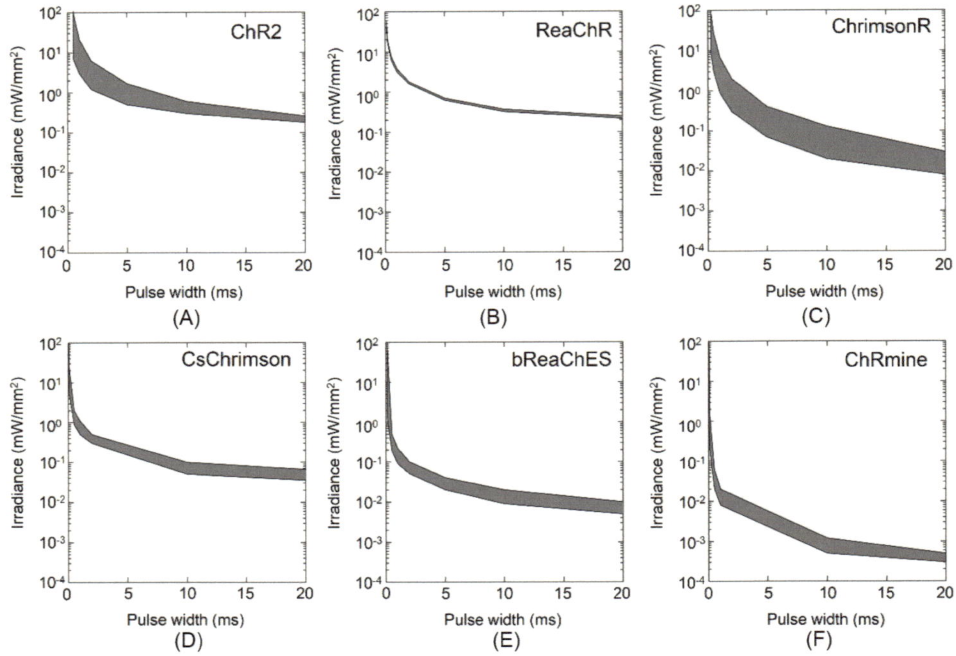

Figure 4.
Tolerance for maintaining single spike resolution by different opsin-expressing neurons against fluctuations in irradiance and pulse width. Variation of minimum (lower boundary of the shaded region) and maximum (lower boundary of the shaded region) irradiance thresholds with pulse-width to evoke 100% spiking at 10 Hz for 2 s in (A) ChR2, (B) ReaChR, (C) ChrimsonR, (D) CsChrimson, (E) bReaChES, and (F) ChRmine-expressing retinal ganglion neurons. © IOP Publishing. Reproduced with permission. All rights reserved [38].

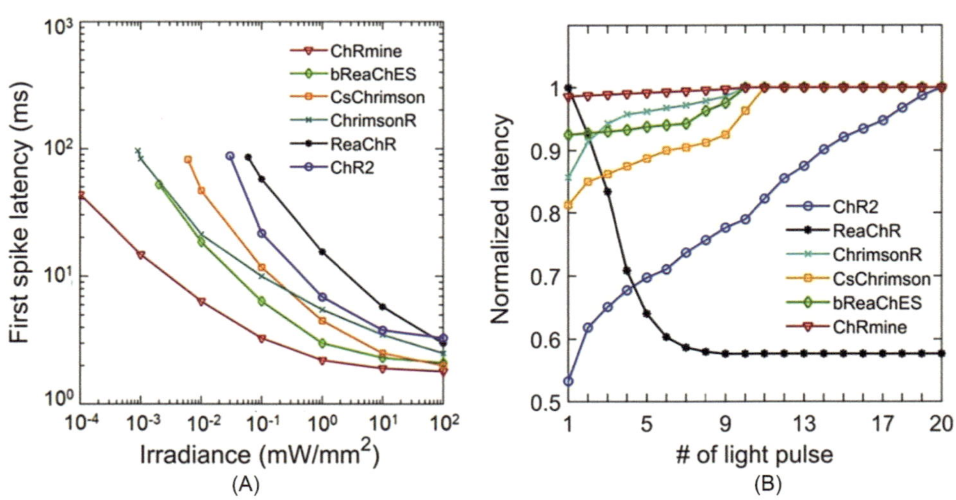

Figure 5.
Latency of spikes in opsin-expressing retinal ganglion neurons in response to light stimulus. (A) Variation of first spike latency with pulse irradiance, and (B) variation of normalized spike latency with sequential position of light pulse each of 5 ms for ChR2, 4 ms for ChrimsonR, 1.8 ms for CsChrimson, 6 ms for ReaChR, 0.4 ms for bReaChES, and 0.13 ms for ChRmine in the stimulus train at 10 Hz and 0.6 mW/mm². © IOP Publishing. Reproduced with permission. All rights reserved [38].

in different opsin-expressing RGNs (**Figure 5A**). Further, latencies of subsequent spikes were also determined to check consistency on illuminating with a light pulse train (**Figure 5B**). Theoretical simulations revealed that under sustained excitation of RGNs, ChRmine exhibits the most stable and shortest latency during the entire stimulus train (**Figure 5B**).

For accurate information processing to higher visual centers of the brain, it is essential to drive RGNs up to their natural firing rates. Thus, it was important to determine high-frequency limits of each opsin-expressing RGNs. From MIT-irradiance graph, it is clear that there is a trade-off between pulse-width and required irradiances to evoke spike. However, the light pulse cannot be increased beyond a certain limit at a particular frequency (*e.g.,* 5 ms for 100 Hz). On the other hand, higher irradiance above its saturating value is totally waste of energy. Thus, a systematic study of the effect of photostimulation conditions was carried out to determine the high-frequency limit with each opsin under pulsed stimulation.

Further, the high-frequency limit was determined with each opsin. The variation of spiking frequency with stimulation frequency at optimized photostimulation conditions is shown in **Figure 6A**. Each opsin maintains 100% spike fidelity up to a certain frequency limit. The spiking patterns at the high-frequency limit are shown in **Figure 6B**. Among these opsins, ChrimsonR is the only opsin that allows 100% spiking fidelity up to 100 Hz. However, the required photon flux density with ChrimsonR ~8.3×10^{15} photons. mm^{-2} s^{-1} at 590 nm is beyond the safety threshold for the human retina [38, 41]. On the other hand, ChRmine maintains single-spike resolution up to 40 Hz, which is sufficient for RGNs, it needs pulses of the lowest light power (**Figure 6**) [38].

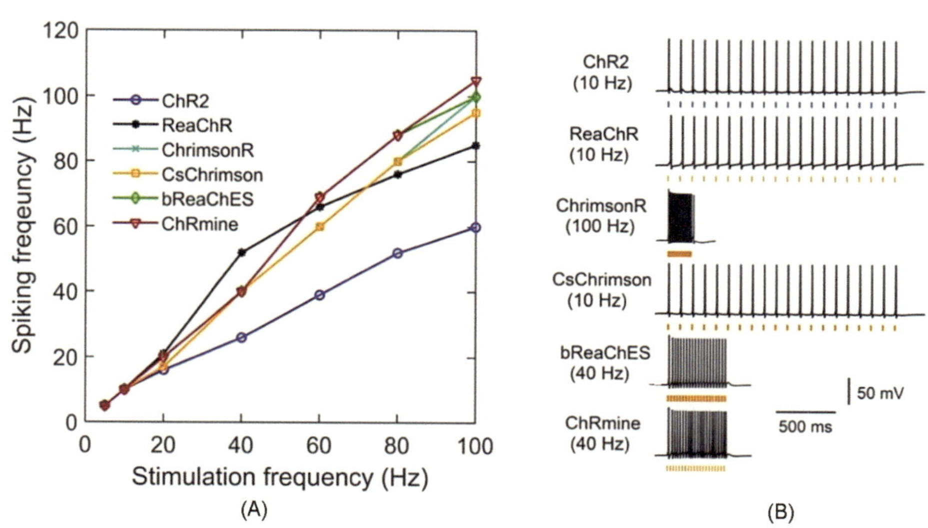

Figure 6.
Frequency response of different opsin-expressing retinal ganglion neurons. (A) Variation of spiking frequency with stimulation frequency on illuminating with 20 light pulses at different frequencies and at different irradiances and pulse widths as follows: 5 mW/mm² and 2.5 ms for ChR2, 2.8 mW/mm² and 1.2 ms for ChrimsonR, 0.13 mW/mm² and 5 ms for CsChrimson, 5 mW/mm² and 1 ms for ReaChR, 0.02 mW/mm² and 6 ms for bReaChES, and 0.013 mW/mm² and 0.93 ms for ChRmine, and (B) corresponding spiking patterns at the high-frequency limit with 100% spike fidelity. ©IOP Publishing. Reproduced with permission. All rights reserved [38].

7. Conclusion

Optogenetic retinal prostheses fundamentally has the potential to restore quality vision in the human retina. Although there are certain limitations and challenges associated with opsin characteristics and delivery methods, in the coming years, repetitive clinical trials with new opsins and safe delivery methods would allow the efficient design of optogenetic retinal prosthetic devices and circuits. Theoretical studies in optogenetics have the potential to guide future experiments with reduced irradiance and enhanced visual contrast. Future experiments by co-expressing excitatory and inhibitory or spectrally orthogonal opsins into different retinal neurons *e. g.,* ON and OFF type of RGNs, would significantly improve the quality of restored vision.

Conflict of interest

The authors declare no conflict of interest.

Nomenclature

AAV	Adeno-associated virus
ChR2	Channelrhodopsins
NpHR	*Natronomonas pharaonis*
RGN	Retinal ganglion neuron
RP	Retinitis pigmentosa
RTB	Return to baseline

Author details

Himanshu Bansal and Sukhdev Roy
Department of Physics and Computer Science, Dayalbagh Educational Institute, Agra, India

*Address all correspondence to: sukhdevroy@dei.ac.in

References

[1] Flaxman SR, Bourne RR, Resnikoff S, Ackland P, Braithwaite T, Cicinelli MV, et al. Global causes of blindness and distance vision impairment 1990-2020: A systematic review and meta-analysis. The Lancet Global Health. 2017;**5**(12):e1221-e1234

[2] Mitchell P, Liew G, Gopinath B, Wong TY. Age-related macular degeneration. Lancet. 2018;**392**(10153):1147-1159

[3] Cross N, van Steen C, Zegaoui Y, Satherley A, Angelillo L. Current and future treatment of retinitis pigmentosa. Clinical Ophthalmology. 2022;**16**:2909-2921

[4] Baker CK, Flannery JG. Innovative optogenetic strategies for vision restoration. Frontiers in Cellular Neuroscience. 2018;**12**:316. DOI: 10.3389/fncel.2018.00316

[5] Kleinlogel S, Vogl C, Jeschke M, Neef J, Moser T. Emerging approaches for restoration of hearing and vision. Physiological Reviews. 2020;**100**(4):1467-1525

[6] Margalit E, Maia M, Weiland JD, Greenberg RJ, Fujii GY, Torres G, et al. Retinal prosthesis for the blind. Survey of Ophthalmology. 2002;**47**(4):335-356

[7] Humayun MS, Dorn JD, Da Cruz L, Dagnelie G, Sahel JA, Stanga PE, et al. Interim results from the international trial of Second Sight's visual prosthesis. Ophthalmology. 2012;**119**(4):779-788

[8] Jacobson SG, Sumaroka A, Luo X, Cideciyan AV. Retinal optogenetic therapies: Clinical criteria for candidacy. Clinical Genetics. 2013;**84**(2):175-182

[9] Chaffiol A, Caplette R, Jaillard C, Brazhnikova E, Desrosiers M, Dubus E, et al. A new promoter allows optogenetic vision restoration with enhanced sensitivity in macaque retina. Molecular Therapy. 2017;**25**(11):2546-2560

[10] Lorach H, Goetz G, Smith R, Lei X, Mandel Y, Kamins T, et al. Photovoltaic restoration of sight with high visual acuity. Nature Medicine. 2015;**21**(5):476-482

[11] Makin S. Four technologies that could transform the treatment of blindness A decade ago, clinicians had nothing to offer most people affected by retinal degeneration. Breakthroughs in genetics, bionics and stem-cell therapy are changing that. Nature. 2019;**568**:S1. DOI: 10.1038/d41586-019-01107-8

[12] Zrenner E. Fighting blindness with microelectronics. Science Translational Medicine. 2013;**5**(210):210ps16

[13] Singh RK, Nasonkin IO. Limitations and promise of retinal tissue from human pluripotent stem cells for developing therapies of blindness. Frontiers in Cellular Neuroscience. 2020;**14**:179

[14] Cabrera FJ, Wang DC, Reddy K, Acharya G, Shin CS. Challenges and opportunities for drug delivery to the posterior of the eye. Drug Discovery Today. 2019;**24**(8):1679-1684

[15] Boyden ES, Zhang F, Bamberg E, Nagel G, Deisseroth K. Millisecond-timescale, genetically targeted optical control of neural activity. Nature Neuroscience. 2005;**8**(9):1263-1268

[16] Deisseroth K. Optogenetics: 10 years of microbial opsins in neuroscience. Nature Neuroscience. 2015;**18**(9):1213-1225

[17] Guru A, Post RJ, Ho YY, Warden MR. Making sense of optogenetics.

The International Journal of Neuropsychopharmacology. 2015;**18**(11):pyv079

[18] Pan ZH, Lu Q, Bi A, Dizhoor AM, Abrams GW. Optogenetic approaches to restoring vision. Annual Review of Vision Science. 2015;**1**:185-210

[19] Marc R, Pfeiffer R, Jones B. Retinal prosthetics, optogenetics, and chemical photoswitches. ACS Chemical Neuroscience. 2014;**5**(10):895-901

[20] Roska B, Sahel JA. Restoring vision. Nature. 2018;**557**(7705):359-367

[21] Klapper SD, Swiersy A, Bamberg E, Busskamp V. Biophysical properties of optogenetic tools and their application for vision restoration approaches. Frontiers in Systems Neuroscience. 2016;**10**:74

[22] Ferrari U, Deny S, Sengupta A, Caplette R, Trapani F, Sahel JA, et al. Towards optogenetic vision restoration with high resolution. PLOS Computational Biology. 2020;**16**(7): e1007857

[23] Farnum A, Pelled G. New vision for visual prostheses. Frontiers in Neuroscience. 2020;**14**:36

[24] Entcheva E, Kay MW. Cardiac optogenetics: A decade of enlightenment. Nature Reviews. Cardiology. 2021;**18**(5):349-367

[25] Sahel JA, Boulanger-Scemama E, Pagot C, Arleo A, Galluppi F, Martel JN, et al. Partial recovery of visual function in a blind patient after optogenetic therapy. Nature Medicine. 2021;**27**(7):1223-1229

[26] Barrett JM, Berlinguer-Palmini R, Degenaar P. Optogenetic approaches to retinal prosthesis. Visual Neuroscience. 2014;**31**(4-5):345-354

[27] Mattis J, Tye KM, Ferenczi EA, Ramakrishnan C, O'shea DJ, Prakash R, et al. Principles for applying optogenetic tools derived from direct comparative analysis of microbial opsins. Nature Methods. 2012;**9**(2):159-172

[28] Bansal H, Gupta N, Roy S. Theoretical analysis of low-power bidirectional optogenetic control of high-frequency neural codes with single spike resolution. Neuroscience. 2020;**449**:165-188

[29] Ferenczi EA, Tan X, Huang CL. Principles of optogenetic methods and their application to cardiac experimental systems. Frontiers in Physiology. 2019;**10**:1096

[30] Shen Y, Campbell RE, Côté DC, Paquet ME. Challenges for therapeutic applications of opsin-based optogenetic tools in humans. Frontiers in Neural Circuits. 2020;**14**:41

[31] Santos A, Humayun MS, de Juan E, Greenburg RJ, Marsh MJ, Klock IB, et al. Preservation of the inner retina in retinitis pigmentosa: A morphometric analysis. Archives of Ophthalmology. 1997;**115**(4):511-515

[32] Engelhard C, Chizhov I, Siebert F, Engelhard M. Microbial halorhodopsins: Light-driven chloride pumps. Chemical Reviews. 2018;**118**(21):10629-10645

[33] Bansal H, Gupta N, Roy S. Comparison of low-power, high-frequency and temporally precise optogenetic inhibition of spiking in NpHR, eNpHR3. 0 and Jaws-expressing neurons. Biomedical Physics & Engineering Express. 2020;**6**(4):045011

[34] Greenberg KP, Pham A, Werblin FS. Differential targeting of optical neuromodulators to ganglion cell soma and dendrites allows dynamic

control of center-surround antagonism. Neuron. 2011;**69**(4):713-720

[35] Busskamp V, Roska B. Optogenetic approaches to restoring visual function in retinitis pigmentosa. Current Opinion in Neurobiology. 2011;**21**(6):942-946

[36] Thyagarajan S, van Wyk M, Lehmann K, Löwel S, Feng G, Wässle H. Visual function in mice with photoreceptor degeneration and transgenic expression of channelrhodopsin 2 in ganglion cells. The Journal of Neuroscience. 2010;**30**(26):8745-8758

[37] Reinhard K, Münch TA. Visual properties of human retinal ganglion cells. PLoS One. 2021;**16**(2):e0246952

[38] Bansal H, Gupta N, Roy S. Theoretical analysis of optogenetic spiking with ChRmine, bReaChES and CsChrimson-expressing neurons for retinal prostheses. Journal of Neural Engineering. 2021;**18**(4):0460b8

[39] Gauvain G, Akolkar H, Chaffiol A, Arcizet F, Khoei MA, Desrosiers M, et al. Optogenetic therapy: High spatiotemporal resolution and pattern discrimination compatible with vision restoration in non-human primates. Communications Biology. 2021;**4**(1):1-15

[40] Bi A, Cui J, Ma YP, Olshevskaya E, Pu M, Dizhoor AM, et al. Ectopic expression of a microbial-type rhodopsin restores visual responses in mice with photoreceptor degeneration. Neuron. 2006;**50**(1):23-33

[41] Sengupta A, Chaffiol A, Macé E, Caplette R, Desrosiers M, Lampič M, et al. Red-shifted channelrhodopsin stimulation restores light responses in blind mice, macaque retina, and human retina. EMBO Molecular Medicine. 2016;**8**(11):1248-1264

[42] Soltan A, Barrett JM, Maaskant P, Armstrong N, Al-Atabany W, Chaudet L, et al. A head mounted device stimulator for optogenetic retinal prosthesis. Journal of Neural Engineering. 2018;**15**(6):065002

[43] Wu J, Seregard S, Algvere PV. Photochemical damage of the retina. Survey of Ophthalmology. 2006;**51**(5):461-481. DOI: 10.1016/j.survophthal.2006.06.009

[44] Degenaar P, Grossman N, Memon MA, Burrone J, Dawson M, Drakakis E, et al. Optobionic vision—A new genetically enhanced light on retinal prosthesis. Journal of Neural Engineering. 2009;**6**(3):035007

[45] Kleinlogel S, Feldbauer K, Dempski RE, Fotis H, Wood PG, Bamann C, et al. Ultra light-sensitive and fast neuronal activation with the Ca^{2+}-permeable channelrhodopsin CatCh. Nature Neuroscience. 2011;**14**(4):513-518

[46] Ganjawala TH, Lu Q, Fenner MD, Abrams GW, Pan ZH. Improved CoChR variants restore visual acuity and contrast sensitivity in a mouse model of blindness under ambient light conditions. Molecular Therapy. 2019;**27**(6):1195-1205

[47] Lin JY, Knutsen PM, Muller A, Kleinfeld D, Tsien RY. ReaChR: A red-shifted variant of channelrhodopsin enables deep transcranial optogenetic excitation. Nature Neuroscience. 2013;**16**(10):1499-1508

[48] Mager T, Lopez de la Morena D, Senn V, Schlotte J, Feldbauer K, Wrobel C, et al. High frequency neural spiking and auditory signaling by ultrafast red-shifted optogenetics. Nature Communications. 2018;**9**(1):1-4

[49] Marshel JH, Kim YS, Machado TA, Quirin S, Benson B, Kadmon J, et al.

Cortical layer–specific critical dynamics triggering perception. Science. 2019;**365**(6453):eaaw5202

[50] International Commission on Non-Ionizing Radiation Protection. ICNIRP guidelines on limits of exposure to incoherent visible and infrared radiation. Health Physics. 2013;**105**(1):74-96

[51] Klapoetke NC, Murata Y, Kim SS, Pulver SR, Birdsey-Benson A, Cho YK, et al. Independent optical excitation of distinct neural populations. Nature Methods. 2014;**11**(3):338-346

[52] ClinicalTrials.gov 2015. RST-001 Phase I/II Trail for Advanced Retinitis Pigmentosa. Available from: https://clinicaltrials.gov/ct2/show/study/NCT02556736

[53] McGregor JE, Kunala K, Xu Z, Murphy PJ, Godat T, Strazzeri JM, et al. Optogenetic therapy restores retinal activity in primate for at least a year following photoreceptor ablation. Molecular Therapy. 2022;**30**(3):1315-1328

[54] Tomita H, Sugano E, Murayama N, Ozaki T, Nishiyama F, Tabata K, et al. Restoration of the majority of the visual spectrum by using modified Volvox channelrhodopsin-1. Molecular Therapy. 2014;**22**(8):1434-1440

[55] Nirenberg S, Pandarinath C. Retinal prosthetic strategy with the capacity to restore normal vision. Proceedings. National Academy of Sciences. United States of America. 2012;**109**(37):15012-15017

[56] Lagali PS, Balya D, Awatramani GB, Münch TA, Kim DS, Busskamp V, et al. Light-activated channels targeted to ON bipolar cells restore visual function in retinal degeneration. Nature Neuroscience. 2008;**11**(6):667-675

[57] Doroudchi MM, Greenberg KP, Liu J, Silka KA, Boyden ES, Lockridge JA, et al. Virally delivered channelrhodopsin-2 safely and effectively restores visual function in multiple mouse models of blindness. Molecular Therapy. 2011;**19**(7):1220-1229

[58] Macé E, Caplette R, Marre O, Sengupta A, Chaffiol A, Barbe P, et al. Targeting channelrhodopsin-2 to ON-bipolar cells with vitreally administered AAV restores ON and OFF visual responses in blind mice. Molecular Therapy. 2015;**23**(1):7-16

[59] Chen F, Duan X, Yu Y, Yang S, Chen Y, Gee CE, et al. Visual function restoration with a highly sensitive and fast Channelrhodopsin in blind mice. Signal Transduction and Targeted Therapy. 2022;**7**(1):104

[60] Gaub BM, Berry MH, Holt AE, Isacoff EY, Flannery JG. Optogenetic vision restoration using rhodopsin for enhanced sensitivity. Molecular Therapy. 2015;**23**(10):1562-1571

[61] Vandenberghe LH, Bell P, Maguire AM, Cearley CN, Xiao R, Calcedo R, et al. Dosage thresholds for AAV2 and AAV8 photoreceptor gene therapy in monkey. Science Translational Medicine. 2011;**3**(88):88ra54

[62] Ivanova E, Hwang GS, Pan ZH. Characterization of transgenic mouse lines expressing Cre recombinase in the retina. Neuroscience. 2010;**165**(1):233-243

[63] Kim CK, Yang SJ, Pichamoorthy N, Young NP, Kauvar I, Jennings JH, et al. Simultaneous fast measurement of circuit dynamics at multiple sites across the mammalian brain. Nature Methods. 2016;**13**(4):325-328

[64] Kishi KE, Kim YS, Fukuda M, Inoue M, Kusakizako T, Wang PY, et al.

Structural basis for channel conduction in the pump-like channelrhodopsin ChRmine. Cell. 2022;**185**(4):672-689

[65] Mardinly AR, Oldenburg IA, Pégard NC, Sridharan S, Lyall EH, Chesnov K, et al. Precise multimodal optical control of neural ensemble activity. Nature Neuroscience. 2018;**21**(6):881-893

[66] Sridharan S, Gajowa MA, Ogando MB, Jagadisan UK, Abdeladim L, Sadahiro M, et al. High-performance microbial opsins for spatially and temporally precise perturbations of large neuronal networks. Neuron. 2022;**110**(7):1139-1155

[67] Kim CK, Adhikari A, Deisseroth K. Integration of optogenetics with complementary methodologies in systems neuroscience. Nature Reviews. Neuroscience. 2017;**18**(4):222-235

[68] Chen R, Gore F, Nguyen QA, Ramakrishnan C, Patel S, Kim SH, et al. Deep brain optogenetics without intracranial surgery. Nature Biotechnology. 2021;**39**(2):161-164

[69] Williams JC, Xu J, Lu Z, Klimas A, Chen X, Ambrosi CM, et al. Computational optogenetics: empirically-derived voltage-and light-sensitive channelrhodopsin-2 model. PLoS Computational Biology. 2013;**9**(9):e1003220

[70] Nikolic K, Grossman N, Grubb MS, Burrone J, Toumazou C, Degenaar P. Photocycles of channelrhodopsin-2. Photochemistry and Photobiology. 2009;**85**(1):400-411

[71] Grossman N, Nikolic K, Toumazou C, Degenaar P. Modeling study of the light stimulation of a neuron cell with channelrhodopsin-2 mutants. IEEE Transactions on Biomedical Engineering. 2011;**58**(6):1742-1751

[72] Grossman N, Simiaki V, Martinet C, Toumazou C, Schultz SR, Nikolic K. The spatial pattern of light determines the kinetics and modulates backpropagation of optogenetic action potentials. Journal of Computational Neuroscience. 2013;**34**(3):477-488

[73] Foutz TJ, Arlow RL, McIntyre CC. Theoretical principles underlying optical stimulation of a channelrhodopsin-2 positive pyramidal neuron. Journal of Neurophysiology. 2012;**107**(12):3235-3245

[74] Arlow RL, Foutz TJ, McIntyre CC. Theoretical principles underlying optical stimulation of myelinated axons expressing channelrhodopsin-2. Neuroscience. 2013;**248**:541-551

[75] Saran S, Gupta N, Roy S. Theoretical analysis of low-power fast optogenetic control of firing of Chronos-expressing neurons. Neurophoton. 2018;**5**(2):025009

[76] Gupta N, Bansal H, Roy S. Theoretical optimization of high-frequency optogenetic spiking of red-shifted very fast-Chrimson-expressing neurons. Neurophoton. 2019;**6**(2):025002

[77] Bansal H, Pyari G, Roy S. Co-expressing fast channelrhodopsin with step-function opsin overcomes spike failure due to photocurrent desensitization in optogenetics: A theoretical study. Journal of Neural Engineering. 2022;**19**(2):026032

[78] Pyari G, Bansal H, Roy S. Ultra-low power deep sustained optogenetic excitation of human ventricular cardiomyocytes with red-shifted opsins: A computational study. The Journal of Physiology. 2022;**600**(21):4653-4676. DOI: 10.1113/JP283366

[79] Sadeh S, Clopath C. Patterned perturbation of inhibition can reveal

the dynamical structure of neural processing. eLife. 2020;**9**:e52757

[80] Mahrach A, Chen G, Li N, van Vreeswijk C, Hansel D. Mechanisms underlying the response of mouse cortical networks to optogenetic manipulation. eLife. 2020;**9**:e49967

[81] Schlag J, Schlag-Rey M. Through the eye, slowly; Delays and localization errors in the visual system. Nature Reviews. Neuroscience. 2002;**3**(3):191